D1242844

Handbook of
Percutaneous Central Venous
Catheterisation

Handbook of
Percutaneous Central Venous Catheterisation

SECOND EDITION

MICHAEL ROSEN CBE, MB, ChB, FRCA, FRCOG
Professor in Anaesthetics, University of Wales College of Medicine, Cardiff
Consultant Anaesthetist, University Hospital of Wales, Cardiff

IAN P. LATTO MB, BS, FRCA, DA
Clinical Teacher, University of Wales College of Medicine, Cardiff
Consultant Anaesthetist, University Hospital of Wales, Cardiff

W. SHANG NG MB, BCh, FRCA
Clinical Teacher, University of Wales College of Medicine, Cardiff
Consultant Anaesthetist, University Hospital of Wales, Cardiff

with contributions by

PETER L. JONES MB, BCh, FRCA
Clinical Teacher, University of Wales College of Medicine, Cardiff
Consultant Anaesthetist, University Hospital of Wales, Cardiff

PAUL WEINER MRCS, LRCP, FRCA
Clinical Teacher, University of Wales College of Medicine, Cardiff
Consultant Anaesthetist, University Hospital of Wales, Cardiff

W. B. Saunders Company Ltd
London Philadelphia Toronto Sydney Tokyo

W.B. Saunders Company Ltd

24–28 Oval Road
London NW1 7DX, England

The Curtis Center
Independence Square West
Philadelphia, PA 19106–3399, USA

55 Horner Avenue
Toronto, Ontario M8Z 4X6, Canada

Harcourt Brace Jovanovich (Australia) Pty Ltd
30–52 Smidmore St
Marrickville, NSW 2204, Australia

Harcourt Brace Jovanovich Japan Inc.
Ichibancho Central Building, 22–1 Ichibancho
Chiyoda-ku, Tokyo 102, Japan

© 1992 W. B. Saunders Company Ltd

Foreign language versions:
Italian (1983), French (1984), Russian (1986)

This book is printed on acid free paper.

A catalogue record for this book is available from the British Library.

ISBN 0–7020–1539–3

Typeset by J&L Composition Ltd, Filey, North Yorkshire
Printed in Great Britain by The Bath Press, Avon

Contents

7 The External Jugular Vein

PART 2   PAEDIATRIC PROCEDURES

Foreword

The central vein serves as the route to information which is essential for the scientific management of many patients in anaesthesia and acute medicine as well as being a crucial pathway for intravenous therapy. Any doctor who bears the responsibility of treating such patients knows that he has to be able to produce the requisite technical skill when required.

Unfortunately, nature is not kind: the venous system is extremely variable where catheterisation might otherwise be relatively easy, and where the anatomy is reasonably constant there is a considerable risk of injury to vital structures. The doctor who wishes to combine minimum hazard with maximum certainty of success needs to be eclectic: it cannot be sufficient just to learn one technique.

However, eclecticism cannot be promoted without the opportunity for extensive practice, which is generally unavailable.

Several techniques have been developed and shown to be practicable and safe in the hands of the originators, and it is not yet possible to say that one technique is unequivocally better than another. In these circumstances, clear guidance on all the established published techniques is what the practitioner needs to have available and that is what my colleagues in Cardiff have attempted to provide. Only time will show whether they have succeeded, but I predict that many practitioners (including the already skilled) will be glad to have this book readily to hand.

M. D. Vickers
FRCAnaes.
Professor in Anaesthetics,
University of Wales College of Medicine, Cardiff

Preface to the 1st Edition

Catheterisation of the great veins has become an important manoeuvre both for measuring the central venous pressure and for carrying out long-term intravenous alimentation. Furthermore, in an emergency – as after acute haemorrhage with peripheral vasoconstriction – it may be impossible to catheterise a peripheral vein percutaneously and only a central vein may be available for the rapid restoration of blood volume. Most hospital doctors will be faced with this situation at some time. Even clinicians who work regularly in the cardiovascular and neurosurgical fields, in which central venous catheterisation is frequently employed, may find their usual techniques unsuccessful. In such circumstances they have to perform an unfamiliar technique quickly yet safely, perhaps without the benefit of previous experience. At that time it is often difficult to call to mind all the details of the numerous techniques available, which is our justification for bringing together the major methods of percutaneous central venous catheterisation in a practical handbook, using a systematic format and illustrating each technique by diagrams.

Our presentation of the major methods is not exhaustive and the basis of our selection is discussed in Chapter 1, 'Choosing the vein'. The principles governing the choice of equipment are described in Chapter 2, but, once again, it has proved impractical to discuss the whole range available.

In the remaining six chapters, we have made what we hope is the most useful selection from the different approaches to each vein, including a number of variations on some; for example, eleven techniques for cannulating the internal jugular vein are described, although, even then, a number of minor variations have had to be excluded. The techniques chosen have not been selected on the results of controlled comparative trials; rather they reflect our opinions based on personal experience and a review of the literature. Since we have not tested each method personally, the original authors' descriptions of their techniques have been retained, although the anatomical terminology has, in some cases, been altered for the sake of uniformity. When it seemed helpful to clarify the description, we have done so in italics. The text also indicates when a technique was adopted by the original authors specifically for neonates or infants.

We hope this handbook will prove useful to those who work in the operating theatre, intensive therapy unit, casualty department, obstetric unit and all other units where central venous catheterisation may be required.

Michael Rosen
Ian P. Latto
W. Shang Ng

Preface to the 2nd Edition

The first edition has been found to be of practical value to many specialists in addition to anaesthetists and surgeons since the use of central venous cannulation has spread widely into other areas of medical practice. Complications abound but excellent technique can reduce their incidence.

The arm veins still constitute the safest and probably the most popular approach. The axillary vein is underused in spite of being a relatively safe vein to puncture; it will almost certainly increase in popularity. The use of the subclavian route in anaesthetic practice has certainly declined except for long term catheterisation. Most anaesthetists have come to rely upon the internal jugular vein, and with proper technique, virtually all serious complications should be avoidable. The use of the external jugular vein has received impetus through the introduction of J-tipped guide wires which ensure high success in a visible, and easily punctured, vein.

This edition introduces a paediatric section. Although many of the techniques used in adults are applicable to children the detailed management may be different. The requirement for central venous access in infants and small children appears to be increasing.

Advances in equipment design have increased the variety of apparatus available to the clinician. Since the first edition the demise of catheter-through-needle devices seems complete. New materials are becoming available with favourable antithrombogenic and antimicrobial characteristics. These, together with good technique, will ensure safer short and long term catheterisation.

Michael Rosen
Ian P. Latto
W. Shang Ng

PART 1

General Considerations and Adult Procedures

1

Choosing the Vein

Before 1960 peripheral venous pressure was frequently used to judge the state of intravascular volume.[1] This technique was abandoned with the introduction of central venous pressure measurement. Surprisingly though no longer used, peripheral venous pressure has been shown to reflect central venous pressure quite accurately under controlled circumstances.[1] The history of central venous catheters from the time of Stephan Hales in 1733 to the pioneering work of Bleichroder in 1905 and Forssmann in 1929 has been carefully reviewed by Kalso.[2]

The great majority of central venous catheters are used for measuring trends in central venous pressure or for infusing drugs or alimentation fluid into the central circulation. Small diameter catheters are satisfactory for this purpose. In a small number of cases (probably less than 1%) a Seldinger technique with a vein dilator may be used to insert a large diameter catheter into a central vein in order to facilitate rapid infusion of crystalloid or colloid solutions in shocked patients.

CLINICAL TRENDS

Cubital and femoral vein routes were reported to be most popular during the early years of central venous catheterisation.[2] Until the late 1970s in anaesthesic practice in the United Kingdom many clinicians appeared to use only the arm veins. In an unpublished survey in Cardiff in 1979 it was shown that 30 clinicians questioned used arm veins as their first choice route. Other routes were considered only if cannulation through arm veins was unsuccessful. If this was the case some anaesthetists attempted an alternative percutaneous route whilst others called for the assistance of a surgeon to perform a cut-down. Surgical cut-downs were certainly much more widely used 10 years ago than they are today. However, with improved clinical skills and the availability of a wider range of equipment, it is now very rare in anaesthetic practice for an experienced clinician to fail with percutaneous techniques in adult patients. Since publication of the first edition of this book in 1981 one of the outstanding trends in central venous catheterisation practice has been the increasing use of the internal jugular vein. Indeed this is now used routinely in most centres for cardiac anaesthesia. With the advent of the J-wire, which facilitates successful cannulation, it can be confidently predicted that there will be a trend towards more frequent use of the external jugular vein. At the same time there appears to be a marked decrease in the use of the subclavian route in anaesthetic practice although this route is still widely used in the field of intensive care especially for the administration of parenteral nutrition.

The Cardiff anaesthetic records (approximately 20 000 patients per year between 1972 and 1977) show some trends in the overall use of central venous lines. In 1972 the incidence was 4·1% of all anaesthetics and in 1977 it was 6·7%. These figures have remained roughly constant, the rates between 1985 and 1988 (approximately 23 000 patients per year) being 6·8%, 6·8%, 6·9% and 7% respectively.

Local anaesthesia is usually adequate for cannulating superficial veins; whilst some clinicians cannulate deep veins under local anaesthesia, many wait until the patient has been anaesthetised. One report showed significant cardiovascular stimulation during percutaneous insertion of arterial and pulmonary artery catheters prior to induction of anaesthesia in patients with coronary artery disease,[3] although a later study did not substantiate this finding.[4] However, it was recommended that these patients should be sedated and treated with anti-angina drugs if required. Clinicians carrying out such techniques in these patients should be adequately supervised if they have limited skill and experience.

THE LEARNING CURVE

Whilst experienced clinicians rarely fail in attempts to insert internal jugular vein catheters, many central venous catheters are inserted by inexperienced clinicians. In a 1982 study from Dallas, Texas, the success rate of medical house officers using jugular and subclavian veins was 363 out of 470 attempts (77%).[5] The success rate was improved if the attempt was made under elective circumstances and if the vein was initially located with a small seeker needle. Only 62% of attempts were successful when catheterisations were carried out during cardiopulmonary resuscitation. The authors recommended that no more than three attempts should be permitted with a large needle at the same site.

In another study involving intensive care patients the failure rate for subclavian and internal jugular routes was 19·4% for inexperienced and 10·1% for experienced clinicians.[6] The complication rate was 11% for inexperienced and 5·4% for experienced clinicians. Inexperienced clinicians caused fewer complications when attempts were carried out whilst patients were anaesthetised and mechanically ventilated than in conscious patients breathing spontaneously. The success rate for central venous cannulation is higher for experienced clinicians under elective circumstances in the operating theatre than when performed by inexperienced clinicians under emergency circumstances.

In yet a further study, house officers attempting to insert catheters in patients receiving intensive care had a success rate of only 74%.[7] A wide variety of insertion sites were used and both elective and emergency cases were studied. Their complication rate was 6·1%. Pleural complications were the most serious and insertion of chest drains was commonly needed. These authors recommended that the internal jugular vein should be used in preference to the external jugular or subclavian vein. Other authors have suggested that a medial

antecubital vein should be used in emergency conditions to reduce the number of complications.[8] A Seldinger technique for arm veins with a vein dilator could be an added help. In seriously ill patients arm veins may be too small to successfully use a needle/cannula method. Manufacturers were urged to make suitable Seldinger guide wire equipment available.

INITIAL TRAINING

How should the junior doctor acquire skills at central venous cannulation? It has been recommended that the trainee should practise initially on manikins or cadavers.[8] This advice does not however appear to be followed in many hospitals. In addition the trainee should be carefully supervised and possibly make his early attempts on anaesthetised rather than conscious patients. When learning a subclavian technique the ideal clinical situation would be an anaesthetised or unconscious patient with a chest drain already *in situ*. It was stressed that clinicians should acquire expertise with both an internal jugular and a subclavian technique. Trainees should be taught to avoid if possible, but also to recognise, and treat any complications that might arise. The superficial veins of the arm and neck require less skill than the subclavian and internal jugular routes and the 'see one, do one, teach one' method of training is often used. Indeed techniques using these veins may even fit into the 'do one (under supervision), teach one' mould.

THE ROUTES

A number of routes have been described for cannulating central veins, and for each of these routes a variety of techniques have been used. This wide choice often makes it difficult to determine the most suitable route and technique for a particular patient. In practice, decisions are commonly taken on empirical grounds, but a consideration of certain relevant factors would enable a more rational approach to be made. Such factors include the objectives of the cannulation, whether the patient is awake or unconscious, the expertise and experience of the operator, the success and complication rates of the technique, and the availability of

Table 1.1. Indications for the various routes

Route	Indication
Arm	
Basilic vein	For short-term
Cephalic vein	use. Safe for
Forearm vein	the beginner
Axillary vein	
Proximal basilic vein	A rarely used alternative
Cephalic vein in	to distal arm veins
deltopectoral groove	
Chest	
Subclavian vein	Long-term access, e.g.
supraclavicular	parenteral nutrition,
infraclavicular	chemotherapy,
	haemodialysis
Neck	
External jugular vein	A safe alternative to arm
	veins
Internal jugular vein	For cardiac anaesthesia and
	major surgical procedures
Leg	
Femoral vein	Rarely used but a useful
	technique in paediatrics
Scalp	
Threaded through	A technique used in
superficial veins	neonates which avoids a
	cut-down

Table 1.2. Factors influencing the choice of method for central venous cannulation

Patient
   Time cannula likely to be required:
      long term
      intermediate
      short term
   Suitability of vein for technique chosen

Operator
   Theoretical knowledge of the technique
   Practical knowledge of the technique
   Expertise in the technique

Technique characteristics
   Success rate for vein cannulation
   Success rate for central placement
   Complication rate
   Applicability to different ages of patient
   Ease of learning
   Venepuncture of a visible and/or palpable vein or
   'blind' venepuncture (especially important for the
   inexperienced clinician)

Apparatus
   Availability of suitable apparatus
   Cost
   Suitability of material for long-term cannulation

Choice of cut-down or percutaneous technique
   Cut downs are now rarely required by
   experienced clinicians for adult patients
   (only used if percutaneous techniques fail)

suitable apparatus. The main indications for the different routes and techniques are shown in Table 1.1, and those factors to be considered when choosing a suitable route are detailed in Table 1.2.

Peripheral arm veins

The basilic, cephalic, or forearm veins may be the first choice for the inexperienced clinician since their use avoids the risk of the major complications associated with blind puncture of the internal jugular or subclavian veins. The peripheral approach is often indicated in patients undergoing short operative procedures under general anaesthesia. In a patient whose peripheral veins are constricted it may be helpful to await the vasodilation induced by anaesthesia. The basilic vein should be chosen in preference to the cephalic as central placement is more frequently successful in the former.[9] If the catheter is likely to be left in for a few days, the non-dominant arm should be chosen. Cannulation of superficial arm veins is specifically indicated in patients who are having anti-coagulant therapy or who have a bleeding diathesis, as the development of a haematoma can be easily seen and compression applied.

Peripheral veins are, however, not always readily available, particularly in ill patients requiring long-term intravenous therapy. The veins may be thrombosed, inflamed, covered in plaster or dressings, or the preferred site may be burnt or infected. Sometimes veins are thrombosed as a result of previous surgical cut-down and ligation. In some patients, especially the obese, veins may be difficult to find. It may in some cases be useful to identify the vein either with a temperature-change strip or by a Doppler ultrasonic detector.

If percutaneous cannulation of arm veins is unsuccessful, an alternative route should be used.

Proximal arm veins

The proximal portion of the basilic vein and the distal portion of the axillary vein have been used

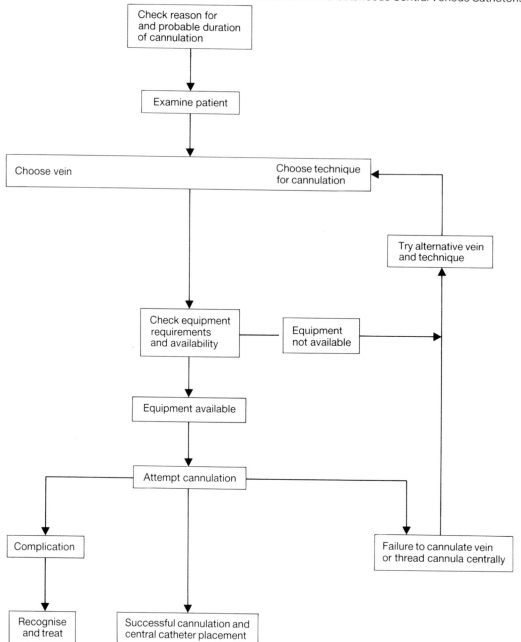

Figure 1.1. Central venous cannulation when operator is familiar with technique chosen.

successfully.[10,11] The cephalic vein, where it lies in the deltopectoral groove, has also been used for long-term catheterisation.[12]

The indications for selecting the proximal arm veins are the same as for the more distal veins, but there is the additional advantage of a larger vein. However, as these veins are usually not visible, venepuncture is more difficult than with distal arm veins. These sites are not commonly used perhaps because of the paucity of references to the technique in the literature.

The external jugular vein

The external jugular vein is usually visible and easy to cannulate. It is, therefore, a useful superficial

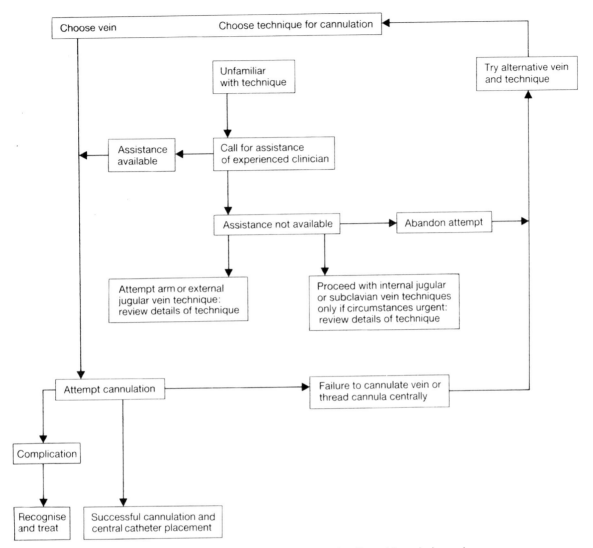

Figure 1.2. Central venous cannulation when operator is not familiar with technique chosen.

vein for the clinician unskilled in internal jugular techniques. Success appears to be related largely to the type of equipment used. Flexible catheters pass more easily around acute bends at the external jugular subclavian vein junction than do rigid catheters: rigid catheters are also more likely to penetrate the vein wall.[13] Blitt *et al.*[14] in 1974 used a modified Seldinger technique with a flexible J-shaped wire originally described by Judkins *et al.*[15] The J-wire was threaded through the external jugular vein and manipulated into the superior vena cava, enabling the central venous catheter to be inserted into a central vein over the J-wire. Successful central venous placement was reported in 96% of attempts. The experiences of other

authors with J-wires and other catheters is described in Chapter 7.

Stoelting[16] showed that the readings from a short (50 mm) catheter introduced into the external jugular vein reflected right atrial pressure in anaesthetised patients, both with controlled and spontaneous ventilation. A round ended-catheter that is placed just above the junction of the subclavian and external jugular vein will give accurate central venous pressure readings.[17] These are unaffected by head movement.

There are no specific contraindications, apart from local infection, to the use of the external jugular vein.

The internal jugular vein

The internal jugular vein now appears to have become the accepted route of choice for major surgical cases. However, the long-term nursing management of neck catheters can be difficult, particularly if the patient requires to be turned regularly. Contraindications include aneurysm of the carotid artery and local sepsis.

Internal jugular techniques can be arbitrarily divided into high and low approaches, according to their position in relation to the apex of the lung. A high approach should avoid the risk of pneumothorax. In the low approaches of English et al.[18] and Rao et al.[19] the reported incidences of pneumothorax were 0·2% and 0·3% respectively. Although some deaths have been associated with cannulation of the internal jugular vein,[20,21] many more have been reported following use of the subclavian vein route. In the young child the technique is more difficult to perform and the success rates may be reduced.[22] Ullman and Stoelting[23] suggest using a blood flow detector for localising the internal jugular vein. This could be especially helpful in young or obese patients, in whom anatomical landmarks may be difficult to locate. If failure occurs on one side the other can be used.

The subclavian vein

The subclavian vein has a wide calibre (1–2 cm in diameter in adults) and is held open by surrounding tissue even in severe circulatory collapse. The vein is usually easily accessible to the anaesthetist during a surgical operation. In shocked patients there is a choice between the subclavian and the internal jugular vein because the latter can also be successfully cannulated using a guide wire technique. Its size allows for rapid infusion of fluid. The subclavian vein is the route most commonly adopted for long-term parenteral nutrition.

Use of the subclavian vein allows the catheter to be securely fixed on the chest wall with minimal subsequent movement, thus decreasing the risk of infection. Most authors report a high success rate for central placement, but serious complications occur much more frequently than with other routes. Pneumothorax is one of the most common, so the technique should be used with caution, if at all, in patients with severe lung disease. Attempts at cannulation on both sides are best avoided because of the risk of producing a bilateral pneumothorax. In patients in whom a thoracotomy is planned, ipsilateral cannulation is recommended as a chest drain will be used postoperatively.

This route is unsuitable for the inexperienced operator unless adequately supervised.

Table 1.3. Features of the different routes of central venous cannulation

Feature	Arm veins	External jugular vein	Internal jugular vein	Subclavian vein
Ease of venepuncture for the inexperienced clinician	+ + +	+ + +	+	+
Complications relating to insertion of catheter	0	0	+	+ + +
Central placement success rate (%)	50–98 (normally approximately 80)	50–98 (depends on use of J-wire)	90–100 (does *not* depend type of catheter used)	90–98
Suitability for long-term parenteral nutrition	+	+	+ +	+ + +

CENTRAL VENOUS CATHETERISATION IN INFANTS AND CHILDREN

The Report of the National Confidential Enquiry into Perioperative Deaths (CEPOD)[24] published in 1989 was unable to comment on the minimal requirements of training and current practice in anaesthesia for children. The authors however recognised that there was a problem that needed to be addressed urgently.

A clinician should not feel obliged to anaesthetise a child of less than 5 years of age on an occasional basis. Such young children should ideally be anaesthetised by clinicians regularly involved in paediatric anaesthesia. Similarly it is inappropriate for a clinician to be involved in inserting central venous catheters in such children on an occasional basis. These catheters should ideally be inserted by the designated paediatric anaesthetist. Some paediatric patients are however still anaesthetised by clinicians on an occasional basis. These patients are generally not high risk cases and are very unlikely to need a central venous catheter. It is almost unheard of for clinicians to fail with percutaneous techniques on the jugular or arm veins in adults. This is however not the case with children. Under these circumstances some clinicians attempt cannulation of the subclavian veins, others ask for a surgical cut down.

Inserting a central venous catheter into a small peripheral arm vein in a child is technically more difficult than in an adult. Suitable guide wire equipment is not usually available, therefore it is usual to attempt to cannulate other veins. The external jugular vein can be cannulated with minimal risk. Experience with internal jugular vein techniques should, however, first be obtained in adults. Prince et al.[25] compared their results of internal jugular vein cannulation in children with those of subclavian vein cannulation by Groff and Ahmed[26] in children less than 2 years old, and concluded that the use of the subclavian vein in patients of that age should be condemned. Our practice is to use a subclavian vein only as a last resort when attempts at internal and external jugular veins have failed. Alternatively a surgical cut-down may be used. In small infants, scalp veins have been used and catheters threaded through a needle into the superior vena cava.[27,28]

THE OPERATOR

No individual can be equally familiar with all the techniques described. Most anaesthetists have considerable experience with arm and jugular veins. The inexperienced clinician should select a technique that is intrinsically safe although possibly yielding a lower success rate. If a particular route is strongly indicated, the assistance of someone experienced in that technique should be sought unless circumstances are urgent. All trainee physicians should initially be supervised in the practical aspects of performing a technique until sufficient expertise is acquired.

It is an important ethical issue whether a technique with a known incidence of major complications should be employed solely to gain experience when alternative and less dangerous methods would suffice. This is justifiable only if the inexperienced operator is carefully supervised and facilities are readily available to institute effective treatment of complications.

The operator is ultimately limited in his choice of routes by the equipment available to him. This may be a particular problem in the management of children. Flow diagrams showing the steps in central venous cannulation when the operator is experienced or inexperienced in the chosen technique are shown in Figures 1.1 and 1.2. Important features of the different routes are shown in Table 1.3.

REFERENCES

1. Joseph, D. M., Philip, B. K. and Philip, J. H. (1985). Peripheral venous pressure can be an accurate estimate of central venous pressure. *Anesthesiology* **65**, A166.
2. Kalso, E. (1985). A short history of central venous catheterization. *Acta Anaesthesiologica Scandinavica* **81**, 7.
3. Lunn, J. K., Stanley, T. H., Webster, L. R. and Bidwai, A. V. (1979). Arterial blood-pressure and pulse-rate responses to pulmonary and radial arterial catheterization prior to cardiac and major vascular operations. *Anesthesiology* **51**, 265.
4. Waller, J. L., Zaidan, J. R., Kaplan, J. A. and Bauman, D. I. (1982). Hemodynamic responses to preoperative vascular cannulation in patients with coronary artery disease. *Anesthesiology* **56**, 219.
5. Bo-Linn, G. W., Anderson, D. J., Anderson, K. C., McGoon, M. D. and the Osler Medical House Staff

(1982). Percutaneous central venous catheterization performed by medical house officers: a prospective study. *Catheterization and Cardiovascular Diagnosis* **8**, 23.

6. Sznajder, J. I., Zveibil, F. R., Bitterman, H., Weiner, P. and Bursztein, S. (1986). Central vein catheterization. Failure and complication rates by three percutaneous approaches. *Archives of Internal Medicine* **146**, 259.

7. Sessler, C. N. and Glauser, F. L. (1987). Central venous cannulation done by house officers in the intensive care unit: a prospective study. *Southern Medical Journal* **80**, 1239.

8. *Lancet* (1986). Central vein catheterisation. Editorial, **2**, 669.

9. Webre, D. R. and Arens, J. F. (1973). Use of cephalic and basilic veins for introduction of central venous catheters. *Anesthesiology* **38**, 389.

10. Spracklen, F. H. N., Niesche, F., Lord, P. W. and Besterman, E. M. M. (1967). Percutaneous catheterisation of the axillary vein. *Cardiovascular Research* **1** 297.

11. Ayim, E. N. (1977). Percutaneous catheterisation of the axillary vein and proximal basilic vein. *Anaesthesia* **32**, 753.

12. Jacobs, P. and Jacobson, J. (1978). Placement of central feeding catheters. *British Medical Journal* **2**, 1789.

13. Guest, J. and Leiberman, D. P. (1976). Late complications of catheterisation for intravenous nutrition. *Lancet* **2**, 805.

14. Blitt, C. D., Wright, W. A., Petty, W. C. and Webster, T. A. (1974). Central venous catheterization via the external jugular vein. A technique employing the J-wire. *Journal of the American Medical Association* **229**, 817.

15. Judkins, M. P., Kidd, H. J., Frische, L. H. and Dotter, C. T. (1967). Lumen-following safety J-guide for catheterization of tortuous vessels. *Radiology* **88**, 1127.

16. Stoelting, R. K. (1973). Evaluation of external jugular pressure as a reflection of right atrial pressure. *Anesthesiology* **38**, 291.

17. Shah, M. V., Swai, E. A. and Latto, I. P. (1986). Comparison between pressures measured from the proximal external jugular vein and a central vein. *British Journal of Anaesthesia* **58**, 1384.

18. English, I. C. W., Frew, R. M., Pigott, J. F. and Zaki, M. (1969). Percutaneous catheterisation of the internal jugular vein. *Anaesthesia* **24**, 521.

19. Rao, T. L. K., Wong, A. Y. and Salem, M. R. (1977). A new approach to percutaneous catheterization of the internal jugular vein. *Anesthesiology* **46**, 362.

20. Ayalon, A., Anner, H., Berlatzky, Y. and Schiller, M. (1978). A life threatening complication of the infusion pump. *Lancet* **i**, 853.

21. Wisheart, J. D., Hassan, M. A. and Jackson, J. W. (1972). A complication of percutaneous cannulation of the internal jugular vein. *Thorax* **27**, 496.

22. Vaughan, R. W. and Weygandt, G. R. (1973). Reliable percutaneous central venous pressure measurement. *Anesthesia and Analgesia: Current Researches* **52**, 709.

23. Ullman, J. I. and Stoelting, R. K. (1978). Internal jugular vein location with the ultrasound Doppler blood flow detector. *Anesthesia and Analgesia Current Researches* **57**, 118.

24. Campling, E. A., Devlin, H. B. and Lunn, J. N. (1989). The Report of the National Confidential Enquiry into Perioperative Deaths.

25. Prince, S. R., Sullivan, R. L. and Hackel, A. (1976). Percutaneous catheterization of the internal jugular vein in infants and children. *Anesthesiology* **44**, 170.

26. Groff, B. D. and Ahmed, N. O. (1974). Subclavian vein catheterization in the infant. *Journal of Pediatric Surgery* **9**, 171.

27. Shaw, J. C. L. (1973). Parenteral nutrition in the management of sick low birth weight infants. *Pediatric Clinics of North America* **20**, 333.

28. Cockington, R. A. (1979). Silicone elastomer for naso jejeunal intubation and central venous cannulation in neonates. *Anaesthesia and Intensive Care* **7**, 248.

2

Choosing the Equipment

The basic equipment required is a needle and a catheter of sufficient length to reach a central vein. The catheter can be introduced either through or over the introducing needle (Table 2.1). In a development of the technique, a *cannula* is first inserted into the vein over a needle; then, after removal of the needle, the catheter is threaded through the cannula. The guide wire or Seldinger[1] technique also starts with a needle being introduced into the vein; a matching guide wire is then passed through the needle, and, after removal of the needle, the catheter is introduced into the vein over the guide wire. A modification of this technique makes use of a tapered vein dilator with a wide-bore cannula, through which a large-sized catheter (e.g. a Swan–Ganz) can be inserted into a small vein. The terms 'cannula' and 'catheter' are not clearly defined in the medical literature. Shorter lengths, such as are commonly used for peripheral intravenous infusions, are usually, but not always, referred to as cannulae. Longer lengths (usually over long needles), intended for cannulation of subclavian or internal jugular veins, are sometimes referred to as cannulae and sometimes as catheters according to the manufacturer. Very long tubing is always referred to as a catheter. Since there is no agreement on definitions, the terms for the shorter lengths of tubing are used interchangeably in this book.

Table 2.1. Basic types of equipment

1. Catheter-through-needle
2. Catheter-over-needle
3. Catheter-through-cannula
4. Catheter-over-guide wire

BASIC TYPES OF EQUIPMENT

Catheter-through-needle devices

The catheter-through-needle equipment was the first to become widely available for introducing a long venous catheter although rarely used now. The device is easy to use because, once the needle tip is successfully inserted into the lumen of the vein, the catheter can be advanced through the needle tip without difficulty. It is also easy to see 'flashback' of blood into the hub of the needle immediately the vein is entered. Since the catheter lies inside the introducing needle it does not have to be pushed through the skin and deeper tissues; consequently the catheter can be constructed of a soft, pliant material and the tip need not be sharp. The long catheters of this type are usually protected by a transparent sleeve, so facilitating a 'no touch' technique during insertion of the catheter.

A drawback with this technique is that there may be leakage of blood, because the catheter is smaller than the hole made by the needle. The main disadvantage, however, is that the catheter may shear if attempts are made to withdraw it while the needle tip is still in the vein. Reports of sheared catheters nearly always relate to the use of catheter-through-needle devices.[2,3] Since the needle cannot usually be removed from the catheter because there is a fixed hub on the catheter, a protective sheath is supplied to prevent the sharp needle tip from damaging or cutting the catheter. The catheter may still be sheared through, however, if the protective sheath is incorrectly applied or becomes dislodged. A solution to this problem is to deliberately cut off the fixed hub from the catheter and so enable the needle to be removed. A suitable adaptor, such as a

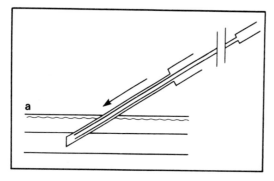

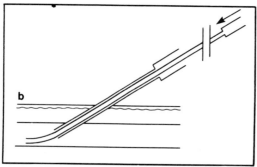

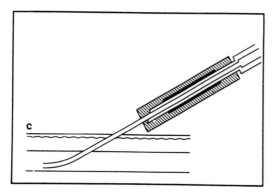

Figure 2.1. Catheter-through-needle devices: technique of use.

Touhy Borst connector, is then attached to the cut end of the catheter.

Technique (Figure 2.1)

(a) A percutaneous venepuncture is performed.
(b) The catheter is threaded through the needle and advanced along the vein. If the passage of the catheter is obstructed, both catheter and needle should be withdrawn from the vein and catheterisation attempted again. The catheter should on no account be pulled back through the needle.
(c) The needle is withdrawn over the catheter,

and the protective device to prevent the needle cutting the catheter is attached.

This type of device has been universally condemned[4,5] and is no longer produced by leading suppliers.

Catheter-over-needle devices

The catheter-over-needle device was developed to eliminate the risk of the needle cutting through the catheter. The needle is inside the catheter and both are inserted together when the vein is punctured. The needle is then withdrawn and the catheter advanced along the vein. Long and short versions of the catheter-over-needle device are available (Figure 2.2). In the long catheter, such as is used for catheterisation through arm veins, a syringe cannot be attached to aspirate blood and accelerated 'flashback' is the only reliable indication of entry into the vein. Furthermore, the needle tip protrudes beyond the catheter and so, although blood in the catheter may indicate that the needle tip is in the vein, it does not guarantee that the catheter tip is also in the vein.

The shorter catheter is simply an extra-long cannula (Figure 2.2a) intended for cannulation of the subclavian or internal jugular vein. A syringe can be attached to the needle so that blood can be aspirated to indicate successful venepuncture. Again this does not guarantee that the cannula tip is also inside the vein.

In both long and short types the catheter tip has to be fairly sharp and rigid since it must be pushed through the skin. It can therefore injure the vein as it is advanced or later, when in position. One advantage is that the hole made in the vein by the needle is smaller than the size of the catheter, so leakage of blood is less likely than with catheter-through-needle devices. Because the long cannula with long needle device is flexible, the operator may have to grasp the cannula near its distal end in order to push it through the skin and deeper tissues.

Because of its length, the long cannula on long needle has, not unexpectedly, been associated with inadvertent injury to most superior mediastinal structures.

Technique (Figure 2.3)

(a) A percutaneous venepuncture is made with the needle and closely fitting catheter. The

(a)

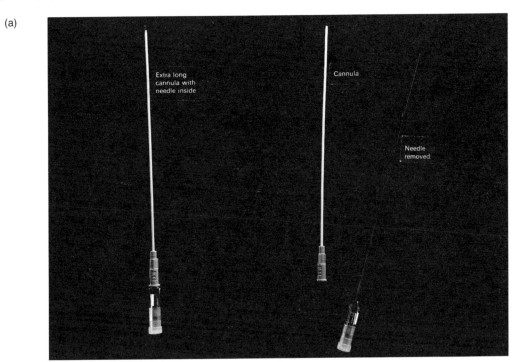

(b)

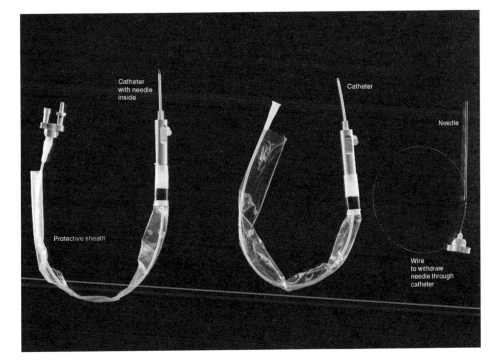

Figure 2.2. Catheter-over-needle devices.

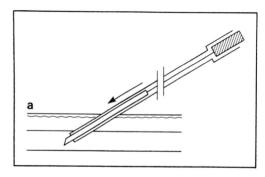

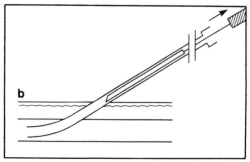

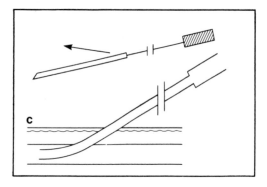

Figure 2.3. Catheter-over-needle devices: technique of use.

needle tip is advanced a further short distance (3–4 mm) to ensure that the catheter tip is also in the vein.
(b) The needle is withdrawn into the catheter, which is advanced into the vein.
(c) The needle is then completely removed and discarded.

Catheter-through-cannula devices (Figure 2.4)

The catheter-through-cannula device was devised to preserve the advantages of both the catheter-through-needle and catheter-over-needle devices whilst overcoming their drawbacks.

Venepuncture is performed with a short cannula with the needle inside. A syringe can therefore be attached to the needle and successful venepuncture easily detected. The cannula tip must still be fairly sharp and rigid since it has to be pushed through the skin and wall of the vein, but the catheter tip that is subsequently inserted through the cannula can be of a much safer material and design. The needle is removed before the catheter is inserted to eliminate the risk of damaging the catheter.

Certain disadvantages remain. It is still possible that the cannula tip does not lie within the lumen of the vein with the needle tip. Furthermore, the catheter is smaller than the hole in the vein so blood may leak around the catheter. The syringe must usually be detached from the cannula to insert the catheter, and at this point there is a risk of air embolism and bacterial contamination (Figure 2.4).

In all these types, if the introducing cannula is left in the lumen of the vein and the proximal end is open to atmosphere, there is a danger of serious air embolism.[6] The cannula tip should always be withdrawn from the vein, even if only to lie subcutaneously, where it can protect the catheter from kinking.

The catheter-through-cannula device is recommended for general use in catheterisation of veins at any site.

Technique (Figure 2.5)

(a) A percutaneous venepuncture is made with the short needle and introducing cannula.
(b) The needle is withdrawn completely and the catheter inserted through the cannula into the vein.
(c) The cannula should be withdrawn from the vein to be outside the skin *or* (d) at least withdrawn from the vein but left subcutaneously.

Catheter-over-guide wire devices

The catheter-over-guide wire technique, originally described for arterial cannulation,[1] can also be used for central venous catheterisation of any route, but is particularly indicated for subclavian or jugular vein techniques. The catheter is inserted into the vein over a guide wire. The guide wire is flexible and has an even more flexible leading end with a rounded tip. Obviously, a kinked or otherwise damaged wire should not be used. The main advantage of this technique is that the initial 'blind' needling of the vein can be performed with a

(a)

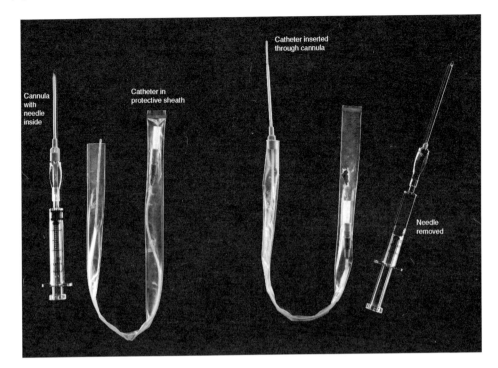

(b)

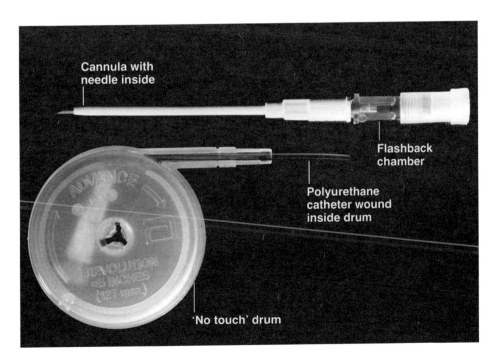

Figure 2.4. Catheter-through-cannula devices.

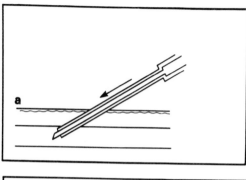

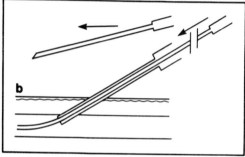

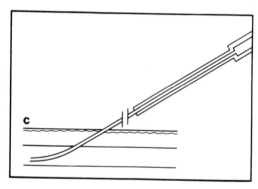

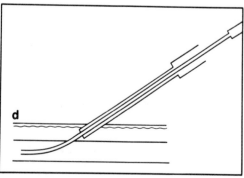

Figure 2.5. Catheter-through-cannula devices: technique of use.

smaller gauge needle (just wide enough to admit the appropriate guide wire). Trauma to important structures, including inadvertent arterial puncture with haematoma formation, is thus minimised. The guide wire technique is especially suited to catheterisation of the small deep veins of infants and children. Although this is a through-the-needle technique, there is no risk of damage to the catheter since the needle is completely removed before the catheter is introduced.

Inserting a long guide wire with its accompanying catheter from a peripheral arm vein is often difficult because of obstruction by valves or branching of veins. Therefore the guide wire method would be indicated only rarely when a peripheral arm vein is used, being more suited to cannulation of the subclavian, internal jugular, or femoral vein. Nevertheless, the guide wire technique may be used with advantage.[7] Since the catheter has to be pushed through the skin, it must be fairly rigid, sharp and tapered and is thus likely to damage the wall of the vein as it is advanced and subsequently when it lies in the vein. A recent and useful development is first to insert a short tapered cannula (vein dilator) over the guide wire; this vein dilator carries a shorter, wide-bore cannula. The taper dilates the vein and so allows the large cannula to be inserted. After removing the vein dilator (and guide wire) a catheter with a soft tip can easily be advanced through the wide-bore cannula. This technique is advocated for inserting the Swan–Ganz catheter.

In the basic guide wire technique the hole made by the needle is smaller than the catheter so leakage of blood is unlikely. Of course this advantage is absent when an introducing cannula is used. Full aseptic precautions including adequate towelling of the area are essential, because a 'no touch' technique cannot be applied.

This technique can be used to insert single and multilumen catheters and is the method advocated for inserting a Swan–Ganz catheter. The technique is not only potentially safer, but can also increase the success rate.[8] It is safer for two reasons. First, there is less risk of harm to deep structures. Second, the method eliminates the danger of air embolisation which is an inherent hazard of through-cannula devices when an open-ended introducer cannula is inadvertently allowed to communicate with the vein.[9,10]

Some clinicians may be deterred from using a guide wire method because of its apparent expense. However, the cost of the equipment is outweighed by the advantage of successful and safer catheterisation.

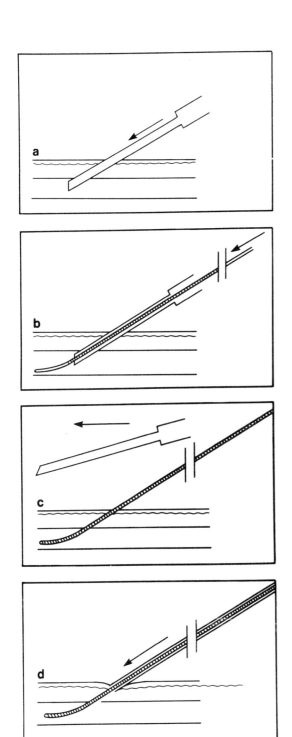

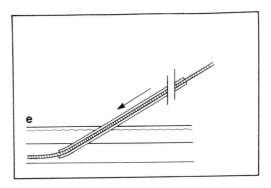

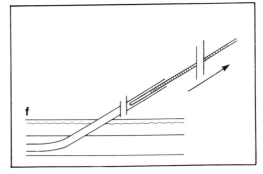

Figure 2.6. Catheter-over-guide wire devices: technique of use without a vein dilator.

Technique without a vein dilator (Figure 2.6)

(a) The guide wire must be smooth (unkinked) and able to pass through the needle. The more flexible end is identified by palpation. The catheter must fit closely over the wire without too much free movement. The guide wire must be at least 100 mm longer than the catheter. A percutaneous venepuncture is made with the needle attached to a syringe. The syringe is removed and steps taken to avoid air embolism.

(b) The flexible guide wire (lubricated with a heparinised saline solution to prevent clotting) is inserted through the needle with the more flexible end leading, a short distance (4–5 cm) into the vein.

(c) The needle is removed over the wire and discarded.

(d) The catheter is inserted over the wire, which is again lubricated, until the wire protrudes through the outside end. Both catheter and wire are pushed through the skin. A small incision made with a scalpel assists the passage of the catheter through the skin.

(e) The catheter and wire together are passed into the vein for a sufficient distance to ensure that the catheter tip lies in the desired position.

(f) The guide wire is removed carefully, retaining the catheter in position.

A useful 'extra' gained from the guide wire technique is the correlation between guide wire distortion and misplacement of the catheter tip when introduced through the infraclavicular sub-clavian vein route. If the wire is seen to be deviated cranially when it is withdrawn, then the inference is that the catheter has been misplaced into a neck vein.[11]

Technique with a vein dilator (Figure 2.7)

(a) and (b) are followed as above (and illustrated in Figure 2.6).

(c) The needle is removed over the guide wire and discarded. A tapered vein dilator carrying a cannula is inserted over the wire, which is again lubricated with heparinised saline. The wire and vein dilator are pushed through the skin into the lumen of the vein.

(d) The wide-bore outer cannula is pushed over the vein dilator, through the skin and into the lumen of the vein.

(e) The guide wire and vein dilator are removed, allowing a catheter (e.g. a Swan–Ganz) to pass readily through the wide-bore cannula.

(f) The tip of the large cannula is withdrawn outside the vein to act as a protective sheath, or is withdrawn completely outside the skin.

In a simpler progression the vein dilator is removed and the catheter inserted over the guide wire, along the dilated passage, into the vein.

A combined guide wire and vein dilator can increase the success rate of central venous catheter-isation through antecubital fossa veins.[12] Cathe-terisation through tributaries of the basilic vein has a far better chance of reaching a satisfactory central position than those inserted through the cephalic vein. However, an operator may be deterred from using a very small basilic vein to insert a large (13 gauge) cannula and opt for a larger cephalic vein which results in a poorer chance of successful central positioning. With the wire/dilator tech-nique a small gauge needle (18 gauge) is used to puncture the vein and to introduce a wire. Over this wire a vein dilator is then inserted progressing to the introduction of a large introducer allowing the

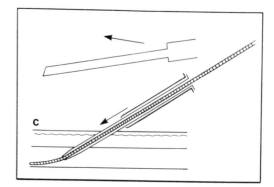

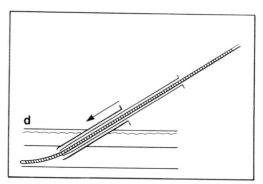

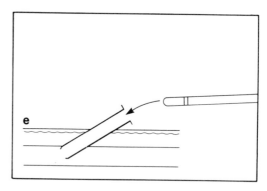

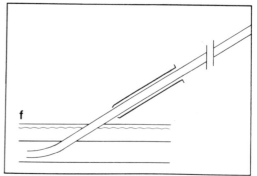

Figure 2.7. Catheter-over-guide wire devices: technique of use with a vein dilator.

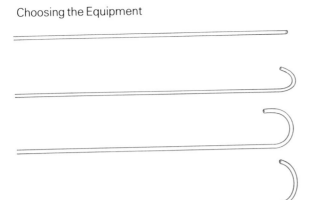

Figure 2.8. Flexible wire catheter guides. Straight and a variety of J-tipped wires. Reproduced with kind permission of Blitt *et al.* (1982).[17]

long catheter to be advanced centrally. This technique then permits successful catheterisation through a basilic vein even if it is quite small.

GUIDE WIRES (Figure 2.8)

Flexible but straight guide wires were originally used to facilitate percutaneous vascular catheterisation[1] and are still used extensively in angiographic techniques.

J-tipped guide wires were developed to overcome the difficulties encountered with the straight wire in negotiating tortuous or atheromatous arteries.[13,14] At the same time less damage to endothelial structures seemed likely. The smooth convexity of the J facilitates smooth advancement and enables the wires to 'turn corners' where a straight wire would be stopped by engagement of the tip in the wall of the vessel (Figure 2.9).

Blitt pioneered the use of the J-tipped wire in venous cannulation in 1974[15] when he described its advantage in obtaining virtually complete success in external jugular vein catheterisation. With conventional catheter devices, experience with this route is often disappointing, failure usually being attributed to tortuosity and acute angulation of the course of this vein together with the obstruction presented by venous valves. Similar success with the J-wire has not always been found by others[16,18] but many other workers have found the J-tipped wire advantageous and Blitt's further studies reinforce its value.[17]

The J-wire has also been used to significantly increase successful central venous catheter positioning when antecubital fossa veins are used. When the wire could be introduced into the basilic vein, all catheters reached a satisfactory position; 78% success was gained through the cephalic vein.[7]

Guide wires are not without their own hazards. Straight wires have been implicated in perforation of central vessel walls leading to pericardial tamponade.[18] Other complications have been reported.[19]

One of the causes of failure with the guide wire technique is displacement of the introducing needle tip out of the lumen of the vessel due to movement when a firmly fitted syringe is disconnected from the needle hub. In addition air embolism is a danger with the needle hub open to the atmosphere. These dangers have been eliminated by an ingenious device (Figure 2.10) now commercially available (Safety Syringe®–Arrow International Inc). The J-wire is introduced into the vein through a channel in the specially constructed syringe plunger without the need to disconnect the syringe.

Precautions when using guide wires

A straight guide wire may be selected for vessels having a linear configuration. A J-tipped wire is indicated for veins which have a tortuous course such as the external jugular vein. Some authorities advise the routine use of J-tipped wires to minimise endothelial damage.[20] This would seem to be sound advice.

Technical complications which can occur with the wire include knotting of the most flexible portion of the straight wire, separation of the helical portion of a straight wire and displacement of the rounded tip of a J-wire.

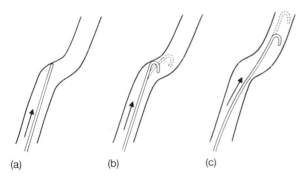

(a)   (b)   (c)

Figure 2.9. Schematic representation of obstruction to guide wire tip and advantage of J-tipped (b and c) over the straight tip (a).

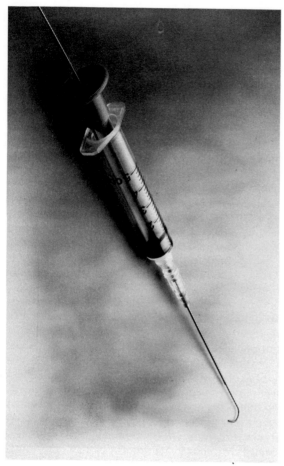

Figure 2.10. Arrow–Raulerson Syringe with the guide wire passing through the syringe. Reproduced with kind permission of Arrow International Inc. (Europe).

Complications can be avoided if the following precautions are taken:

(a) Inspect the wire for defects before insertion.
(b) Consider a guide wire to be a delicate and fragile instrument.
(c) When resistance to insertion is met, remove and inspect the wire for damage; reposition the introducer so that no resistance to its passage is felt.
(d) Enlarge the skin puncture with a pointed scalpel blade to enable smooth one step passage of the catheter insertion over the wire.
(e) If multiple manipulations are needed, re-inspect the wire and replace if necessary.
(f) Always inspect the wire for complete removal at the end of the procedure.
(g) Do not reuse disposable guide wires.

MULTILUMEN CATHETERS

A multilumen catheter is a central venous catheter with more than one completely separate channel. They may be double or triple lumen, the latter appearing to be most popular (Figure 2.11). Only double lumen catheters are available for paediatric use. They are necessarily large catheters with external diameters of 2·3 mm or more compared with single lumen catheters which are not usually more than 2 mm (14 gauge) across. A typical arrangement of the channels in a triple lumen catheter as seen longitudinally is shown in Figure 2.12.[21] The distal ports of the three channels are staggered along a short length of catheter to minimise mixing of infusates as they exit.

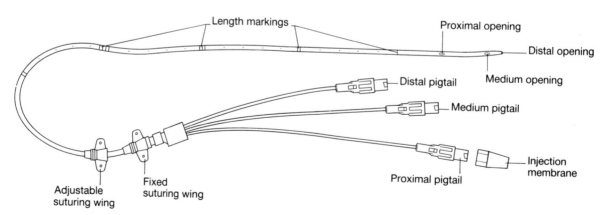

Figure 2.11. Features of a triple lumen catheter.

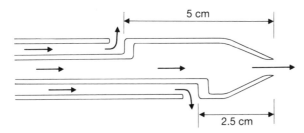

Figure 2.12. Diagram of longitudinal section of distal end of a triple lumen catheter. Reproduced by kind permission of Coe and Coates (1988).[21]

Manufacturers produce a variety of ways in which the separate lumens are disposed in cross section (Figure 2.13). A typical arrangement for double lumen catheters is shown in Figure 2.13a. The most common arrangement in triple lumen catheters is one large lumen (16 gauge) and two smaller (18 gauge) ones (Figure 2.13c, d). The lumen diameter determines the flow rate through the channel. The wall thickness determines to some extent the catheter's strength. Any particular configuration of lumen diameters therefore represents a compromise.

Catheter lengths available are 15 and 20 cm for right-sided internal jugular and subclavian vein entry sites whilst longer catheters (25 and 30 cm) cater for left-sided attempts. Most catheters incorporate distance markings.

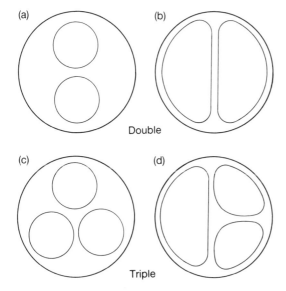

Figure 2.13. Cross section of double and triple lumen catheters showing how lumen size can vary.

Paradoxically, the first of what is essentially a multi-lumen central venous catheter produced commercially was the most complex. This was the pulmonary artery flotation catheter which, although a single device, incorporated not only a thermistor and balloon-tipped pulmonary artery catheter but also a separate catheter with its own lumen opening into the right atrium for injecting an indicator solution for estimating cardiac output. The nature of its construction prevents the flotation catheter itself from being guided into the vein over a flexible wire, so the introduction of the flotation catheter spawned a number of introducer kits which facilitated insertion of the large-bore catheter. The introducer and vein dilator themselves necessitated a guide wire for their insertion. There appears therefore to have developed from this available technology the production of the simpler multi-lumen catheter. The first double and triple lumen venous catheters were made available in 1982 (Arrow–Howes Multi-Lumen Central Venous Catheter, Arrow International Inc.). Similar designs are now widely available from all leading manufacturers.

Multi-lumen central venous catheters provide several benefits in those situations where several routes of venous access are needed for the effective management of the patient. For example, in many patients undergoing intensive therapy, central venous access is needed for drug administration, blood sampling, pressure measurements and intravenous infusions of both crystalloids and parenteral nutrition fluids. If all these functions are being carried out through a single lumen catheter there are obvious hazards resulting from the constant interruption of and surges in drug delivery and the mixing of infusates, apart from the practical inconvenience. In addition, the advantage of the multi-lumen catheter is very apparent in reducing the hazards inherent in making several separate venepunctures into deep neck veins to secure several individual venous channels.[22]

The main disadvantages appear to be cost and the risk of interaction of the different infusates as they emerge from the exit ports which must necessarily be close together. Catheter infection and catheter-related sepsis is well documented in relation to single lumen catheters[23–26] and an increased incidence might have been expected with multi-lumen catheters. Critical appraisal of such reports suggests that catheter-related sepsis is more likely to be expected in patients with multi-lumen catheters because they are more ill and require more handling of their catheter and connections.[27]

Breach of catheter management protocol is also an important contributing factor.[28] However, several careful prospective studies indicate that multi-lumen catheters may be safely used in severely ill patients requiring total parenteral nutrition provided that the care protocol is adhered to.[27,29–31] Prospective comparative studies with single lumen catheters support the safety of multi-lumen catheters although the risk of catheter sepsis is no less.[32] With these conflicting reports in mind it is probably wise to use a channel of a triple lumen catheter for parenteral nutrition only in the short term if such a catheter has been deemed necessary for the overall management of the patient. If intravenous feeding is likely to be long term, then at a later stage a dedicated tunnelled single lumen catheter can be inserted. A practical disadvantage of relying on venous access only through a multi-lumen catheter is that 'all one's eggs are in one basket'. If the multi-lumen catheter has to be removed, all venous access is lost in one move.

Insertion of multi-lumen catheters

The recommended method of inserting these catheters is with the Seldinger guide wire technique and vein dilator (see p. 18).

Before proceeding examine the catheter and identify each channel with its own proximal pigtail (usually colour coded). Irrigate each channel with heparinised saline.

(a) Perform venepuncture of the chosen vein using the small-gauge wire introducer needle.
(b) Insert guide wire to the SVC and remove the needle. Allow a length of wire outside the skin sufficient to thread the whole length of the catheter plus an extra 2–3 cm to hold the wire as the catheter is slid into the vein over the wire.
(c) Enlarge the puncture with a sharp-pointed scalpel blade.
(d) Advance the vein dilator over the wire into the vein.

Table 2.2. Sizes of needles, catheters and guide wires (adults).

Route of insertion	Introducer and long catheter			Long cannula with long needle	Introducer, guide wire and catheter			
	Outside diameter of introducing needle or cannula (G)	Minimum length of introducing needle or cannula (mm)	Minimum length of catheter* (mm)	Minimum length[†] (mm)	Outside diameter of introducing needle for guide wire (G) (mm)	Outside diameter guide wire (mm)	Minimum length of catheter (mm)	Length of guide wire
Arm veins	14 or 16	Short (40)	600	Not applicable	18(1·2)	0·77	600	
Internal jugular vein	14 or 16	Short (40) Some techniques require 70	200	130	18(1·2)	0·77	200	Must exceed length of catheter by at least 100 mm
Subclavian vein	14 or 16	Mid-clavicular insertion 60. More lateral 70	200	130	18(1·2)	0·77	200	
External jugular vein	14 or 16	Short (40)	200	130	18(1·2)	0·77	200	
Femoral vein	14	Short (40)	600	Not applicable	18(1·2)	0·77	600	

* The catheter length allows for surplus catheter outside the skin for secure fixation.
[†] The design precludes excess length for fixation of catheter.

(e)   Remove vein dilator.
(f)   Thread the catheter tip over the wire and insert it to its required length.
(g)   Remove the wire and confirm satisfactory positioning by easy aspiration of blood from each channel, flushing each lumen with heparinised saline.
(h)   Secure and apply a dressing to the puncture site.
(i)   Confirm position of catheter tip with a chest x-ray.

Some catheters are inserted using a catheter-through-cannula technique (see p. 14). The introducer cannula can be peeled apart and removed so eliminating any danger of air embolism which may exist with a through the cannula technique where the introducer cannula is left in the vein. This technique is probably only necessary for inserting the very soft silicone elastomer multi-lumen catheters.

SIZE OF NEEDLES, CATHETERS AND GUIDE WIRES

Table 2.2 gives some guidance in the selection of suitably sized equipment.

The introducing needle and cannula

Length

For puncturing visible superficial veins the introducing needle and cannula can be short (about 40 mm). When attempting puncture of deep veins the length must be adequate to reach the vein – something that may be difficult to estimate accurately in an obese patient. An introducer may need to be up to 70 mm long to gain entry to the subclavian vein, although a shorter length (40–60 mm) is adequate for puncture of the internal jugular vein.

In the case of the long cannula over the long needle, a sufficient length of cannula must be inserted into the vein for its tip to reach a satisfactory central venous position. This requirement determines the minimum length of the needle. Since the long needle is flexible it is difficult to control the tip accurately when attempting to puncture a vein. The risk of traumatic complications may thus be increased.

Diameter

Peripheral veins in particular can vary widely in size and may not even be visible or palpable in states of circulatory collapse, whereas the subclavian vein is always held open by its surrounding tissues. Veins can usually be distended by adopting aids such as a tourniquet or nitroglycerine ointment in the case of peripheral arm veins or a head-down position in the case of internal jugular and subclavian veins. Generally, in adults, a 14 or 16 gauge outside diameter (O.D.) introducing needle or introducing cannula is appropriate for central venous cannulation through large proximal veins. In the case of superficial veins the operator can make his decision only after inspecting the veins. Whenever the chosen vein is constricted or small, a guide wire technique will allow the use of a smaller gauge introducing needle and the subsequent insertion of a large diameter catheter, using a vein dilator if necessary. Much smaller introducing needles or cannulae (18 gauge or smaller) have to be used in infants.

Cannulae and catheters

Length

The minimum length of a central venous cannula or catheter should equal the distance from the skin puncture to the desired central venous position with sufficient length outside the skin to facilitate secure fixation. This distance should be estimated on the skin surface of the patient when selecting equipment.

Diameter

The outside diameter of the catheter in a through-needle or -cannula device must be related to the type of introducer, as it must obviously be smaller than the needle or introducing cannula in order to pass through it. If the catheter is to be inserted over the needle, the inside diameter of the catheter is also relevant. In most commercially available equipment the introducing needle and catheter are closely matched. In a guide wire technique the wire must pass easily through the introducing needle; furthermore, the internal diameter of the catheter and the outside diameter of the wire must be such as to form a close fit.

Table 2.3. Choice of material for catheter

Type of material	Thrombogenic	Stiffness	Short-term use (48 h)	Long-term use
Polyethylene PVC or nylon	+ +	+ +	Suitable	Unsuitable
Polypropylene	+ +	+ + +	Suitable	Unsuitable
Fluorocarbons Teflon TFF	+	+	Suitable	Uncertain
Teflon FEP	+	+	Suitable	Uncertain
Polyurethane	+	0/+	Suitable	Suitable
Hydromer-coated polyurethane	0	0 (when wet)	Suitable	Alternative material of choice
Silicone elastomer	0	0 (pliable but difficult to insert. Stylet needed)	Suitable	Material of choice based on long experience

CATHETER MATERIAL

The ideal catheter material is chemically inert, non-thrombogenic, flexible, radiopaque, and transparent (Table 2.3).

Most plastics contain various additives which may produce chemical phlebitis. These additives may comprise as much as 50% of the plastic material[33] and include plasticisers, stabilising agents, antioxidants, barium or tungsten salts for radiopacity, and colouring material. The only way to determine whether these substances may leach out in the body is by subjecting the catheter material to biological implant tests. Most British and American manufacturers use only tested materials. Silicone elastomer catheters have been generally considered to be the most biologically inert but the validity of this has been questioned.[34]

Physical characteristics

Physical damage to the wall of the vein is related to the stiffness of the catheter. Stiff catheters generate thrombosis by pressure on the vein wall,[35] whilst flexible catheters that float in the bloodstream are less likely to produce injury.[36] Catheters made of polyethyl and polypropylene are relatively stiff and thrombogenic.[35-40] Fluorocarbons represent some improvement over the earlier materials, and fluoro-

ethylene propylene (Teflon FEP) in particular has been shown to cause fewer venous complications than the older materials and tetrafluoroethylene (Teflon TFE).[41,42] Teflon FEP was widely used in the manufacture of cannulae. Most of these materials have now been dropped by most manufacturers in favour of polyurethane (PU). PU catheters have superior mechanical properties (tensile strength, wearing resistance many times that of silicone elastomer, ability to recover original shape after deformation). In addition PU is resistant to oils, oxidation hydrolysis and thermal degradation. In practice, these properties confer advantages in resisting kinking, bending and deformation compared with the plastics that were previously popular (Teflon, polyethylene and PVC). The softest and most flexible material is silicone elastomer, and is still generally regarded as the least thrombogenic and traumatic of currently available catheter materials. However, silicone elastomer catheters are so soft that they are difficult to insert into veins unless a stylet is employed. SE catheters are much more fragile than PU catheters and are relatively easily ruptured when distended.[34]

Thrombogenicity

Whilst catheter stiffness has been implicated in the initiation of thrombus formation, making silicone elastomer with its soft characteristics preferable, it is possible that the chemical composition of the catheter is a more important factor in determining the incidence of clinical thrombophlebitis. Comparing equally soft PU and SE catheters, thrombophlebitis occurred significantly less often with the PU catheter.[34] Other experimental studies show a wide range of thrombogenicity between different materials. Comparing PU, Hydromer (TM)-coated PU, PVC, and SE catheters, Hydromer (TM)-coated PU appeared the best, followed by SE. Plain PU was the worst.[43]

Hydromer is a polymer made from polyvinylpyrrolidone (PVP) and an isocyanate prepolymer. PVP is widely used in medical practice which includes its role as a plasma expander. The Hydromer (TM) polymer so formed is a hydrophilic substance (i.e. it absorbs water) and forms a gel. When a Hydromer (TM)-coated catheter is wetted, water is adsorbed onto the coating and the resulting gel acts as a barrier between the blood flowing past in the vessel and the catheter material (a foreign substance which would normally lead to platelet deposition).

Thus any tendency for the initiation of thrombosis is inhibited. A practical advantage of a Hydromer-coated catheter is that when wetted by body fluids including blood, the catheter becomes exceptionally slippery which assists easy passage of the catheter thus producing less trauma to the blood vessel.

Heparin coating and bonding have proved disappointing for protecting catheters against the risk of thrombogenesis in long-term catheterisation. Studies show no benefit compared with uncoated catheters.[44,45]

Catheters should be radiopaque since it has been shown by many authors that an x-ray is the only reliable method of determining the position of the catheter tip. Radiopaque catheters constructed of all the materials mentioned above are now commercially available. Catheters of transparent material allow air bubbles and particles to be easily seen. The older materials are transparent but some Teflon and silicone elastomer catheters are opaque.

Table 2.4. Long-term central venous catheter devices

Catheter type	Description	Examples
Tunnelled silicone catheter	Silicone catheter tunnelled subcutaneously exiting the skin medial to the nipple. Dacron cuff around catheter at least 3 cm away from the skin entry site	Hickman— single or double lumen Broviac— smaller lumen Quinton—double lumen Grosshong— single or double lumen, special sealing valve at tip allowing saline instead of heparin to maintain patency
Subcutaneous infusion port	Silicone catheter tunnelled subcutaneously ending in a self-sealing silicone reservoir implanted beneath the skin	Mediport Infus-a-Port Port-a-Cath Vascuport

Most catheter materials are suitable for short-term catheterisation (up to 48 hours) and selection is therefore determined by availability, ease of insertion, and cost. For long-term use, non-thrombogenicity, flexibility, and chemical inertness are paramount and override the requirements for ease of insertion and radiopacity. Silicone elastomer catheters are therefore recommended for longer-term catheterisation, especially for prolonged intravenous alimentation. Of the other materials, polyurethane- and hydromer (TM)-coated polyurethane catheters are to be preferred for long term use.

APPARATUS USED IN LONG-TERM CENTRAL VENOUS ACCESS

Long-term central venous access has become an integral requirement in the management of an increasingly wide spectrum of disease. The needs of patients in this category has led to the development of special devices to avoid the shortcomings of simpler catheter systems which include the frequent occurrence of catheter-related pain, phlebitis and infections.[46] With repeated treatments some patients have simply run out of accessible veins.

The components of these specialised systems comprise a suitable catheter which has been invariably of silicone elastomer. In recent years newer materials such as Hydromer-coated polyurethane have been advocated for long-term catheters. Traditionally, the catheter has been inserted into a suitable vein (usually the subclavian) using a surgical cut-down procedure. Catheters can, however, also be inserted satisfactorily with percutaneous techniques although it appears that surgical cut-down retains its popularity in these special cases. The catheter is then tunnelled subcutaneously to a distal site where it terminates in two possible ways (Table 2.5).

Where the catheter is led through a skin exit site, a Dacron cuff surrounds the catheter before it emerges. The Dacron cuff is designed to encourage local fibrosis, which acts as a physical barrier to the entry of bacteria along the track of the catheter as well as to anchor the catheter securely.

In the second type of device (Figures 2.14 and 2.15), the catheter ends in a reservoir (e.g. Port-a-Cath) which has been implanted subcutaneously. The reservoir has a self-sealing silicone diaphragm through which entry is made into the reservoir by

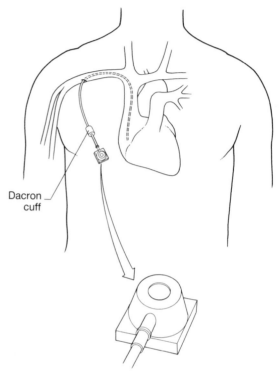

Figure 2.14. The long-term central venous catheter with a subcutaneously implanted reservoir (Port-a-Cath type). Note Dacron cuff. Reproduced with kind permission of Clarke and Raffin (1990).[51]

percutaneous puncture. A needle with a special Huber point is available (Viggo Products, Swindon, UK). The tip of this needle is designed to displace rather than tear the fibres of the silicone diaphragm of the reservoir.[47] A Dacron cuff is again often incorporated in this system.

A recent innovation has been the introduction of a cuff made of biodegradable collagen to which silver ion has been chelated.[48] The cuff has been developed to be used with percutaneously inserted catheters. It is attached to the catheter prior to insertion into the vein. Subsequently, subcutaneous tissue grows into the collagen and as with the Dacron cuff, provides a barrier to bacteria and secures the catheter. In addition, the silver ion acts as a chemical barrier to the passage of organisms. Studies give encouraging results in the reduction of catheter-related sepsis and the enhanced life span of catheters.

Unfortunately, even these sophisticated techniques have not fully prevented a significant incidence of catheter-related problems, especially catheter infections. Nevertheless, experience over many years confirms the value of these specialised devices in long-term central venous catheter survival, but only if strict recommendations concerning their insertion and maintenance are adhered to (see Ch. 3).

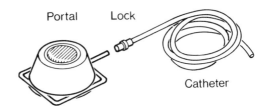

DOUBLE LUMEN CENTRAL VENOUS HAEMODIALYSIS CATHETERS

These were introduced to provide permanent access for renal dialysis and to spare peripheral vessels for the creation of more durable arterio-venous fistulae. The method of insertion is identical to any guide wire technique. It is crucial to place both distal orifices of the catheter in a large diameter vein to obtain adequate flows for the dialysis machine. Full patency and adequate free flow of blood through both lumens of the catheter must be established before the catheter is fixed in position.

These catheters have integral clamping devices to prevent air embolism. When not in use the catheter is regularly flushed with heparinised saline. The majority of these catheters will function for up to two months. Replacement of the catheter can be performed over a guide wire provided that the original catheter is not the source of sepsis and is not blocked by thrombus.[49,50]

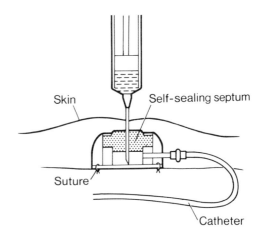

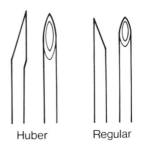

Figure 2.15. The Port-a-Cath system and diagram showing percutaneous access to the portal using the Huber-point needle. Reproduced with kind permission of Soo *et al.* (1985).[52]

REFERENCES

1. Seldinger, S. I. (1953). Catheter replacement of needle in percutaneous arteriography: new technique. *Acta Radiologica* 39, 368.
2. Taylor, F. W. and Rutherford, C. E. (1963). Accidental loss of plastic tube into venous system. *Archives of Surgery* 86, 177.
3. Bennett, P. J. (1963). Use of intravenous plastic catheters. *British Medical Journal* 2, 1252.
4. John, G. E. (1972). Serious accidents involving intravenous catheters. DHSS DS (Supply) 6/72. DHSS Circular.
5. Farman, J. V. (1978). Which central venous catheter? *British Journal of Clinical Equipment* 32, 210.
6. Ross, S. M., Freedman, P. S. and Farman, J. V. (1979). Air embolism after accidental removal of intravenous catheter. *British Medical Journal* 1, 987.
7. Smith, S. L., Albin, M. S., Ritter, R. R. and Bunegin, L. (1984). CVP catheter replacement from the antecubital veins using a J-wire catheter guide. *Anesthesiology* 60, 238.
8. Belani, K. G., Buckley, J. J., Gordon, J. R. and Castenda, W. (1980). Percutaneous cervical central venous line placement: a comparison of the internal and external jugular vein routes. *Anesthesia and Analgesia* 59, 40.
9. Peters, J. L. and Armstrong, R. (1978). Air embolism occurring as a complication of central venous catheterization. *Annals of Surgery* 187, 375.
10. *Lancet* (1986). Central venous catheterisation. Editorial. 2, 669.

11. Miller, J. D. B. and Broom, J. (1983). Early non-radiological recognition of misplacement of central venous catheter. *British Medical Journal* **287**, 95.

12. Bowdle, T. A. (1984). Improved technique for placement of Sorenson CVP catheter. *Anesthesia and Analgesia* **63**, 1143.

13. Baum, S. and Abrams, H. L. (1964). A J-shaped catheter for retrograde catheterization of tortuous vessels. *Radiology* **83**, 436.

14. Judkins, M. and Kidd, H. J. *et al.* (1967). Lumen-following J-guide for catheterization of tortuous vessels. *Radiology* **88**, 1127.

15. Blitt, C. D., Wright, W. A., Petty, C. P. and Webster, T. A. (1974). Central venous catheterization via the external jugular vein. A technique employing the J-wire. *Journal of the American Medical Association* **229**, 817.

16. Blyth, P. L. (1985). Evaluation of the technique of central venous catheterisation via the external jugular vein using the J-wire. *Anaesthesia and Intensive Care* **13**, 131.

17. Blitt, C. D., Carlson, G. L., Wright, W. A. and Otto, C. W. (1982). J-wire versus straight wire for central venous system cannulation via the external jugular vein. *Anesthesia and Analgesia* **61**, 536.

18. Wilkie, M. and Hughes, M. (1988). Complications of central venous cannulation. *British Medical Journal* **297**, 1126.

19. Schwartz, A. J., Harrow, J. C., Jobes, D. R. and Ellison, N. (1981). Guide wires – a caution. *Critical Care Medicine* **9**, 347.

20. Kaye, C. G. and Smith, D. R. (1988). Complications of central venous cannulation. *British Medical Journal* **297**, 572.

21. Coe, A. J. and Coates, D. P. (1988). Triple lumen catheters. *British Journal of Hospital Medicine* **3**, 313.

22. Powell, H. (1988). Safety first with triple lumen. *Murmurs (Lilly Cardiac Care)* **5**.

23. Mogenson, J. V., Frederiksen, W. and Jensen, J. K. (1972). Subclavian vein catheterization and infection: a bacteriological study of 130 catheterization insertions. *Scandinavian Journal of Infectious Disease* **4**, 31.

24. Bernard, R. W., Stahl, W. M. and Chase, R. M. Jr. (1971). Subclavian vein catheterization: a prospective study. II. Infectious complications. *Annals of Surgery* **173**, 191.

25. Applefield, J. A., Carruthers, T. E., Reno, D. J. *et al.* (1978). Assessment of the sterility of long-term cardiac catheterization using the thermodilution Swan–Ganz catheter. *Chest* **74**, 377.

26. Michel, L., Marsh, M., McMichan, J. C. *et al.* (1981). Infection of pulmonary artery catheters in critically ill patients. *Journal of the American Medical Association* **245**, 1032.

27. Payne-James, J. J., Doherty, J., Rees, R. G. and Silk, D. B. A. (1989). A prospective evaluation of a multi-lumen central venous catheter in patients requiring total parenteral nutrition. ITCM Aug/Sept. **89**, 213.

28. Clarke, P. J., Ball, M. J., Tunbridge, A. and Kettlewell, M. G. W. (1988). The total parenteral nutrition service: an update. *Annals of the Royal College of Surgeons* **70**, 296.

29. Kelly, C. S., Ligas, J. R., Smith, C. A., Madden, G. M.,

Ross, K. A. and Becker, D. R. (1986). Sepsis due to triple lumen central venous catheters. *Surgery, Gynecology and Obstetrics* **163**, 14.

30. Paterson-Brown, S., Parry, B. R. and Sim, A. J. W. (1987). The role of double-lumen catheters in intravenous nutrition. *Intensive Therapy and Clinical Monitoring* **8**, 54.

31. Kaufman, J. L., Rodriguez, J. L., McFadden, J. A. and Brolin, R. E. (1986). Clinical experience with the multi lumen central nervous catheter. *Journal of Parenteral and Enteral Nutrition* **10**, 487.

32. Miller, J. J., Venus, B. and Mathru, M. (1984). Comparison of the sterility of long-term central venous catheterization using single lumen, triple lumen, and pulmonary artery catheters. *Critical Care Medicine* **12**, 634.

33. Mitchell, D. C. (1975). Putting up a drip. *Info* No. 12. Queensborough, Kent: Abbott Laboratories.

34. Linder, L., Curelaru, I., Gustavsson, B., Hansson, H., Stenqvist, O. and Wojciechowski, J. (1984). Material thrombogenicity in central venous catheterization: a comparison between soft, antebrachial catheters of silicone elastomer and polyurethane. *Journal of Parenteral and Enteral Nutrition* **8**, 399.

35. Indar, R. (1959). The danger of indwelling polyethylene cannulae in deep veins. *Lancet* **1**, 284.

36. Hoshal, V. L., Ause, R. G. and Hoskins, P. A. (1971). Fibrin sleeve formation on indwelling subclavian central venous catheters. *Archives of Surgery* **102**, 353.

37. Wyatt, R., Glaves, I. and Cooper, D. J. (1974). Cannulation of the radial artery. *Lancet* **2**, 156.

38. Frazer, I. H., Eke, N. and Laing, M. S. (1977). Is infusion phlebitis preventable? *British Medical Journal* **2**, 232.

39. Pottecher, T., Forrier, M., Picardat, R. and Krause, D. (1984). Central venous catheter thrombogenicity. *European Journal of Anaesthesia* **1**, 361.

40. Stenqvist, O., Curelaru, I., Linder, L. and Gustavsson, B. (1983). Stiffness of central venous catheters. *Acta Anaesthesiologia Scandinavica* **27**, 153.

41. Dinley, R. J. (1976). Venous reactions related to indwelling plastic cannulae: a prospective clinical trial. *Current Medical Research and Opinion* **3**, 607.

42. Thomas, F. W., Evers, W. and Racz, B. G. (1970). Post infusion phlebitis. *Anesthesia and Analgesia: Current Researches* **49**, 150.

43. Borow, M. and Crowley, J. G. (1985). Evaluation of central venous catheter thrombogenicity. *Acta Anaesthesiologia Scandinavica, Suppl.* **81**, 59.

44. Bennegard, L., Curelaru, I., Gustavsson, B., Linder, L. E. and Zachrisson, B. F. (1982). Material thrombogenicity in central venous catheterization. I. A comparison between uncoated and heparin-coated, long, antebrachial polyethylene catheters. *Acta Anaesthesiologica Scandinavica* **26**, 112.

45. Mollenholt, P., Eriksson, I. and Andersson, T. (1987). Thrombogenicity of pulmonary–artery catheters. *Intensive Care Medicine* **13**, 57.

46. Peters, J. L., Belsham, P. A., Taylor, B. A. and Watt-Smith, S. (1984). Long-term venous access. *British Journal of Hospital Medicine* **32**, 230.

47. Shanbhogue, L. K. R., Bruce, J. and Bianchi, A. (1990). Implantation of a central venous access device. *Journal of the Royal College of Surgeons, Edinburgh* **35**, 252.

48. Maki, D. G., Cobb, L., Garman, J. K. and Shapiro, J. M. (1988). An attachable silver-impregnated cuff for prevention of infection with central venous catheters: a prospective randomized multicenter trial. *American Journal of Medicine* **85**, 307.

49. Dunn, Y., Nylander, W. and Richie, R. (1987). Central venous dialysis access: experience with dual lumen silicone rubber catheters. *Surgery* **102**, 784.

50. Schwab, S. J., Buller, G. L. and McCann, R. L. *et al.* (1986). Prospective evaluation of a Dacron cuffed haemodialysis catheter for prolonged use. *American Journal of Kidney Disease* **11**, 166.

51. Clarke, D. E. and Raffin, A. (1990). Infectious complications of indwelling long-term central venous catheters. *Chest* **97**, 966.

52. Soo, K. C., Davidson, T. I., Selby, P. and Westbury, G. (1985). Long-term venous access using a subcutaneous implantable drug delivery system. *Annals of the Royal College of Surgeons of England*, **67**, 264.

3

Practical Aspects of Technique

Each technique of central venous catheterisation is described separately below, but there are a number of important practical procedures which can increase the likelihood of a successful and safe cannulation in all methods. Guidance in these procedures is presented in roughly the sequence in which an operator may need them during central venous catheterisation.

IDENTIFICATION OF ANATOMICAL PLANES

In many of the techniques described in this book it is necessary to relate the direction in which the needle is advanced to conventional anatomical planes (Figure 3.1). This is important in order to avoid ambiguity in the descriptions.

PREVENTION OF AIR EMBOLISM

There is a risk of air embolism whenever a vein is cannulated and particularly when it is a large vein such as the internal jugular or subclavian. This complication can occur through a leak or a disconnection (deliberate or accidental) which opens the system to the atmosphere. It has been estimated that a fatal dose of air – 100 ml – can enter through a 14 gauge cannula in 1 second. Attention to the following points can greatly diminish the danger.

Position

If the venous pressure at the site of the venepuncture can be increased by correct positioning of the patient the risk of aspiration of air is diminished. For instance, in approaches to the subclavian and

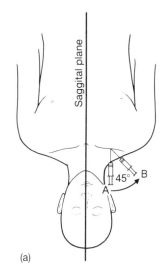

(a)

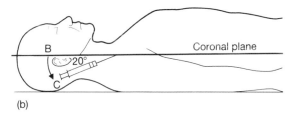

(b)

Figure 3.1. Identification of anatomical planes. (a) Needle and syringe moved 45° away from *sagittal* plane (A to B). (b) Needle and syringe depressed 20° below the *coronal* plane (B to C).

How the FLO●SWITCH® works

Push switch forward,
ball bearing presses
onto tube.

Move switch back
and fluid pathway
is opened.

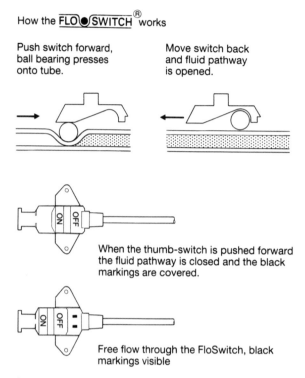

When the thumb-switch is pushed forward
the fluid pathway is closed and the black
markings are covered.

Free flow through the FloSwitch, black
markings visible

Figure 3.2.　FloSwitch.

jugular veins a head-down tilt (10–30°) is necessary – besides distending the vein and facilitating successful venepuncture this also prevents air embolism. The same advantages follow the use of a tourniquet during puncture of the arm veins. It is important to remember, however, that when the tourniquet is released the open hub on the needle or catheter must be kept below the level of the patient's right atrium until it is closed by means of a stopcock or connected to an infusion system. These precautions also apply when catheterising the femoral vein.

Air leaks

Most techniques employ a syringe attached to a needle. It is essential to check that the joint between syringe and needle (or introducing cannula) is airtight. Some cannulae incorporate an on/off switch at the hub (FloSwitch, Viggo-Spectramed, Swindon, UK, Figure 3.2) or a flexible hub (Flexihub, H. G. Wallace Ltd, Colchester, U.K., Figure 3.3) which can be compressed between the fingers. These types of device help to prevent the entry of air during cannulation and when connections are being made.

A less obvious danger of air embolism exists when a catheter is introduced into the vein through a wide-bore cannula which is left with its tip in the vein,[2] for air can pass through the space between the catheter and the wide-bore cannula. If the catheter is accidentally withdrawn, there is a very wide passage for air to reach the vein. It is therefore essential to withdraw the introducing cannula completely from the interior of the vein.

Split introducer cannulae, as their name suggests, can be peeled apart and removed entirely from the vein after successful insertion of a catheter with a fixed hub (Figure 3.4).

Patient's respiration

If the patient is inhaling deeply when the system is open to the air, the subatmospheric pressure within the thorax may suck air into the venous system. Therefore, a conscious patient should be instructed not to breathe deeply during the procedure. If an anaesthetised or unconscious patient is attached to a breathing circuit the venous pressure should be increased by holding the lungs briefly in inflation at any critical time.

INITIAL LOCATION OF THE VEIN WITH A SMALL-GAUGE NEEDLE

The technique of using a small-gauge needle to locate the vein can be employed usefully in any approach in which venepuncture is 'blind'. Exploration with a small-gauge needle minimises

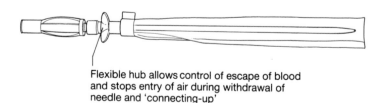

Flexible hub allows control of escape of blood
and stops entry of air during withdrawal of
needle and 'connecting-up'

Figure 3.3.　Flexihub.

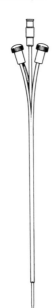

Figure 3.4. Split introducer. Reproduced with kind permission of Wood (1985).[113]

injury and haematoma formation should an artery be inadvertently punctured.

This technique has been advocated for the internal jugular route,[3,4,5] and the subclavian route.[6]

Directional guide

A 21 or 22 gauge outside diameter needle of suitable length is attached to a syringe. If local anaesthetic is being infiltrated subcutaneously, the same needle can be introduced more deeply to locate the vein.[7] A slight negative pressure is maintained on the syringe as the needle is advanced until a 'flashback' of blood indicates entry into the vein. The position of the vein is noted, the small needle removed (or left in position as a guide) and venepuncture with the larger needle attempted along a parallel track.

Guide wire technique

If a guide wire technique is used, the small gauge wire introducer needle can serve also as the locating needle. However, in many commercially available kits, the introducer needle is sometimes, it seems, unnecessarily long and large (18 or 16 gauge). In these cases a small gauge 21 or 22 short needle is recommended to find the vein first.

An ingenious method has been described which makes use of apparatus which is freely available and represents a modified guide wire method. This technique was used in internal jugular vein cannulation.[3] An adult 22 gauge spinal needle is threaded through a large (14 gauge) but shorter needle. The lumen of the vein is first located with the spinal needle and the needle advanced 2–3 mm into the vein. The wider bore needle is then inserted into the vein using the longer spinal needle as a guide. It is essential before using this method to ensure that the spinal needle is long enough to allow a sufficient length to protrude through the wider needle to reach the vein. Now that guide wire kits are widely available it is unlikely that this method will be used because it suffers the inherent dangers of puncturing deep veins with long rigid needles.

FIXATION OF THE CATHETER

The catheter must be securely fixed in position as soon as it has been successfully inserted. This is necessary for two reasons. First, the catheter will not be lost into the vein if it is inadvertently cut across outside the skin. This complication is usually associated with catheter-through-needle devices[8,9] but any catheter may fracture or be accidentally cut.[10,11] A 'lost' catheter must be removed because of the high risk of infection; if the fragment has entered the heart it can be removed either by the Dormia-type catheter device[12] passed into the heart or, if unsuccessful, by open heart surgery. Second, securing the catheter prevents any movement, which will produce mechanical and chemical irritation of the intima of the vein encouraging local thrombophlebitis.[13] Furthermore, preventing movement reduces the chance of infection produced by the inward migration of bacteria proliferating at the site of skin puncture.

Adhesive tape can be used when the catheter is to be in position for a short time only (for example, during an operation). Tape soon loses its adhesiveness and skin reactions commonly occur. For anchoring the catheter for a long period a skin suture is especially recommended. In comparison with adhesive tape, it is likely to be more effective in reducing the risk of catheter embolism if the catheter is accidentally cut across.

Adhesive tape

Narrow (1 cm) adhesive tape is passed beneath the catheter, adhesive side facing upwards, crossed over above the catheter, ensuring that the catheter is gripped firmly, and attached to the skin. Tincture of benzoin applied to the skin before the tape is attached improves its adhesion and may also reduce damage to the underlying skin.[14]

Skin suture[7]

A 3–0 silk or fine wire stitch is inserted through the skin and subcutaneous tissue and tied loosely over the catheter. The two ends of the suture are then passed around the catheter and firmly tied. In this way the catheter is securely fastened without any direct pressure by the catheter on the skin.

Bio-occlusive dressing

Recently, the use of thin transparent adhesive dressings has gained popularity following claims that it prevents contamination at the point of entry of the cannula, isolates the catheter from the surrounding area whilst allowing frequent inspection without the need to remove the dressing. Some of these occlusive dressings are available ready impregnated with iodine compounds.

CORRECT POSITIONING OF THE CATHETER TIP

The tip of a central venous catheter inserted for the measurement of central venous pressure or for long-term parenteral nutrition should lie in a large intrathoracic vein. The preferred position[15] (Figure 3.5a) is in the upper part of the superior vena cava above the pericardial reflection, so as to avoid any danger of perforation or erosion of the lower portion of the superior vena cava, right atrium, or right ventricle, which could lead to pericardial haemorrhage and cardiac tamponade.[16,17] In one study there was an 87% mortality rate among 16 patients who developed cardiac tamponade following the use of a central venous catheter.[15] An additional reason for ensuring that a catheter does not enter the heart is the risk of provoking dysrhythmias.[10] Even with the catheter tip positioned above the pericardial reflection, perforation of the subclavian or innominate veins can still

give rise to the serious complications of hydromediastinum or hydrothorax.[18,19] There are occasional indications for deliberately placing a catheter in the right atrium – for instance, to aspirate air which may reach the heart from the site of operation in certain neurosurgical procedures.[20] If the catheter is inserted through the femoral vein, the tip should lie in the inferior vena cava below the diaphragm.

Numerous investigations have shown that if the catheter tip is placed blindly it may settle in an unsatisfactory site, irrespective of the route of insertion.[21-28] The position of the catheter tip is deemed unsatisfactory if it lies in a peripheral vein (Figure 3.5b), in an internal jugular vein (Figure 3.5c), or in the heart (Figure 3.5d).

Even when a sufficient length of catheter has been advanced into the vein, the tip may still not have reached a central position. The catheter may curl on itself and pass retrogradely. A catheter inserted through an arm vein may traverse the intrathoracic veins and emerge in the other arm vein. A catheter can find its way into the internal jugular vein from any route of insertion (other than through the femoral vein), but this most frequently happens with catheters inserted through arm veins.[21,26,27,29,30] Inserting too great a length of catheter so that it enters the right atrium or right ventricle is a common occurrence. The catheter may even enter the pulmonary artery.[10] A catheter lying in the internal jugular vein may be satisfactorily repositioned by withdrawing an appropriate length, but the catheter should not be reinserted as the portion withdrawn is no longer sterile. Withdrawing the appropriate length of a catheter that has entered the heart results in a perfectly positioned catheter in the superior vena cava.

The following steps should be taken when any central venous catheter is inserted:

1. The catheter (kept in the sterile coverings) should be placed against the skin and the length from the intended skin puncture site to a satisfactory central position roughly estimated. This length can later be rechecked using the stylet (if provided) after inserting the catheter. In many commercially available kits, distance markings are printed on the catheter which enables the precise length inserted to be known.

2. When the catheter is in place it should be possible to aspirate and reinject blood freely without undue resistance.

3. When connected to a manometer, oscillations should be seen which are synchronous with respiration and pulse.

(a)

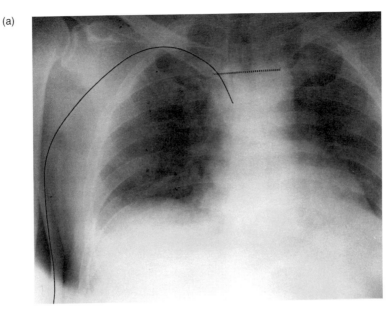

(b)

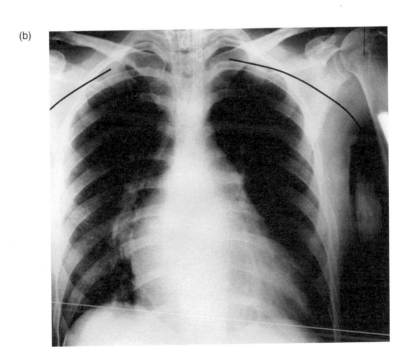

Figure 3.5. (a) Correct positioning of the catheter tip in the upper part of the superior vena cava. (b) Incorrect positioning of the catheter tip in a peripheral vein.

(c)

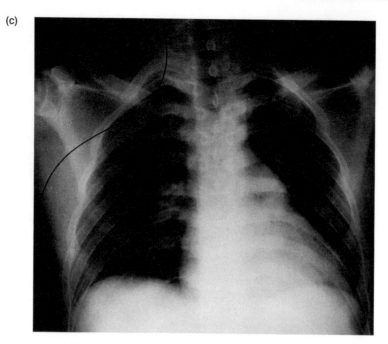

(d)

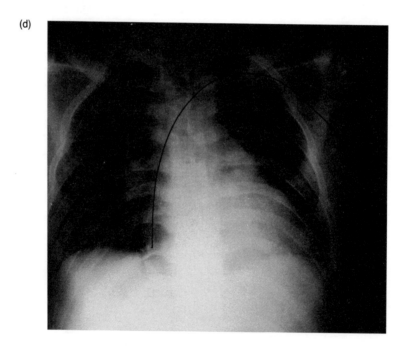

Figure 3.5 (c) Incorrect positioning of the catheter tip in an internal jugular vein. (d) Incorrect positioning of the catheter tip in the heart.

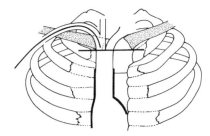

Figure 3.6. Outline diagram of central veins superimposed on skeletal appearance of posteroanterior chest radiograph. Line is drawn below lower surface of each clavicle (shaded), and we suggest that tip of catheter should lie no more than 2 cm below this. Heavy lines represent pericardial reflections around superior vena cava. Reproduced with kind permission of Grennall et al. (1975).[15]

4. A chest x-ray is the only certain method of identifying the position of the tip and should be taken as soon as possible. However, if the catheter is not made of radiopaque material, it must be filled with a radiopaque medium[14] such as Urografin 60% (sodium diatrizoate injection). In adults the catheter tip should lie no more than 2 cm below a line joining the lower surfaces of the ends of the clavicle on a posteroanterior chest x-ray (Figure 3.6).[15] This line corresponds to the division of the superior vena cava into a portion well above and a portion below the pericardial reflection (Figure 3.5a). If the catheter has been inserted into the inferior vena cava, its tip should lie below the level of the diaphragm.

Only after ascertaining the position of the catheter tip should the administration of intravenous fluid be started.

Ultrasound aided central venous catheterisation

An ultrasound apparatus, if available, can facilitate and make the insertion of a central venous catheter safer under direct imaging. The method gives immediate and accurate confirmation of correct positioning of the catheter tip. Ultrasound techniques have been used in catheterisation through subclavian and internal jugular vein routes.[32,33,34]

Several suppliers now offer compact, portable ultrasound apparatus suitable for aiding central venous cannulation. One particular device has been specifically designed for central venous cannulation.

The miniature ultrasound scanner is dedicated to internal jugular vein puncture (Site-Rite (R), Dymax Corporation, Pittsburgh, USA). The scanner incorporates a needle guide enabling accurate advancement of the needle tip into the vein as the operator watches a clear display (Figure 3.7).[115]

Visualisation of the procedure in this way can reduce the number of attempts required to gain satisfactory entry into the vein and increase the rate of successful cannulation. This is accompanied by a convincing reduction in the incidence of complications.[115,116]

ECG guided placement of central venous catheters

This technique was first used in helping position the tip of a ventriculoatrial catheter being inserted for the treatment of hydrocephalus.[35] Precise positioning in the right atrium was crucial to the proper functioning of the catheter. The method eliminated the need for a confirmatory x-ray during the operation. Furthermore there appeared to be few complications and yet the method does not appear to have been taken up outside neurosurgery. In this particular field, the technique has also been employed to accurately position a central venous catheter tip to aspirate air embolism[20] and for venous pressure measurement.[36] It is likely that uncertainty about the methodology has deterred its gaining wider popularity.

The key to the technique is recognition of the large negative or biphasic P wave of the ECG trace as the fluid-filled catheter acting as an exploring electrode is advanced into the right atrium (Figure 3.8).

A good success rate of 81% has been achieved using a catheter filled with electrolyte connected through a metal stopcock and wire to the V5 lead of the ECG monitor. The conducting fluids used were 8·4% sodium bicarbonate (readily available) and 4% saline (made up). The time taken was between 5 and 15 minutes.[36]

Other authors have made useful recommendations.[37] Their usual ECG configuration consisted of:

    right arm lead to the right shoulder
    left arm lead to the left shoulder
    left leg lead to the upper half of the sternum.

When ECG guided central venous catheterisation was needed, the following adjustments were made:

    right arm as above
    left leg lead to the left shoulder

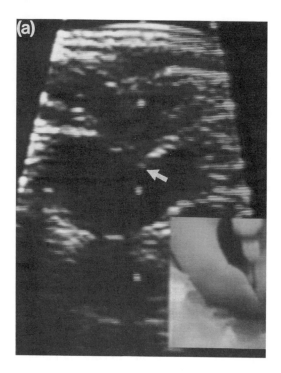

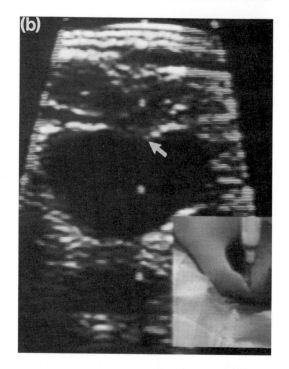

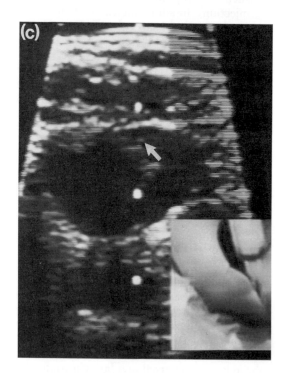

Figure 3.7. Ultrasound display of venepuncture of
internal jugular vein using the Site-Rite(TM) scanner.
(a) Arrow shows the vein wall being invaginated as the
needle approaches the vein. (b, c) Vein wall springs
back as the needle penetrates and is advanced into the
lumen.

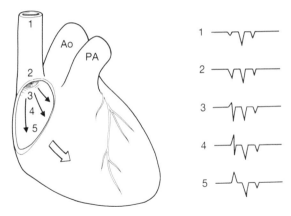

Figure 3.8. The P wave which is negative at first becomes progressively more negative as it approaches the SA node in the atrium. When the tip of the catheter enters the atrium and lies near the SA node, the P wave becomes large and biphasic. As the tip is advanced further into the atrium the wave becomes positive. Ao, aorta; PA, pulmonary artery. Reproduced with kind permission of Cucchiara *et al.* (1980).[112]

left arm lead was clipped to the distal end of the guide wire inside the catheter. Alternatively, if the catheter had no metal stylet or wire, the catheter was filled with saline and attached to a saline drip. The left arm lead was then clipped to a metal needle inserted into the drip tubing.

A purpose-made device is commercially available.[38] The Arrow-Johans RAECG Adapter is a disposable 20 mm long plastic Luer-Lock adaptor which has a steel nipple pressed through its wall so permitting contact with the intravascular conductive electrolyte fluid path.

MOVING THE SITE OF ENTRY OF A CENTRAL VENOUS CATHETER

Normally, the sites where the skin and the vein are punctured lie close to each other. In consequence the track can easily become infected, especially in longer-term catheterisation. This risk can be reduced by widely separating the two puncture sites by means of a subcutaneous tunnel. The technique has been used with catheters inserted for intravenous alimentation through the subclavian vein[39-41] as well as through the internal and external jugular vein[14,40] routes in both adults and children.[14] Particularly strong indications for using a subcutaneous tunnel are the presence of skin

infection, burns, or a tracheostomy wound near the point where the catheter enters the skin.[40] Moving the entry point of the catheter could be especially advantageous in the case of catheters inserted into the subclavian vein by the supraclavicular route. The supraclavicular fossa tends to collect secretions and perspiration and is difficult to keep dry; furthermore, because of the irregular contour, it is not easy to secure the catheter with adhesive tape or to hold a dressing in place. For similar reasons, the use of the technique in femoral vein catheterisation could reduce the high rate of infection associated with the route. However, contradictory reports have questioned the value of tunnelling in the reduction of catheter-related sepsis.[42] Nevertheless, the technique remains widely practised.

There are now many commercially available composite long-term catheter/tunnelling kits which are both convenient and effective. Hickman–Broviac catheters are widely used for longer-term central venous catheterisation. They are universally tunnelled and have the advantage of a Dacron cuff around the catheter as it lies subcutaneously. Over a period of several weeks, fibrous tissue grows into and around the Dacron cuff anchoring it and acting as a barrier to the spread of infection from the skin entry site.[43] These long-term catheters have customarily been inserted by surgical cut-down procedures, but apparatus for percutaneous insertion is now available from leading manufacturers (see Choosing the Equipment, p. 26).

PERCUTANEOUS INSERTION OF LONG-TERM CENTRAL VENOUS CATHETER WITH TUNNELLING PROCEDURE

Insertion of guide wire (Figure 3.9)

1. Perform the procedure under aseptic conditions.
2. Locate central vein with small gauge needle (22 gauge).
3. Enlarge skin puncture site with scalpel blade.
4. Perform venepuncture with the introducer needle and cannula or needle alone guided by the locater needle.
5. Insert guide wire through the introducer and advance to a satisfactory central position confirmed by fluoroscopy if available. Hold guide wire firmly in place.

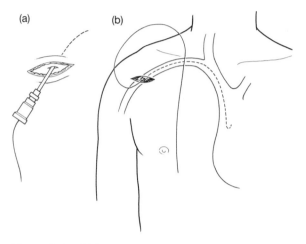

Figure 3.9. (a) Introduction of spring wire guide. (b) Final position of wire guide after removal of introducer.

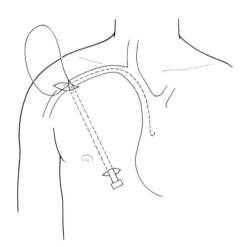

Figure 3.10. Insertion of wire guide through tunnel dilator.

Forming a subcutaneous tunnel (Figure 3.10)

6. Infiltrate local anaesthetic just below and medial to the nipple and make incision for tunnel.
7. Insert tunnelling needle with its dilator into this skin incision and advance the assembly, so creating a subcutaneous tunnel, until the tip protrudes through the upper incision. Remove the tunnel needle leaving the tunnel dilator in place.
8. Insert the guide wire into the tip of the tunnel

dilator and push it through until it emerges at the lower end. Grasp the wire and pull it through the dilator leaving a 5 cm loop of wire at the upper incision. Grasping this loop firmly, remove the dilator.

9. Thread the tip of the central venous catheter over the guide wire and advance it upwards through the tunnel until it emerges in the upper incision. Guide it over the wire loop, whilst maintaining the loop, into the vein until the correct length has been inserted into the superior vena cava (Figures 3.11 and 3.12). Traction on the lower end of the catheter will now straighten out the redundant loop by pulling it into the tunnel.

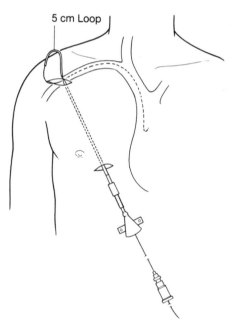

Figure 3.11. Threading catheter over spring wire guide in subcutaneous tunnel.

Placing a Dacron cuff around the catheter

1. Dilate the lower incision by blunt dissection with an artery forceps to about 3 cm into the tunnel.
2. Position the Dacron cuff by pushing the silicone sleeve, on which it is mounted, along the catheter so that it lies no less than 3 cm inside the tunnel. Tie the cuff firmly to the catheter by means of a suture around the silicone sleeve. Remove the guide wire.
3. Secure the catheter with the temporary catheter clamp provided until fibrosis into the

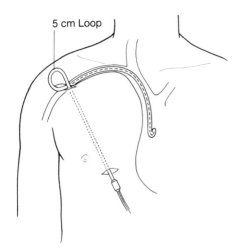

Figure 3.12.

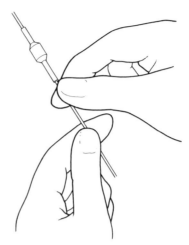

Figure 3.12. Maintaining 5 cm loop during introduction of the catheter into the superior vena cava.

Figure 3.13. The Dacron cuff over silicone sleeve can be repositioned along the catheter by firmly grasping the catheter and pushing on the proximal end of the silicone sleeve (not cuff).

Dacron cuff fixes the catheter (about 10–14 days).

4. Close the two incisions with sutures and apply suitable dressings.

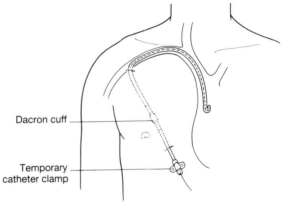

Figure 3.14. Completed procedure showing position of Dacron cuff and temporary catheter clamp.

PREVENTION OF INFECTION DURING CATHETERISATION

Aseptic technique

Meticulous aseptic technique is essential when undertaking central venous catheterisation and is particularly important when a catheter may be required for long-term use. Infection at the puncture site may lead to thrombophlebitis, venous thrombosis, embolism, or septicaemia. If any of these complications develops, the intravenous catheter may have to be removed. This could be a serious matter if there are few alternative sites suitable for cannulation. The operator should therefore scrub his hands and wear mask, gown, and gloves. The skin need not be shaved unless hair obscures the vein.[44] The skin is first scrubbed with soap or a detergent compound in water and then with an antiseptic preparation. Suitable preparations are 2% tincture of iodine, followed by 70% alcohol; povidone iodine surgical scrub; or 0.5% chlorhexidine in 70% alcohol (allowing one minute for drying to take place).[45] The skin area is then isolated with sterile towels. It is wise to include these aseptic precautions as a routine, even when using a system incorporating a 'no touch' sheath or drum; such devices may often be inserted without contamination, but sometimes it is necessary to manipulate the catheter in order to pass it successfully along the vein. Obviously, in an emergency, the operator must use his discretion on which sterile precautions are practicable.

Fixing the catheter

The catheter should be fixed securely to prevent it from moving, which encourages infection (see above). A subcutaneous tunnelling technique should be considered if long-term use of the catheter is foreseen (see above).

Sterile dressing

Before applying a sterile dressing to the puncture site a topical antimicrobial preparation may be applied, but this is not without potential complication (see below).

The dressing should not usually be completely occlusive[45] as some studies have shown a more rapid bacterial and fungal growth under such conditions.[46,47] However, an occlusive, waterproof dressing should certainly be used if the puncture site is close to an open wound, a burn, or a tracheostomy incision.[48]

LONG-TERM CARE: PREVENTION OF THROMBUS FORMATION AND INFECTION

Central venous catheters have been kept patent and free from infection for months and even years.[7,14,41,48-51] This has been accomplished by following a strict protocol covering all aspects of the management of the catheter, which includes aseptic technique when the catheter is inserted, and subsequently when the catheter, dressing, or fluid administration system is changed. Similar precautions are taken when injections into or withdrawals from the fluid administration system are made. If the strict regimen is not enforced, infection becomes inevitable.[13,52,53] The protocol must include instructions on the following points.

Catheter material

Catheters made of silicone elastomer are preferred for long-term intravenous alimentation. This material has been advocated by most authors to reduce the incidence of catheter-related thrombus formation and subsequent infection.[7,39,41,50,51,54-56] However, silastic catheters are difficult to insert because of the softness and flexibility of the material and they may not be radiopaque. Therefore catheters of other plastic material are still used for intravenous alimentation.[13]

Currently, catheters made of polyurethane are the most popular as they are comparatively non-thrombogenic and soft. Nitrates are not absorbed as they are with PVC catheters. There is some evidence that Hydromer-coated polyurethane catheters (Viggo) are superior in that fibrin sleeve formation is inhibited.

It is possible to incorporate heparin into the catheter material and this, it has been suggested, will reduce the formation of a fibrin sheath.[54,57] It is doubtful whether heparin bonding of catheters is advantageous in reducing fibrin sleeve formation as was originally thought.[54,57] Fibrin sleeves have been found equally in heparin-coated and plain catheters at post-mortem.[58]

Antibiotic-coated catheters are designed to reduce catheter-related sepsis. This is likely to be of little value as the surfactant–antibiotic complex is broken down by the sterilisation process; soaking the catheter in antibiotic solution prior to use has been recommended.[59]

Change of dressing

There are differences of opinion on the frequency with which the dressings over the skin puncture site should be changed. Many authors suggest a change every two to four days,[45] but one group changed the dressings once per week to avoid undue disturbance of the catheter at the puncture site,[60] while yet others practised daily dressing changes.[61,62] It would seem reasonable to change the dressing immediately should it become moist.[45] Transparent bio-occlusive film (e.g. Op-Site (TM), Smith & Nephew Medical Ltd, Hull, UK) allows daily inspection of the puncture site and provided the area is not inflamed the dressing need not be changed.

All authors agree that a strict aseptic technique is obligatory when changing the dressing.

Antibiotic and antimicrobial ointment

Topical preparations containing antibiotics such as bacitracin, neomycin, and polymyxin were once popular to prevent infection at the skin puncture site.[63-66] Although these studies suggest that the incidence of catheter-related infection is reduced by applying these antimicrobial ointments, there is an increased risk of fungal infection at the catheter site and the proliferation of bacteria resistant to the antibiotics in the ointment.[65,66] Current opinion is that topical antibiotic preparations should not be used.[26]

An ointment containing povidone iodine, which has both antibacterial and antifungal properties, is an improvement in theory, and povidone iodine ointments are widely recommended at present.[7,13,41,67-69] However, there is no firm evidence for the efficacy of such preparations in reducing fungal infection when applied at the site of insertion of the catheter, and there is clearly room for further investigation into this topic.[45]

Changing the catheter

There are conflicting recommendations on the frequency with which a catheter should be changed. Authors have suggested that this should be done every two days,[44,70,71] every three days,[72] every 14 days,[68] and even every 30 days.[49] It has also been maintained that, not only is it unnecessary to change the catheter frequently, but that this may increase the risk of thrombus formation from repeated venepuncture.[13] There appears to be no strong correlation between the duration of catheterisation and the incidence of catheter-related sepsis.[45] In fact, in some patients it is impracticable to change the catheter regularly because of a lack of suitable veins, and there are, indeed, several studies which demonstrate that a carefully managed catheter can be kept free of infection for many months.[7,69,72-74] It seems reasonable, therefore, to change the catheter only when there is a specific indication such as clinical septicaemia or pyrexia of unknown origin.[45]

The diagnosis of catheter-related sepsis can only be made if the catheter tip culture, peripheral blood culture and culture of blood drawn from the catheter grow the same organisms. The incidence is low (less than 3·5%) and insertion of a fresh catheter in a new site is only really necessary if this diagnosis is positive. In other cases, substituting a new catheter after first inserting a guide wire through a suspect catheter is an acceptable method. It is safer, simpler and can be performed by the relatively inexperienced. However, if *Staphylococcus aureus* or fungi are grown from culture of the insertion site, a new route for catheterisation should be chosen.[75-77]

Other recommendations have been made. If a patient receiving total intravenous alimentation develops signs of sepsis, the catheter is replaced every one to three days for the duration of the infection.[70] Although other workers do not remove the catheter if another source of infection can be found.[72,78] If a patient develops septic shock, the catheter should be removed even before positive blood cultures are found.[13]

Occlusion of the catheter by thrombus accounts for 10–20% of catheter failure. Before changing the catheter, restoration of patency by instilling streptokinase should be considered.[79] A sterile 2 ml syringe can be used to instil a minute aliquot of streptokinase into the catheter; the syringe is left in place for several hours.[80] Another suggestion is to instil a mixture of streptokinase in 0·9% sodium chloride (2000 U/ml) into the catheter dead space and to leave for an hour before flushing with heparinised saline.[81] No force should be used to flush a silicone catheter as they are easily ruptured.

Fluid administration system

Personnel who take part in the care of the fluid administration system must be warned of the hazards of contaminating the system as well as the precautions necessary to reduce the risk.[73,82] When possible, the infusion system should be completely closed; this is essential if it is used for intravenous alimentation.[45] Blood sampling from the line, intravenous injections into the line, and the use of stopcocks with injection ports should be rigorously avoided.[13,83,84] Fluids should be administered at steady rates, avoiding periods of cessation in which clotting may occur. Mechanical infusion devices are recommended, especially when small volumes of viscous fluids are being administered, and are probably essential in infants when infusing fluids through inevitably very fine bore catheters.[14]

Additives to intravenous fluids

Intravenous fluids and any additives should be prepared in the aseptic laboratory of the pharmacy.[41,63,85] Single bag total parenteral nutrition compounding is a service commonly provided by pharmacy aseptic laboratories. If it is necessary to add drugs outside the pharmacy, strict aseptic precautions are essential.

Changing the administration set

Currently accepted practice for total intravenous nutrition is to change the whole fluid administration system down to the catheter every 24 hours.[13,60,61,70]

Bacterial filters

In-line filters have been recommended to prevent infusion of particulate material and bacteria. In addition the filter must be able to prevent the transfer of endotoxins released into the filter medium.[86-88]

Only filters with a pore size of 0·22 microns can be regarded as sterilising grade. They are effective in reducing the incidence of phlebitis, infused particulate matter, pyrogenic reactions and the incidence of the need to change the catheter insertion site. However, infusion devices are necessary to drive fluids through such small-sized pores.

At the time of writing, only the Posidyne N66 filter medium provides such pyrogen retention for over 96 hours of infusion. With this device, infusion sets can be used for longer periods without the risk of bacteria or endotoxins passing into the patient.[89,90]

Heparinisation

Low-dose heparin (1 IU/ml of infusate) has been advocated to keep the catheter tip free of blood clot and thus reduce the incidence of septic complications, especially during long-term parenteral nutrition.[91,92] Heparin prevents the formation of a fibrin sleeve around the catheter tip and therefore prevents the development of a nidus for bacterial colonisation. Intermittent flushing with heparinised saline is an acceptable alternative to constant infusion.

Heparin bonding of polythene catheters has not proved effective in preventing fibrin sheath or thrombus formation.[93]

Bacteriological monitoring

Routine bacteriological monitoring of the site of catheter entry of the intravenous tubing and of the infusion solution is unnecessary and is accompanied by the risk of contaminating the system. However, if the patient develops any evidence of infection, bacteriological investigation should be instituted in consultation with a clinical bacteriologist. Investigations include culture of swabs taken from the entry site in the skin, fluids being administered, patient's blood, and the catheter if this has been removed. Other potential sources of infection such as the genitourinary tract should not be overlooked.

When catheter-related sepsis is suspected the catheter need not necessarily be removed immediately. Quantitative blood cultures enable long-term central venous catheter-related bacteraemia to be definitively diagnosed.[94,95] These techniques permit quantification of colony counts of bacteria in blood cultures taken from the central as well as a peripheral intravenous catheter. A ratio of bacterial colony count greater than 10:1 (central to peripheral) indicates a catheter infection. A ratio of 5:1 is warning of incipient catheter-related sepsis.[96]

The great majority of central venous catheter-related bacteraemias can be successfully treated with antibiotics. Infections around the skin entry site also usually respond to antibiotics and local wound care. Catheter tunnel infections (more than 2 cm from the skin puncture) though can be resistant to treatment especially if the organism is a *Pseudomonas* species.

INSERTION OF A FLOTATION (SWAN–GANZ) CATHETER

The balloon-tipped flotation catheter introduced into clinical practice in 1970 by Swan and Ganz[97] enabled the pulmonary artery to be catheterised for the measurement of pressures without calling on the manipulative skill and radiological control demanded by other methods of cardiac catheterisation. The Swan–Ganz catheter has been further developed for measuring cardiac output by the thermodilution technique,[98] for cardiac pacing,[99] for electrocardiography,[100,101] for pulmonary angiography[102] and for fibreoptic mixed venous blood oximetry[103] and is now used in a wide variety of clinical situations.[104]

The common indications for the insertion of a Swan–Ganz catheter include the management of post-traumatic, surgical and septic shock in order to optimize tissue oxygen transport; in cardiogenic shock to correct pulmonary wedge pressure and to

Table 3.1. Contraindications to insertion of a Swan–Ganz catheter and complications associated with Swan–Ganz catheterisation.

Contraindications
Prosthetic tricuspid or pulmonary valve
Tricuspid and pulmonary valve disease
Cardiac septal defects
Left bundle branch block
Endocardial pacemaker *in situ*
Untreated severe coagulopathy and
　thrombocytopaenia

Complications
Arrhythmias
Arterial punctures and pneumothorax
Pulmonary artery rupture
Pulmonary infarction and thrombosis
Catheter-related sepsis
Damage to tricuspid valve and pulmonary valve by the
　catheter
Endocarditis
Balloon rupture

improve cardiac index; in profound hypoxaemia to improve oxygen delivery and oxygen consumption; in cardiac surgery for coronary artery disease to aid early detection of myocardial ischaemia and to manipulate pre- and afterload.[105] The main contra-indications (Table 3.1) are pathology or prostheses of the valves of the right heart, presence of an endo-cardial pacemaker and severe bleeding disorders.

Choice of vein and technique of cannulation

A Swan–Ganz catheter may be inserted into any vein used for central venous catheterisation. Surgi-cal cut-down on an antecubital fossa vein may be used and cut-down on the proximal basilic vein has also been advocated[106] but percutaneous insertion is easier and is possible in most cases.[107]

Percutaneous cannulation of a vein in the ante-cubital fossa is the most comfortable for the conscious patient[108] but the vein may be too small to admit the larger size Swan–Ganz catheter and it may be difficult to advance the catheter in the shoulder region.[109]

Operators with the appropriate skill may prefer the external jugular, subclavian, or femoral vein routes, but percutaneous insertion through the right internal jugular vein is the most favoured because of its short, direct path to the right atrium.[109,110] The route of insertion selected will depend upon the experience of the operator, the accessibility of the vein, and the equipment available.

A cannula of adequate size has to be inserted into the chosen vein to admit the Swan–Ganz catheter. The cannula can be inserted directly into the vein, although to use a modified Seldinger (guide wire) and vein dilator technique (see p. 18) is preferable and safer, especially in deep veins such as the internal jugular or subclavian.[107,110,111] Because of its construction, the Swan–Ganz catheter cannot be inserted by the conventional guide wire technique.

Equipment

Flotation catheter

For adults a 6 French (1·8 mm O.D.) or 7 French (2·1 mm O.D.) flotation catheter is suitable. For children 5 French (1·5 mm O.D.).

Introducing cannula

The introducing cannula may have to be one size larger than the Swan–Ganz catheter in order to accommodate the deflated balloon.

Catheter (Swan–Ganz)-through-cannula device

Cannula diameter 12 gauge (O.D.) to pass a 7 French Swan–Ganz catheter. Cannula length is appropriate for the chosen vein.

Modified guide wire (Seldinger) technique using a vein dilator

Diameter of final wide-bore cannula is 8 French to admit a 7 French Swan–Ganz catheter, and 6 French to admit a 5 French Swan–Ganz catheter. (Sets containing matching guide wire, vein dilator and wide-bore cannula are now commercially available from several manufacturers.)

Flushing solution

Normal saline (500 ml) containing 500 IU heparin.

General

Trolley equipped for central venous catheterisation using aseptic technique.

Two 20 ml syringes containing heparinised saline. Scalpel to incise skin if a guide wire technique is used.

Pressure recording system. Electrocardiograph. Defibrillator. Cardiac arrest trolley.

Precautions

Do not use a resterilised Swan–Ganz catheter. Use aseptic technique to insert the catheter. Identify the balloon inflating stopcock.

Procedure

1. Check that the balloon is intact by inflating to the recommended volume. Do not inject fluid into this lumen.
2. Fill the lumen of the monitoring catheter with heparinised saline.
3. Cannulate the chosen vein. Insert guide wire and vein dilator. Finally, insert the introducer.
4. Insert the Swan–Ganz catheter into the vein and connect the pressure-monitoring lumen to the recording apparatus.
5. Advance the catheter into the thorax. Its arrival can be recognised by an increased fluctuation in pressure with respiration. When the patient is asked to cough, the pressure rises sharply to about 40 mmHg.

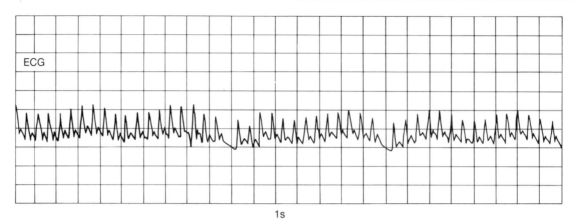

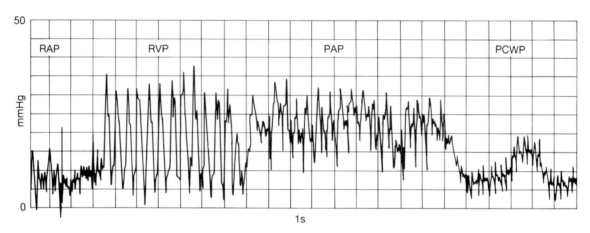

Figure 3.15. Inserting a pulmonary artery flotation catheter: the characteristic pressure trace as the catheter traverses the right atrium (RAP), the right ventricle (RVP) and enters the pulmonary artery (PAP). PCWP = pulmonary capillary wedge pressure. Reproduced with kind permission of George and Banks (1983).[114]

6. Advance the catheter further (into the lower part of the superior vena cava close to the right atrium).

   The length of the catheter inserted will depend on the site of insertion. For an average-sized adult these will be:

right antecubital fossa vein	35–40 cm
left antecubital fossa vein	45–50 cm
internal jugular vein	10–15 cm
subclavian vein	10 cm
femoral vein	35–45 cm

7. Inflate the balloon with the recommended volume and advance the catheter slowly to allow it to be carried along in the main blood flow. Watch the pressure trace and observe the following characteristic changes as the catheter traverses the chambers of the heart (Figure 3.15):

Right ventricle: The atrial trace alters to the large ventricular trace (often accompanied by premature ventricular contractions).

Pulmonary artery: Trace alters. The systolic pressure remains the same but the diastolic pressure rises.

Pulmonary artery wedged position: The trace alters and shows a pressure approximately equal to the pulmonary artery diastolic pressure.

8. As soon as the catheter shows the pulmonary artery wedged pressure (PAWP), stop advancing the catheter. Deflate the balloon and confirm that the trace returns to that of the normal phasic pulmonary artery pressure. From now on, the balloon should be reinflated intermittently and for short periods only in order to measure PAWP.

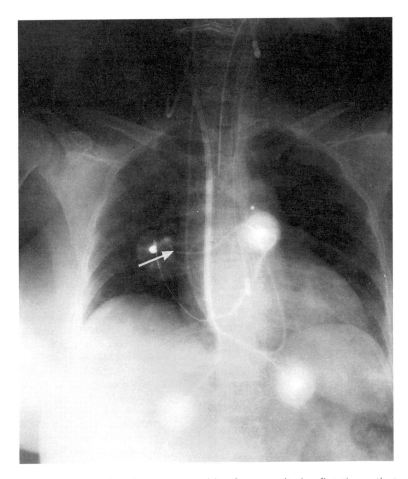

Figure 3.16. Chest radiograph showing the correct position for a monitoring flotation catheter.

If the catheter has not reached the pulmonary artery when about 60 cm of catheter has been inserted, withdraw the catheter to the right atrium and attempt again. The catheter must never be withdrawn whilst the balloon is inflated; serious damage to the heart valves or vessels can occur.

9. Protect the length of catheter outside the puncture site with a sterile dressing and secure it temporarily with adhesive tape.

10. Check the position of the catheter with a chest radiograph. The catheter tip is in an ideal position when it lies in one of the main branches of the pulmonary artery (Figure 3.16).

If intermittent right ventricular complexes appear, the catheter tip has probably 'recoiled' into the right ventricle. The catheter should be advanced 1–2 cm before it is secured.

11. After recording the end expiratory pulmonary capillary wedge pressure deflate the balloon. The pressure measured can only be regarded as valid if the pressure trace then returns to a pulmonary artery pressure wave form.

When satisfactory wedging has been obtained, extend the protective sheath (if supplied) to cover the full length of the catheter outside the skin so that manipulations of the catheter can be made later in a 'no touch' manner. Secure the collar onto the introducer cannula. Fix the catheter with skin sutures and cover with a bio-occlusive dressing.

Problems

Failure to enter the right atrium: The catheter has inadvertently entered the internal jugular vein or contralateral subclavian vein or even coiled up in the superior vena cava. Prevention is probably helped by inserting the catheter through the right internal jugular vein and by pointing the catheter tip in the right direction. Withdraw and reinsert. If persistently unsuccessful it may be necessary to resort to the aid of an image intensifier to guide the catheter along the correct path.

Failure to pass through the tricuspid or pulmonary valve: Reduce the size of the balloon or deflate completely before advancing further.

Failure to enter the pulmonary artery: If the ventricular trace persists or reappears after advancing the catheter 10–20 cm after its first appearance, the catheter is coiling up on itself and there is a danger of knotting. Deflate the balloon and pull back into the atrium and readvance. Several attempts may be made before resorting to the image intensifier.

Catheter obstruction: If the catheter tip appears to be stuck against the wall or at the bifurcation of branches of the pulmonary artery the pressure trace will steadily rise above the expected value. Deflate the balloon and draw back. Wedge again with a smaller volume of air in the balloon.

It is essential that the catheter is free of blood and air and well flushed with heparinised saline before it is connected to a pressure transducer. Omitting these measures can result in a poor trace and inaccurate measurements. Many of the complications of pulmonary artery catheters can be avoided if the catheter is not left *in situ* for more than 48–72 hours. Table 3.1 shows the complications most commonly encountered.

Maintenance of the Swan–Ganz catheter

1. The pulmonary artery pressure trace should be continuously displayed so that 'spontaneous wedging' may be promptly diagnosed. This occurs if the catheter material softens, when the tip migrates into the smaller branches of the pulmonary artery and into a wedged position. If flushing does not remove a wedged trace, withdraw the catheter 1–2 cm.

2. Take careful precautions on reinflating the balloon to measure PAWP. It is possible that the catheter tip may migrate into a more distal branch of the pulmonary artery and inflating the balloon to its full volume may cause local damage. Therefore always reinflate slowly and with increments of 0·1–0·2 ml until the PAWP trace is obtained. If a much smaller volume is required to elicit PAWP, withdraw the catheter

1–2 cm until the full volume is needed to obtain a wedged pressure. Always deflate the balloon prior to moving the catheter.

3. Continuously flush the catheter with heparinised saline, with a 'fast flush' at hourly intervals. If a continuous flush is not available, flush every 10 minutes.

4. Use an aseptic technique during any manipulation or inspection of the catheter.

5. Radiograph the chest at least once a day.

REFERENCES

1. Flanagan, J. P., Gradisar, I. A., Gross, R. J. and Kelly, T. R. (1969). Air embolus – a lethal complication of subclavian venepuncture. *New England Journal of Medicine* **281**, 488.

2. Ross, S. M., Freedman, P. S. and Farman, J. V. (1979). Air embolism after accidental removal of intravenous catheter. *British Medical Journal* **1**, 987.

3. Civetta, J. M., Gabel, J. C. and Gemer, M. (1972). Internal jugular vein puncture with a margin of safety. *Anesthesiology* **36**, 622.

4. Daily, P. O., Griepp, R. B. and Shumway, N. E. (1970). Percutaneous internal jugular vein cannulation. *Archives of Surgery* **101**, 534.

5. Prince, S. R., Sullivan, R. L. and Hackel, A. (1976). Percutaneous catheterization of the internal jugular vein in infants and children. *Anesthesiology* **44**, 170.

6. Haapaniemi, L. and Slatis, P. (1974). Supraclavicular catheterisation of the superior vena cava. *Acta Anaesthesiologica Scandinavica* **18**, 12.

7. Ryan, J. A. Jr. (1976). Complications of total parenteral nutrition. In *Total Parenteral Nutrition* edited by J. E. Fischer, p. 55. Boston; Little, Brown.

8. Bennett, P. J. (1963). Use of intravenous plastic catheters. *British Medical Journal* **2**, 1252.

9. Taylor, F. W. and Rutherford, C. E. (1963). Accidental loss of plastic tube into venous system. *Archives of Surgery* **86**, 177.

10. Farman, J. V. (1978). Which central venous catheter? *British Journal of Clinical Equipment* **32**, 210.

11. Parulkar, D. S., Grundy, E. M. and Bennett, E. J. (1978). Fracture of a float catheter. *British Journal of Anaesthesia* **50**, 201.

12. Zwiauer, K., Grabenwoger, F., Lachmann, D. *et al.* (1987). Non-surgical removal of iatrogenic intracardiac foreign bodies. A study in a 5 month old infant. *Monatsschrift Kinderheilkunde* **135**, 784.

13. Ryan, J. A., Abel, R. M., Abbott, W. M., Hopkins, C. C., Chesney, T. McC., Colley, R., Phillips, K. A. and Fischer, J. F. (1974). Catheter complications in total parenteral nutrition. A prospective study of 200 consecutive patients. *New England Journal of Medicine* **290**, 757.

14. Heird, W. C., Driscoll, J. M., Schullinger, J. N., Grebin, B.

and Winters, R. W. (1972). Intravenous alimentation in pediatric patients. *Journal of Pediatrics* 80, 351.

15. Greenall, M. J., Blewitt, R. W. and McMahon, M. J. (1975). Cardiac tamponade and central venous catheters. *British Medical Journal* 2, 595.

16. Csanky Treels, J. C. (1978). Hazards of central venous pressure monitoring. *Anaesthesia* 33, 172.

17. James, O. F. and Tredarea, C. R. (1979). Cardiac tamponade caused by caval catheter – a radiological demonstration of an unusual complication. *Anaesthesia and Intensive Care* 7, 174.

18. Adar, R. and Mozes, M. (1971). Fatal complications of central venous catheters. *British Medical Journal* 3, 746.

19. Rudge, C. J., Bewick, M. and McColl, I. (1973). Hydrothorax after central venous catheterization. *British Medical Journal* 3, 23.

20. Michenfelder, J. D., Terry, H. R., Dow, E. F. and Miller, R. H. (1966). Air embolism during neurosurgery: a new method of treatment. *Anesthesia and Analgesia: Current Researches* 45, 390.

21. Deitel, M. and McIntyre, J. A. (1971). Radiographic confirmation of site of central venous pressure catheters. *Canadian Journal of Surgery* 14, 42.

22. Gilday, D. L. and Downs, A. R. (1969). The value of chest radiography in the localization of central venous pressure catheters. *Canadian Medical Association Journal* 101, 363.

23. Johnston, A. O. B. and Clark, R. G. (1972). Malpositioning of central venous catheters. *Lancet* 2, 1395.

24. Kellner, G. A. and Smart, J. F. (1972). Percutaneous placement of catheter to monitor 'central venous pressure'. *Anesthesiology* 36, 515.

25. Kuramoto, T. and Sakabe, T. (1975). Comparison of success in jugular versus basilic vein techniques for central venous pressure catheter positioning. *Anesthesia and Analgesia: Current Researches* 54, 696.

26. Langston, C. S. (1971). The aberrant central venous catheter and its complications. *Radiology* 100, 55.

27. Ng. W. Shang and Rosen, M. (1973). Positioning central venous catheters through the basilic vein. A comparison of catheters. *British Journal of Anaesthesia* 45, 1211.

28. Sorensen, T. I. A. and Sonne-Holm, S. (1975). Central venous catheterization through the basilic vein or by infraclavicular puncture?: a controlled trial. *Acta Chirurgica Scandinavica* 141, 322.

29. Bridges, B. B., Carden, E. and Takacs, F. A. (1979). Introduction of central venous pressure catheters through arm veins with a high success rate. *Canadian Anesthetists' Society Journal* 26, 128.

30. Burgess, G. E., Marino, R. J. and Peuler, M. J. (1977). Effect of head position on the location of venous catheters inserted via basilic veins. *Anesthesiology* 46, 212.

31. Williamson, J. (1976). Prevention and early recognition of complications of central venous catheterization. *American Heart Journal* 92, 667.

32. Sukigara, M., Yamazaki, T. *et al.* (1988). Ultrasonic real time guidance for subclavian venepuncture. *Surgery, Gynecology and Obstetrics* 167, 239.

33. Schering, A., Klein, A. and Jantzen, J. P. (1987). Catheterization of the internal jugular vein using sonography. *Anasthesie Intersivtherapie Notfallmedizin* 22, 229.

34. Switzer, D. F., Nanda, N. C., Harris, P. and Bren, W. (1988). The use of two dimensional Doppler technique in facilitating percutaneous catheterization of the subclavian vein. *Pacing and Clinical Electrophysiology* 11, 13.

35. Robertson, J. T., Schick, R. W., Morgan, F. and Matson, D. (1961). Accurate placement of ventriculo–atrial shunt for hydrocephalus under electrocardiographic control. *Journal of Neurosurgery* 18, 225.

36. Colley, P. S. and Artru, A. A. (1984). EKG guided placement of CVP catheters via arm veins: success rate, placement time and optimal conductive solutions. *Anesthesia and Analgesia* 63, 175 (Abstracts p. 200).

37. Farag, H., Gyamfi, Y. A. and Naguib, M. (1983). Non-radiological recognition of misplacement of central venous catheter. *British Medical Journal* 287, 761.

38. On Target (Arrow International Inc.) Vol. 1, No. 1.

39. Broviac, J. W., Cole, J. J. and Scribner, B. H. (1973). A silicone rubber atrial catheter for prolonged parenteral alimentation. *Surgery, Gynecology and Obstetrics* 136, 602.

40. Parsa, M. H., Habit, D. V. and Ferrer, J. M. (1970). Techniques for placement of long-term indwelling superior vena cava catheters. Monograph and film presented at the Fifty-sixth Annual Clinical Congress of the American College of Surgeons, Chicago, October, 1970.

41. Powell-Tuck, J., Nielsen, T., Farwell, J. A. and Lennard-Jones, J. E. (1978). Team approach to long-term intravenous feeding in patients with gastro-intestinal disorders. *Lancet* 2, 825.

42. Moran, K. T., McEntee, G., Jones, B. *et al.* (1987). To tunnel or not to tunnel catheters for parenteral nutrition. *Annals of the Royal College of Surgeons of England* 69, 235.

43. Alfieris, G. M., Wing, C. W. and Hoy, G. R. (1987). Securing Broviac catheters in children. *Journal of Pediatric Surgery* 9, 825.

44. Maki, D. G., Goldmann, D. A. and Rhame, F. S. (1973). Infection control in intravenous therapy. *Annals of Internal Medicine* 79, 867.

45. Allen, J. R. (1977). The incidence of nosocomial infection in patients receiving total parenteral nutrition. In *Advances in Parenteral Nutrition*. Proceedings of an International Symposium held in Bermuda, 16–19th May, 1977, edited by I. D. A. Johnston, p. 339, Lancaster, MTP.

46. Marples, R. R. (1975). Bacterial infections. Section I. Fundamental cutaneous microbiology. In *Dermatology*, edited by S. Moschella, D. M. Pillsbury and H. J. Hurley, Jr., p. 482. Philadelphia; Saunders.

47. Rebora, A., Marples, R. R. and Kligman, A. M. (1973). Experimental infection with Candida albicans. *Archives of Dermatology* 108, 69.

48. Wilmore, D. W. and Dudrick, S. J. (1969). Safe long term venous catheterization. *Archives of Surgery* 98, 256.

49. Durdrick, S. J., Groff, D. B. and Wilmore, D. W. (1969). Long-term venous catheterization in infants. *Surgery, Gynecology and Obstetrics* 129, 805.

50. Filler, R. M. and Coran, A. G. (1976). Total parenteral nutrition in infants and children: central and peripheral approaches. *Surgical Clinics of North America* **56**, 395.

51. Parsa, M. H., Habif, D. V., Ferrer, J. M., Lipton, R. and Yoshimura, N. N. (1972). Intravenous hyperalimentation: indications, technique and complications. *Bulletin of the New York Academy of Medicine* **48**, 920.

52. Freeman, J. B., Lemire, A. and Maclean, L. D. (1972). Intravenous alimentation and septicemia. *Surgery, Gynecology and Obstetrics* **135**, 708.

53. Sanders, R. A. and Sheldon, G. F. (1976). Septic complications of total parenteral nutrition. *American Journal of Surgery* **132**, 124.

54. Hoshal, V. L. (1975). Total intravenous nutrition with peripherally inserted silicone elastomer central venous catheters. *Archives of Surgery* **110**, 644.

55. Jones, M. V. and Craig, D. B. (1972). Venous reaction to plastic intravenous cannulae: influence of cannula composition. *Canadian Anaesthetists' Society Journal* **19**, 491.

56. MacDonald, A. S., Master, S. K. P. and Moffitt, E. A. (1977). A comparative study of peripherally inserted silicone catheters for parenteral nutrition. *Canadian Anaesthetists' Society Journal* **24**, 263.

57. Peters, W. R., Bush, W. H., McIntyre, R. D. and Hill, L. D. (1973). The development of fibrin sheath on indwelling venous catheters. *Surgery, Gynecology and Obstetrics* **137**, 43.

58. Hoshal, V. L., Ause, R. G. and Hoskins, P. A. (1971). Fibrin sleeve formation on indwelling subclavian venous catheters. *Archives of Surgery* **102**, 353.

59. Donetz, A. P., Harvey, R. A. and Greco, R. S. (1984). Stability of antibiotic bound to polytetrafluroethylene with cationic surfactants. *Journal of Clinical Microbiology* **19**, 1.

60. Myers, R. N., Smink, R. D. and Goldstein, F. (1974). Parenteral hyperalimentation five years' clinical experience. *American Journal of Gastroenterology* **62**, 313.

61. Dillon, J. D. Jr., Schaffner, W., Van Way, C. W. III and Meng, H. C. (1973). Septicemia and total parenteral nutrition. *Journal of the American Medical Association* **223**, 1341.

62. Wilmore, D. W. (1975). Parenteral nutrition in the thermally injured patient. In *Total Parenteral Nutrition*, edited by H. Ghadimi, p. 483. New York, Wiley.

63. Goldmann, D. A. and Maki, D. G. (1973). Infection control in total parenteral nutrition. *Journal of the American Medical Association* **223**, 1360.

64. Moran, J. M., Atwood, R. P. and Rowe, M. I. (1965). A clinical and bacteriologic study of infections associated with venous cutdowns. *New England Journal of Medicine* **272**, 554.

65. Norden, C. W. (1969). Application of antibiotic ointment to the site of venous catheterization – a controlled trial. *Journal of Infectious Diseases* **120**, 611.

66. Zinner, S. H., Denny-Brown, B. C., Braun, P., Burke, J. P., Toala, P. and Kass, E. H. (1969). Risk of infection with intravenous indwelling catheters: effect of application of antibiotic ointment. *Journal of Infectious Diseases* **120**, 616.

67. Driscoll, J. D., Heird, W. C., Schullinger, J. N., Gongaware, R. D. and Winters, R. W. (1972). Total intravenous alimentation in low-birth-weight infants: a preliminary report. *Journal of Pediatrics* **81**, 145.

68. McGovern, B. (1972). Septic complications of hyperalimentation. In *Intravenous Hyperalimentation*, edited by C. S. M. Cowan, Jr. and W. L. Scheetz, p. 165. Philadelphia; Lea and Febiger.

69. Riella, M. C. and Scribner, B. H. (1976). Five years' experience with a right atrial catheter for prolonged parenteral nutrition at home. *Surgery, Gynecology and Obstetrics* **143**, 205.

70. Henzel, J. H. and De Weese, M. S. (1971). Morbid and mortal complications associated with prolonged central venous cannulation: awareness, recognition and prevention. *American Journal of Surgery* **121**, 600.

71. Smits, H. and Freedman, L. R. (1967). Prolonged venous catheterization as a cause of sepsis. *New England Journal of Medicine* **276**, 1229.

72. Copeland, E. M., MacFayden, B. V., McGown, C. and Dudrick, S. J. (1974). The use of hyperalimentation in patients with potential sepsis. *Surgery, Gynecology and Obstetrics* **138**, 377.

73. Filler, R. M., Eraklis, A. J., Rubin, V. G. and Das, J. B. (1969). Long term parental nutrition in infants. *New England Journal of Medicine* **281**, 589.

74. Shils, M. E. (1972). Guidelines for total parenteral nutrition. *Journal of the American Medical Association* **220**, 1721.

75. Shanbhogue, L. K. R. (1988). Change of central venous catheters using a guidewire. *Annals of the Royal College of Surgeons of England* **70**, 28.

76. Pettigrew, R. A., Lang, S. D. R., Haydock, D. T. *et al.* (1985). Catheter related sepsis in patients on intravenous nutrition. *British Journal of Surgery* **75**, 52.

77. Bozzetti, F., Terno, G., Bonafanti, G. *et al.* (1983). Prevention and treatment of central venous sepsis by exchange via guidewire. *Annals of Surgery* **198**, 48.

78. Sanderson, I. and Dietel, M. (1973). Nursing care in parenteral nutrition. *Surgery, Gynecology and Obstetrics* **136**, 577.

79. Kondi, E. S., Piertrafitta, J. J. and Barriola, J. A. (1988). Technique for placement of totally implantable venous access devices. *Journal of Surgery and Oncology* **37**, 272.

80. Peters, J. L., Belsham, P. A., Taylor, B. A. and Watt-Smith, S. (1984). Long term venous access. *British Journal of Hospital Medicine* **32**, 230.

81. Gilligan, J. E., Phillips, P. J., Wong, C. H. and Kimber, R. J. (1979). Streptokinase and blocked central venous catheter. *Lancet* **2**, 1189.

82. Phillips, K. J. (1976). The organization of a parenteral nutrition unit. In *Total Parenteral Nutrition*, edited by J. E. Fischer, p. 101. Boston, Little, Brown.

83. Curry, C. R. and Quie, P. G. (1971). Fungal septicemia in patients receiving parenteral alimentation. *New England Journal of Medicine* **285**, 1221.

84. Freeman, J. B. and Litton, A. A. (1974). Preponderance of gram-positive infections during parenteral alimentation. *Surgery, Gynecology and Obstetrics* **139**, 905.

85. National Co-ordinating Committee on Large Volume Parenterals (1975). Recommended methods for compounding intravenous admixtures in hospitals. *American Journal of Hospital Pharmacy* **32**, 261.

86. Stiewstrom, G., Gunnarson, B. and Wikner, H. (1978). Studies on microbiological contamination of in-use I.V. fluids. *Acta Pharmacologica Scandinavica* **15**, 169.

87. Sanders, L. H., Mabadeje, S. A., Avis, K. E. *et al.* (1978). Evaluation of compounding accuracy and aseptic techniques for intravenous admixtures. *American Journal of Hospital Pharmacology* **35**, 53.

88. Holmes, C. J., Kundsin, R. B., Ausman, R. K. *et al.* (1980). Potential hazards associated with microbial contamination of in-line filters during intravenous therapy. *Journal of Clinical Microbiology* **12**, 725.

89. Baumgartner, T. G., Schmidt, G. L., Kamlesh, M. *et al.* (1986). Bacterial endotoxins retention by in-line intravenous filters. *American Journal of Hospital Pharmacology* **43**, 681.

90. Falchuk, K. H., Peterson, L. and McNeil, B. J. (1985). Microparticulate induced phlebitis. *New England Journal of Medicine* **312**, 78.

91. Bailey, M. J. (1979). Reduction of catheter-associated sepsis in parenteral nutrition using low-dose intravenous heparin. *British Medical Journal* **1**, 1671.

92. Feiler, E. M. and de Acva, W. E. (1969). Infraclavicular percutaneous subclavian vein puncture: a safe technique. *American Journal of Surgery* **118**, 906.

93. Bennegard, K., Curelaru, I., Gustavsson, B. and Linder, L. E. (1982). Material thrombogenicity in central venous catheterization. *Acta Anaesthiologia Scandinavica* **26**, 112.

94. Raucher, H. S., Hyatt, A. C., Barzilai, A. *et al.* (1984). Quantitative blood cultures in the evaluation of septicaemia in children with Broviac catheters. *Journal of Pediatrics* **104**, 29.

95. Weightman, N. C. and Speller, D. C. E. (1986). Pour plate blood cultures to detect bacteremias related to indwelling central venous catheters. *Journal of Hospital Infection* **8**, 23.

96. Flynn, P. M., Shenep, J. L., Stokes, D. C. and Barrett, F. F. (1987). In situ management of confirmed central venous catheter related bacteremia. *Pediatric Infectious Diseases* **6**, 729.

97. Swan, H. J. C., Ganz, W., Forrester, J., Marcus, H., Diamond, G. and Chonette, D. (1970). Catheterisation of the heart in man with use of a flow directed balloon-tipped catheter. *New England Journal of Medicine* **283**, 447.

98. Forrester, J. S., Ganz, W., Diamond, G., McHugh, T., Chonette, D. W. and Swan, H. J. C. (1972). Thermodilution cardiac output determination with a single flow-directed catheter. *American Heart Journal* **83**, 306.

99. Meister, S. G., Banka, V. S. and Helfant, R. H. (1973). Transfemoral pacing with balloon-tipped catheters. *Journal of the American Medical Association* **225**, 712.

100. Meister, S. G., Banka, V. S., Chadda, K. D. and Helfant, R. H. (1974). A balloon tipped catheter for obtaining His bundle electrograms without fluoroscopy. *Circulation* **49**, 42.

101. Chatterjee, K., Swan, H. J. C., Ganz, W., Gray, R., Loebel, H., Forrester, J. S. and Chonette, D. (1975). Use of a balloon-tipped flotation electrode catheter for cardiac monitoring. *American Journal of Cardiology* **36**, 56.

102. Wilson, J. E. III and Bynum L. J. (1976). An improved pulmonary angiographic technique using a balloon-tipped catheter. *American Review of Respiratory Diseases* **114**, 1137.

103. Woodcock, T. C., Murray, S. and Ledingham, I. (1984). Mixed venous oxygen saturation changes during tension pneumothorax and its treatment. *Anaesthesia* **39**, 1004.

104. Pace, N. L. (1977). A critique of flow-directed pulmonary arterial catheterisation. *Anesthesiology* **47**, 455.

105. Pierce, T. and Woodcock, T. (1989). How to insert a pulmonary arterial flotation catheter. *British Journal of Hospital Medicine* **42**, 484.

106. Mandel, S. and Barash, P. (1976). The proximal basilic vein: a new approach for introduction of a flow-guided catheter into the pulmonary artery. *Journal of Thoracic and Cardiovascular Surgery* **71**, 376.

107. Swan, H. J. C. and Ganz, W. (1975). Use of balloon flotation catheters in critically ill patients. *Surgical Clinics of North America* **55**, 501.

108. George, R. J. D. (1980). How to insert a flotation catheter. *British Journal of Hospital Medicine* **23**, 296.

109. Civetta, J. M. and Gabel, J. C. (1972). Flow directed-pulmonary artery catheterization in surgical patients: indications and modifications of technic. *Annals of Surgery* **176**, 753.

110. Kaplan, J. A. and Miller, E. D. (1976). Insertion of the Swan–Ganz Catheter. *Anesthesiology Review* **1**, 22.

111. Ellertson, D. G., McGough, E. C., Rasmussen, B., Sutton, R. B. and Hughes, R. K. (1974). Pulmonary artery monitoring in critically ill surgical patients. *American Journal of Surgery* **128**, 791.

112. Cucchiara, R. F., Messick, J. M., Gronert, G. G. and Michenfelder, J. D. (1980). Time required and success rate of percutaneous right atrial catheterization: description of a technique. *Canadian Anaesthetists' Society Journal* **27**, 572.

113. Wood, S. R. (1985). Placement of a tunnelled catheter with a fixed hub using a split introducer. *British Journal of Parenteral Therapy* Vol. 6, 96.

114. George, R. J. D. and Banks, R. A. (1983). Bedside measurement of pulmonary capillary wedge pressure. *British Journal of Hospital Medicine* **29**, 286.

115. Denys, B. G., Uretsky, B. F. *et al.* (1990). Access to the internal jugular vein: comparison between the landmark and ultrasound guided method. *Circulation* **82** (Supplement 3).

116. Troianos, C. A., Jobes, D. R. and Ellison, N. (1991). Ultrasound-guided cannulation of the internal jugular vein. A prospective, randomized study. *Anesthesia Analgesia* **72**, 823.

4

The Arm Veins

The most popular technique for inserting central venous catheters has always been through peripheral arm veins, using a puncture site in the antecubital fossa. The main advantage here is that veins are usually easily seen and palpable, and every clinician has previous experience of venepuncture at this site. Furthermore, because no vital structures lie near these veins, there has been a notable absence of reports of complications arising from the venepuncture.

Nevertheless, the approach through a vein in the antecubital fossa has two main drawbacks. First, studies show that only 65–75% of catheters inserted through these veins reach a suitable central position[1–9] (Table 4.1). Second, and in contrast to the safety of the initial venepuncture, thrombophlebitis and inflammation at the site of insertion quickly develop[10,11] and nearly all patients suffer this complication within 24–48 hours.[8]

In spite of the disadvantages, for short-term use central venous catheterisation through visible palpable peripheral arm veins is safe and remains the method of choice for those with little experience of sophisticated techniques.

Some interest has recently centred on the deep brachial veins. When conventional cannulation through visible or palpable antecubital fossa veins is not possible because of obesity or sclerosed veins, deep percutaneous puncture of the venae comitantes of the brachial artery in the antecubital fossa has been used to gain venous access and thereby avoid a venous cutdown.[12] This site of venepuncture has been used for central venous catheterisation although minor injury to the brachial artery is a risk.[13] Following the description of a cut-down technique on the deep brachial vein at the inner edge of the brachial biceps,[14] a percutaneous method of central venous catheterisation through

the deep basilic vein in the groove between the bellies of the biceps and triceps muscles has been successfully tried.[15] These techniques have not yet achieved popular use. They obviously entail more skill than superficial venepuncture and the danger of damage to the brachial artery is ever present.

In 1967 Spracklen et al.[16] described a technique of central venous catheterisation through a percutaneous venepuncture of the proximal basilic or axillary vein. This approach was later described independently by Ayim[17] in 1977. Both papers reported a high success rate with an absence of serious complication.

More recently, a large series involving axillary vein catheterisation in over 300 instances reported favourable results comparable with other techniques.[18] The method was used to insert both central venous lines and pulmonary artery catheters. The authors claim freedom from damage to lung and other structures associated with techniques involving deep veins. The site of insertion was thought to be particularly advantageous in tracheostomised patients as the separation of the catheter from a potentially infected tracheostome reduced the risk of septicaemia. Another more recent study from the same centre found similar success.[19] These workers recommended the use of a Seldinger guide wire technique to insert the catheter.

However, this approach has not gained popularity, probably because of the high degree of skill required to make the initial venepuncture into a vein that is not readily visible.

The axillary vein can also be reached percutaneously from an infraclavicular approach.[20,21] Based on dissection studies, definitive landmarks have been recommended to trace the course of the axillary vein. Whilst the technique claims to perform venepuncture away from the thoracic inlet the method does nevertheless involve deep and therefore blind needling of the vein. Early reports are encouraging but further studies are needed to determine the role of this method.

An interesting approach which seeks on the one hand to avoid the failings of conventional long arm central venous catheters and the external jugular vein method and at the same time eliminate the dangers of deep neck vein puncture is the concept of the 'half-way' venous catheter. The rationale and anatomical basis for using this method have been examined in depth.[22,23]

In this method the catheter tip is placed within the proximal axillary vein or the distal portion of the subclavian vein. The walls of the proximal axillary vein are held apart by expansions of the coracoclavipectoral fascia so the catheter tip would lie within a large vein which cannot collapse and

one which opens into large central veins. The axillosubclavian venous pathway is relatively long so positioning the catheter can be achieved by clinical estimation, so making x-ray control unnecessary. The technique has been validated by extensive clinical testing.[24]

ANATOMY

The venous blood from the arm drains through two intercommunicating main veins, the basilic and the cephalic. The basilic system runs along the medial side of the arm and the cephalic along the lateral side. There is considerable variation in the anatomy of the arm veins, particularly in the cephalic system. The common arrangement is described below (Figure 4.1).

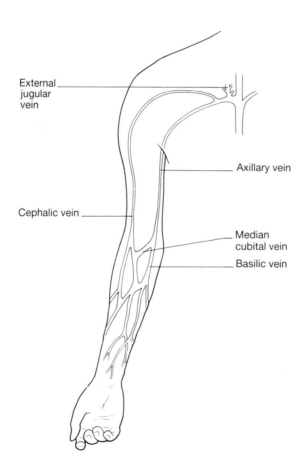

External jugular vein

Axillary vein

Cephalic vein

Median cubital vein

Basilic vein

Figure 4.1. Anatomy of the arm veins.

Basilic vein

The basilic vein ascends from the hand along the medial surface of the forearm, often as two channels which unite before they each the elbow. Near the elbow the vein inclines forwards to run in front of the medial epicondyle, at about which point it is joined by the median cubital vein. It then runs along the medial margin of the biceps to the middle of the upper arm, where it pierces the deep fascia. From here it ascends along the medial side of the brachial artery and becomes the axillary vein on entering the axilla.

Other veins on the posteromedial surface of the forearm ascend to join the basilic vein. Although prominent, they are not firmly supported by the fatty subcutaneous tissue and easily move away from a probing needle point.

Cephalic vein

The cephalic vein ascends on the front of the lateral side of the forearm to the front of the elbow, where it communicates with the basilic vein through the median cubital vein. It then ascends along the lateral surface of the biceps to the lower border of the pectoralis major muscle, where it turns sharply to pierce the clavipectoral fascia and pass beneath the clavicle. It then usually terminates in the axillary vein. The virtual right angle at which the cephalic vein joins the axillary vein is probably one of the main reasons for the obstruction frequently encountered at this point when attempting to pass a catheter through the cephalic vein. Other reasons for obstruction at this site are variations in the anatomy of the termination of the cephalic vein. The vein may join the external jugular vein only or it may bifurcate into two very small veins, one joining the external jugular vein and one the axillary vein. Finally, there are usually valves near its termination.

Axillary vein (Figure 4.2)

The basilic vein continues as the axillary vein on reaching the axilla. Anteriorly, the lateral border of the pectoralis major muscle forms the lateral boundary of the axilla. The axillary vein continues upwards into the apex of the axilla and becomes the subclavian vein on reaching the lower border of the first rib. It usually receives the cephalic vein near its termination.

The axillary vein is divided into three parts by the pectoralis minor muscle, which crosses over the vein to reach its insertion in the coracoid process of the scapula. It is the first (distal) part of the axillary vein which is suitable for venepuncture because it is relatively superficial. This part of the vein is separated from the skin by fascia and aveolar and fatty tissue; the medial cutaneous nerve of the forearm lies on its surface and separates it from the axillary artery, which lies laterally. Other structures of the brachial plexus are more closely related to the artery than the vein and are therefore less likely to be damaged during venepuncture.

Median cubital vein

The median cubital vein is a large communicating vein that springs from the cephalic vein just below the bend of the elbow and runs obliquely upwards to join the basilic vein just above the bend of the elbow. It receives veins from the front of the forearm which themselves may be suitable for catheterisation. It is separated from the brachial artery by a thickened portion of the deep fascia (bicipital aponeurosis). Again, variations in this arrangement are commonly seen.

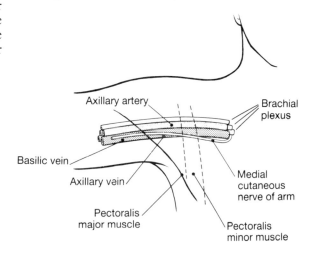

Figure 4.2. Anatomy of the axillary vein.

CHOICE OF TECHNIQUE

A vein in the antecubital fossa is usually the first choice for catheterisation (Figure 4.3). The axillary vein is kept in reserve in case of failure with a more peripheral vein, but may be considered for long-term catheterisation.

Certain recommendations have been made to obtain the best success rate with the peripheral arm vein approach. The advantage of the basilic over the cephalic vein is agreed on by most authors,[1-4,7,26,27] including ourselves, although other studies have revealed no difference in success rate between the two veins.[9,28] With either method the catheter may still not enter the intrathoracic veins. Dietel and McIntyre[3] and Langston[4] suggested turning the head towards the side of venepuncture to reduce the chance of the catheters' entering the ipsilateral internal jugular vein. The value of this manoeuvre was supported by Burgess et al.[29] but not by Woods et al.,[30] though both of these appear to have been careful studies. When the

basilic vein was used, abducting the arm up to 45° from the body improved the success rate.[30]

The value of these various manoeuvres has been assessed whilst inserting catheters into the basilic vein under fluoroscopic control.[31] The findings and recommendations which follow correspond with our experience of many hundreds of catheters inserted through this route.

1. Rotation of the head to the side of venepuncture and supraclavicular digital pressure on the same side alters the anatomy of the veins in such a way as to encourage passage of a catheter centrally. Hyperabducting the arm is least helpful.
2. If resistance is felt after advancing the catheter more than 20 cm then withdrawal of the stylet (if present) 2–3 cm may facilitate the passage of the now more flexible catheter tip.
3. Withdrawal of the stylet combined with injection of a bolus of saline whilst advancing the catheter is also worth trying if the catheter appears held up.

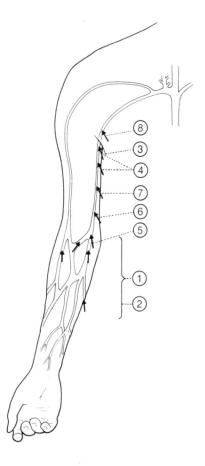

Figure 4.3. Approaches to catheterisation of the arm veins. 1 = Authors'; 2 = Bridges et al. (1979)[33] (basilic vein only); 3 = Spracklen et al. (1967);[16] 4 = Ayim (1977);[17] 5 = Linder et al. (1985);[24] 6 = Saissy et al. (1985);[13] 7 = Koing-Bo et al. (1984);[15] 8 = Nickalls (1987).[20] Adults: methods 1, 2, 3 or 4. Infants: methods 1 or 4.

Kuramota and Sakabe[32] found that they could more satisfactorily position the catheter tip when the right basilic vein was used, but most authors do not agree with this.[6,9]

Lumley and Russell[9] recommended a neck compression test to detect whether a catheter tip is positioned in the internal jugular vein. Neck compression produces a rise of more than 10 cm of water in the venous pressure after inadvertent internal jugular catheterisation, but no such rise occurs when the other side of the neck is compressed. To detect obstruction to the passage of the catheter, Holt[1] measured alterations in the rate of entry of a rapidly running infusion of saline through the catheter. This also indicated whether manoeuvres such as abduction of the arm overcame or reduced the obstruction.

Bridges and his colleagues[33] demonstrated a high success rate when catheterisation was performed with the patient in the sitting position, combined with a special technique for introducing the catheter (described below).

The material or design of the catheter can also influence the success rate. Two groups[6,9] found an improved result with the use of the Drum Cartridge Catheter (Abbott) when compared to the I-Catheter (Bardic). That the type of device used appears to be an important factor in determining the success rate of cannulation through arm veins is emphasised by other workers. Wright and Walker[34] obtained a high success rate again using the (modified) Drum Cartridge Catheter (Abbott Laboratories). The new device eliminates the risk of catheter shearing by adopting a catheter through cannula technique. Comparing their results with those obtained with other products, they attributed their 92% success rate to the soft polyurethane catheter stiffened by a flexible wire stylet throughout its length; the stiffening was thought to be significant.

Method preferred by authors

The authors' preferred technique, both for adults and children, is described immediately below. We have found the selection of a medially placed vein (basilic system) to be the most important factor in obtaining successful catheterisation through an arm vein.

The use of a J-tipped guide wire has been shown to greatly increase the success rate of cannulation through the external jugular vein[35] (see Chapter 7). Similarly, using a J-tipped guide wire when cannulating the antecubital fossa veins, some workers have achieved 100% successful central venous positioning when using the basilic vein and 78% through the cephalic vein;[36] others are not convinced of the advantage of a J-tipped guide wire.[37]

The concept of the 'half-way' catheter does not seem to have achieved widespread appeal in spite of its thorough documentation. All the other techniques described involving the axillary vein and the deep brachial veins require a higher degree of skill and in all these methods a vein is punctured in a blind fashion. These techniques have been described in more recent years so it is too early to fully assess their place in this field.

A useful supplementary technique has been suggested to encourage the use of the relatively safe arm veins when these are very small. A guide wire could be introduced through a small venepuncture needle, followed by a vein dilator and then the introduction of a sufficiently large introducer for a central catheter.[38]

Whatever technique is used to insert a central venous line through a peripheral arm vein, it should be borne in mind that abduction and adduction of the arm can lead to movement of the catheter tip up to, on average, 2–3 cm. Adduction alone can result in the catheter being drawn into the thorax by as much as 9 cm.[39]

Descriptions of the techniques follow

ANTECUBITAL FOSSA APPROACH
Authors' Method

Patient category

Adults and neonates.

Advantages and disadvantages

Venepuncture is made into a visible and palpable vein, so there is a lower risk of immediate complications compared with puncture of deep veins.

Peripheral veins are unsatisfactory for long-term catheterisation.

Preferred side

Either side may be used. Select the arm with the most favourable vein.

Position of patient (Figure 4.4a)

Place the patient in a supine position with the arm to be used held at about 45° from the side of the body. Turn the head towards the side of the puncture.

Position of operator (Figure 4.4a)

Stand on the same side as the puncture site.

Advice on current equipment

Adults. 14 gauge O.D. introducing needle or cannula, length 40 mm (minimum). Catheter length 600 mm (minimum).
Neonates. 18 or 20 gauge O.D. introducing needle or cannula, length 20 mm (minimum). Catheter length 200 mm (minimum).

Anatomical landmarks (Figure 4.4b)

Apply a tourniquet to the upper arm to distend the veins before selecting a suitable vein.

In order of preference, identify:

(i)   A vein on the medial side of the antecubital fossa – the basilic or median cubital vein. Even when not visible, these veins are often easily palpable when engorged.
(ii)   A vein on the posteromedial aspect of the forearm – a tributary of the basilic vein. An assistant may be needed to rotate the arm externally to display these veins.
(iii)   The cephalic vein if the other arm cannot be used.

Preparation

Perform the puncture under sterile conditions using local anaesthesia if indicated.

Precautions and recommendations

Estimate the length of catheter needed by laying the catheter (in its sterile pack) on the surface of the patient, or by measurement with a tape-measure.

Point of insertion of needle

Close to the chosen vein.

Direction of needle and procedure

After puncturing the vein, advance the catheter a short distance (2–4 cm in adults; 1–2 cm in infants) and release the tourniquet. Keep the arm abducted and the head turned to the side of puncture as the catheter is steadily advanced to the distance estimated beforehand.

If the progress of the catheter is held up, do not use force to advance it and do not attempt to retract it if a catheter-through-needle device is used. If other devices are used, the following 'trial and error' manoeuvres may help to advance the catheter: withdraw the catheter 2 or 3 cm and attempt reinsertion; rotate the catheter as it is advanced; withdraw the stylet 1 cm and attempt insertion again.

Other useful measures include digital pressure in the supraclavicular fossa on the ipsilateral side and the injection of a bolus of saline whilst advancing the catheter.

Confirm the position of the catheter tip with a chest x-ray.

Success rate

77·7% (94 catheterisations) using the Drum Cartridge Catheter (Abbott). 52·8% (106 catheterisations) using the I-Catheter (Bardic). No infants were included in this series.

Complications

No complications were associated with the initial venepuncture.

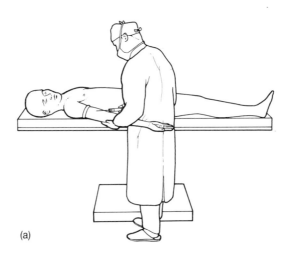

(a)

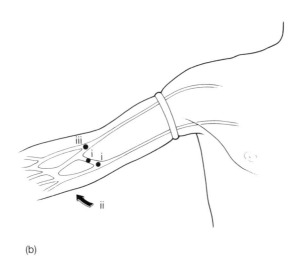

(b)

Figure 4.4. Antecubital fossa approach: authors' method.

ANTECUBITAL FOSSA APPROACH: PATIENT IN THE SITTING POSITION
Bridges et al. *(1979)*[33]

Patient category

Adults. The description of the technique by the original authors did not include its application in children, but this does not necessarily exclude its use in this age group.

Advantages and disadvantages

Because the patient is placed in the sitting position, the catheter is encouraged to bend downwards under the influence of gravity and hence to enter the intrathoracic veins.

Preferred side

Not stated.

Position of patient (Figure 4.5a)

Place the patient in the sitting position (45° to 90° above the horizontal). Turn the head towards the side of the puncture. Abduct the arm to be used 30° away from the patient's side.

Position of operator (Figure 4.5a)

Stand on the same side as the puncture site.

Equipment used in original description

Catheter-through-14 gauge O.D. needle. Bardic catheters were used after testing several catheters for 'softness and tendency to bend'. Bardic, Jelco, Deseret and Sorensen catheters were held at an angle of 45° to the horizontal and allowed to bend under their own weight. The angle to which the catheter bent was then taken as a measure of its softness and tendency to bend.

Advice on current equipment

14 gauge O.D. introducing needle or cannula, length 40 mm (minimum). Catheter length 600 mm (minimum).

Anatomical landmarks (Figure 4.5b)

Apply a tourniquet to the upper arm to distend the veins. Identify a vein on the medial side of the antecubital fossa (basilic or median cubital vein). The vein may be easily palpable even if not visible.

If there is no suitable vein in the antecubital fossa, rotate the arm laterally (an assistant is helpful) and identify a suitable tributary of the basilic vein on the posteromedial surface of the forearm.

Preparation

Perform the procedure under aseptic conditions using local anaesthesia if indicated.

Precautions and recommendations

Estimate the length of catheter needed for its tip to reach:

1. the junction of the cephalic and basilic veins
2. the junction of the internal jugular and innominate veins
3. a satisfactory position in the central veins.

Point of insertion of needle (Figure 4.5b)

Into the chosen vein.

Procedure (Figure 4.5c)

After successful venepuncture, release the tourniquet and insert the catheter until the tip is judged to be in the subclavian vein distal to its junction with the internal jugular vein (Figure 4.5c – position marked x). Withdraw the stylet (if present) 150 mm (6 in) and advance the catheter slowly 12 mm ($\frac{1}{2}$ in) at a time with intervals of 2 seconds between each 12 mm ($\frac{1}{2}$ in) insertion, until it is judged that the catheter has reached its correct intrathoracic position. Confirm the position of the catheter with a chest x-ray.

Success rate

98% (50 cases).

Complications

Not stated.

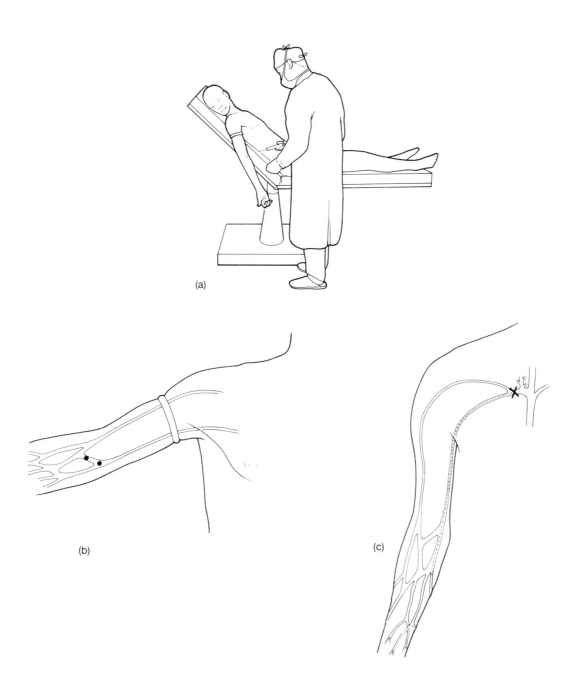

(a)

(b)

(c)

Figure 4.5. Antecubital fossa approach: Bridges
et al. (1979)[33]

ANTECUBITAL FOSSA APPROACH: 'HALF-WAY' VENOUS CATHETERS
Linder et al. (1985)[24]

Patient category

The original description confines this technique to adults only.

Advantages and disadvantages

Venepuncture into a visible vein is easy and free of the possibility of serious trauma. The dangers of intrathoracic catheters – cardiac arrhythmias and perforation of the vena cava and heart are avoided. The rate of misplacement of the catheter tip is less than with conventional long catheters although this only applies when insertion is through the basilic vein. Furthermore, radiological confirmation of the catheter tip is usually unnecessary but again, only if the basilic vein has been used.

The main indication for a 'half-way' catheter is for central venous pressure measurement. They are not suitable for very long-term parenteral alimentation, central venous blood sampling or for aspiration of air embolus.

Preferred side

Either side may be used.

Position of patient (Figure 4.6)

Establish the patient's height. Place the patient in the supine position with the head in the straight ahead position. The arm to be used is abducted 90° away from the body and the forearm fully extended.

Position of operator

Stand on the same side as the puncture site.

Equipment used in original description

Seldinger guide wire technique used exclusively to insert soft polyurethane catheters (Viggo Secalon-Seldy 40 cm long and 1·1/1·7 mm inner/outer diameters).

Advice on current equipment

13 or 14 gauge O.D. introducer cannula. Catheter length 600 mm (minimum). Ensure that it is possible to estimate the length of catheter within the vein, e.g. by inspection and measurement of a used or out-of-date catheter of the same type.

Anatomical landmarks (Figure 4.6)

Apply a tourniquet to the upper arm to distend the veins in the antecubital fossa. Identify the basilic vein (preferable to the cephalic vein). Identify and visualise a line drawn between the epicondyles of the humerus with the arm in the abducted position.

Preparation

Perform the procedure under aseptic conditions using local anaesthesia if indicated.

Precautions and recommendations

Mark off a distance (on the catheter or protective sheath if one is provided) equal to 1/5 of the patient's body height. A useful nomogram is provided (Figure 4.7).

Point of insertion of the needle (Figure 4.8)

Into the basilic vein where it is crossed by a line joining the two epicondyles.

Procedure (Figure 4.8)

Advance the catheter to the marked position on the catheter (1/5 body height). Fix the catheter firmly in this position. If the basilic vein is used and no resistance to advancement is noted and blood can be freely aspirated from the catheter then no radiological confirmation is necessary. However, if in doubt confirm the position with a chest x-ray.

Success rate

113 cases (basilic vein 83, cephalic vein 30): 65% tips in proximal axillary vein; 34% in distal subclavian vein, 1% in internal jugular vein on radiological examination.

Complications

Serious: nil. Minor: temporary interruption of intravenous infusion flow with arm movements, 12 cases; partial/total occlusion of flow, 16; leakage of infusate at puncture site, 1; pain along vein during infusion (potassium solution, cytotoxic drug), 2; thrombophlebitis developing in 2–10 days, 5.

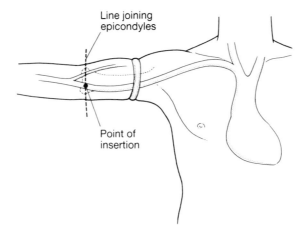

Line joining
epicondyles

Point of
insertion

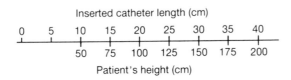

Inserted catheter length (cm)

0   5   10   15   20   25   30   35   40

50   75   100   125   150   175   200

Patient's height (cm)

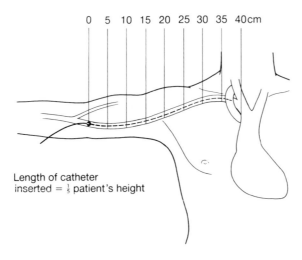

0   5   10 15 20 25 30 35 40cm

Length of catheter
inserted = ⅕ patient's height

Figures 4.6.–4.8.   Antecubital fossa approach:
'Half-way' venous catheters.[24]

DEEP BRACHIAL VEIN: LOWER THIRD OF UPPER ARM
Saissy et al. (1985)[13]

Patient category

The method was described in patients between ages 16 and 70.

Advantages and disadvantages

The technique is indicated when superficial veins are unuseable and deep neck venepuncture is dangerous or impossible. Only a moderate success rate together with the risk of injury to the brachial artery are the main disadvantages.

Preferred side

Either side may be used.

Position of patient

Place the patient in the supine position. Turn the head to the same side as the puncture side. Abduct the arm to be used 45°from the trunk and rotate it externally.

Position of operator

Same side as the puncture site.

Equipment used in original description

Introducer needle 15 gauge; 17 gauge polyethylene catheter of 500 mm length (Centracath Vygon code 135-15).

Advice on current equipment

A Seldinger technique in conjunction with a vein dilator is recommended to minimise potential injury to the artery. Initial needling of vein should be carried out with a small (21–22 gauge) needle.

Anatomical landmarks

Palpate the brachial artery 1 cm above the skin crease in the antecubital fossa. Apply a tourniquet to the upper arm.

Preparation

Perform the procedure under aseptic conditions using local anaesthetic if appropriate.

Precautions and recommendations

Point of insertion of the needle

To the medial side of the palpated brachial artery.

Procedure

Insert the introducer needle to which a 10 ml syringe is attached. Elevate the syringe 45° away from the skin surface. Whilst maintaining a negative pressure on the syringe advance the needle to the medial side of the brachial artery. A flashback of venous blood confirms successful venepuncture. Remove the syringe and insert the catheter. Take a chest x-ray to confirm the position of the catheter tip.

Success rate

Successful venepuncture 88% (50 attempts); successful catheterisation 72%; successful central venous catheterisation 60%.

Complications

Inadvertent puncture of the brachial artery 6 cases (12%) with no serious consequence.

BRACHIAL VEIN: MIDDLE THIRD OF UPPER ARM
Koing-Bo (1984)[15]

Patient category

Adults.

Advantages and disadvantages

Useful when deep neck veins are not suitable. Avoids the need for surgical cut-down. Few complications but the procedure is a blind one so there is a risk of arterial puncture.

Preferred side

Either side.

Position of patient (Figure 4.9)

Patient in the supine position. Abduct the arm to be used 45° away from the side with the hand supinated (palm showing).

Position of operator

Same side.

Equipment used in original description

Guide wire technique. 21 gauge introducer needle to locate vein. A small diameter guide wire to pass through this needle (confirmed by pretesting) is introduced into the vein. The vein is then dilated by inserting an 18 gauge cannula over the wire. A stiffer and larger diameter wire is then introduced over which a large diameter (13 gauge) cannula is advanced into the dilated vein. The catheter (15 gauge) is finally inserted through this large cannula until a central venous position is reached.

Advice on current equipment

The above technique is recommended.

Anatomical landmarks (Figure 4.9)

Identify the groove between the biceps and triceps muscle in the middle third of the upper arm. Palpate the brachial artery. Note from Figure 4.10 the relations of the brachial veins to the brachial artery in this region.

Preparation

Apply a tourniquet high up on the arm. Perform the procedure under aseptic conditions using local anaesthetic if appropriate.

Point of insertion of the needle (Figure 4.9)

In the groove between the muscle bellies in the middle third of the upper arm. If the brachial artery is palpable the needle is inserted slightly lateral to it.

Procedure

Insert the introducer needle and syringe into the point of insertion and move the syringe about 30–45° away from the skin. Advance whilst keeping a slight negative pressure in the syringe until a flashback is obtained. Detach the syringe and introduce the small guide wire into the vein. Release the tourniquet. Proceed as described above under 'Original Equipment'. When the catheter appears successfully placed, take a chest x-ray for confirmation.

Success rate and complications

Not stated. Apparently successful on a number of occasions with no serious complications.

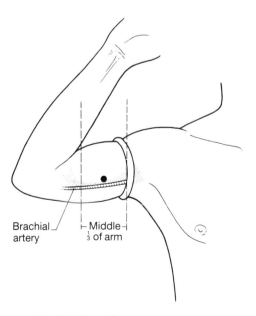

Figure 4.9. Position of the arm for initial venepuncture.

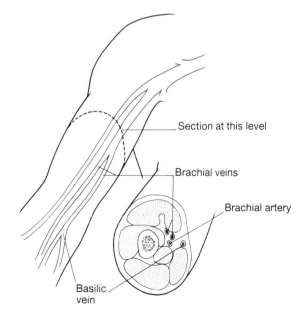

Figure 4.10. Anatomy of veins of the upper arm.

AXILLARY AND PROXIMAL BASILIC VEIN
Spracklen et al. *(1976)*[16]

Patient category
Adults. The description of the technique by the original authors did not include its application in children, but this does not necessarily exclude its use in this age group.

Advantages and disadvantages
Puncture is made in a 'blind' fashion into the axillary vein or proximal basilic vein, using the axillary artery, identified by palpation, as the landmark. This vein may be patent when more peripheral veins are collapsed, as in circulatory failure. The complications of puncture of deep neck veins are avoided.

Preferred side
Either side may be used.

Position of patient (Figure 4.11a)
Place the patient supine with the head in the *straight-ahead* position and resting on one pillow. The arm to be used is abducted away from the patient's side and the hand placed behind the occiput.

Position of operator
Stand on the same side as the puncture site.

Equipment used in original description
Catheter-through-needle, catheter-through-cannula, and guide wire techniques have been used.

Advice on current equipment
14 gauge O.D. introducing needle or cannula, length 40 mm (minimum). Catheter length 600 mm (minimum). Alternatively, a guide wire technique is recommended.

Anatomical landmarks (Figure 4.11b)
Palpate the axillary artery and note its course. Identify the area where the basilic vein continues as the axillary vein.

Preparation
Perform the puncture under sterile conditions using local anaesthesia if indicated.

Precautions and recommendations
None.

Point of insertion of needle (Figure 4.11b)
1 cm medial to the artery in the region of the junction of the basilic and axillary veins.

Direction of the needle and procedure (Figure 4.11c)
Place the point of the needle on the entry site in the skin and elevate the needle 30° above the skin surface. Direct the needle towards the chest wall keeping the needle parallel to the course of the axillary artery. Keep a finger on the artery during venepuncture to act as a landmark and to protect the artery from inadvertent puncture. An assistant (if available) exerting gentle upward pressure in the medial axilla may make venepuncture easier. Maintain a slight negative pressure on the syringe (if used) as the needle is advanced, until the vein is entered. Insert the catheter. Take a chest x-ray to confirm the position of the catheter tip.

Success rate
90% (50 cases). Venepuncture failed at the first attempt in 3 cases but was successful in the opposite arm.

Complications
There were no significant complications. Ten patients (20%) experienced transient local pain or paraesthesiae in the arm. No late neurological injury occurred. Haematomas occasionally formed locally.

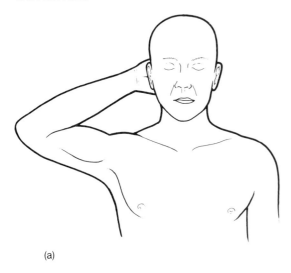

(a)

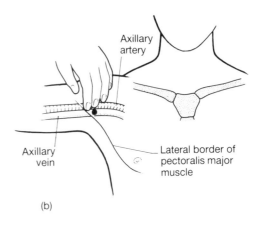

Axillary
artery

Axillary
vein

Lateral border of
pectoralis major
muscle

(b)

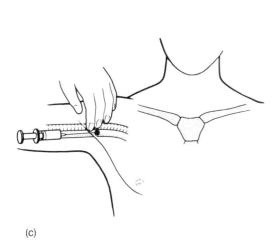

(c)

Figure 4.11. Axillary and proximal basilic vein:
Spracklen *et al.* (1976).[16]

AXILLARY AND PROXIMAL BASILIC VEIN
Ayim (1977)[17]

Patient category

Adults and children. No infants younger than 1 year were included in this study.

Advantages and disadvantages

Puncture is made into a visible or easily palpable vein. This technique is claimed to have a lower failure rate than catheterisation through more peripheral veins whilst avoiding the complications of puncture of the deep neck veins. The relative contraindications to the use of this technique include infection at the site of puncture and gross obesity.

Preferred side

Either side may be used.

Position of patient (Figure 4.12a)

Place the patient supine with the head in the straight-ahead position. Abduct the arm 45°, or more if possible, away from the patient's side and place the hand under the patient's head.

Position of operator

Stand on the same side as the puncture site.

Equipment used in original description

Adults. Catheter-through-cannula and catheter-through-needle (10% of cases).
Infants. 18 gauge O.D. catheter-over-needle.

Advice on current equipment

Adults. 14 gauge O.D. introducing needle or cannula, length 40 mm (minimum). Catheter length 600 mm (minimum).
Infants. 18 or 20 gauge O.D. introducing needle or cannula, length 20 mm (minimum). Catheter length 200 mm (minimum).

Anatomical landmarks (Figure 4.12b)

Identify the lower border of the pectoralis major muscle and the positions of the distal portion of the axillary vein and proximal portion of the basilic vein in the following manner. Palpate the axillary artery; the axillary vein lies medial to the artery. This distal portion of the axillary vein is superficial but becomes inaccessible when it passes deep to a muscle layer in its middle portion. The proximal

portion of the basilic vein, which forms the immediate distal continuation of the axillary vein, also lies superficially and has the same relation to its accompanying artery (brachial artery).

Preparation

Perform the puncture under sterile conditions using local anaesthesia if indicated.

Precautions and recommendations

An assistant may be helpful.

Point of insertion of needle (Figure 4.12c)

In order to distend the vein, apply a narrow (1–2 cm wide) rubber tourniquet as high up in the axilla as possible and instruct the assistant to pull the tourniquet towards the lateral half of the clavicle. If the armpit is hollow, use a pad of gauze under the tourniquet to help compress the vein. Alternatively, use the thumb or third and fourth fingers of the free hand to compress the vein medial to the pulsation of the axillary artery and as high up in the armpit as possible.

Following attempts to distend the vein, enter at the most prominent portion, whether the proximal basilic vein or the axillary vein.

Procedure

Do not proceed with this technique unless one of the veins is visible or easily palpable. Maintain a slight negative pressure in the syringe (if used) as the needle is advanced until the vein is entered. Insert the catheter. Take a chest x-ray to confirm the position of the catheter tip.

Success rate

Axillary vein. 95·9% (73 cases, all adults).
Proximal basilic vein. 93·1% (68 cases, both adults and children).

Complications

Haematoma, 3%.
Probable incipient venous thrombosis, 3·9%.
There were no paraesthesiae or evidence of nerve injury.
The average duration of catheterisation was, for the axillary vein, 7·8 days (range 1–28 days) and, for the proximal basilic vein, 4·3 days (range 1–14 days).

(a)

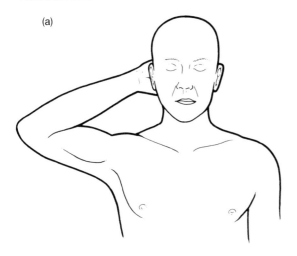

(b)

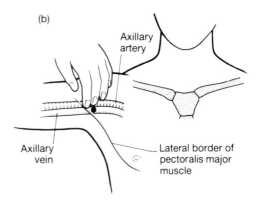

(c)

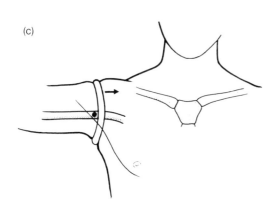

Figure 4.12.   Axillary and proximal basilic vein:
Ayim (1977).[17]

AXILLARY VEIN: INFRACLAVICULAR APPROACH
Nickalls (1987),[20] Taylor and Yellowlees (1990)[21]

Patient category
Adults and children.

Advantages and disadvantages
Avoids dangers of trauma to deep structures of the thoracic inlet. Specific landmarks. Convenience and ease of fixation in the infraclavicular region. Since the tip of the needle is always inferior (below) the clavicle, puncture of the pleura is virtually impossible. Furthermore, in the event of inadvertent trauma to a blood vessel, direct pressure is easily applied and surgical exploration is facilitated if this were to become necessary.

Preferred side
No preferred side but diagrams indicate a right sided approach.

Position of patient (Figure 4.13a and b)
Place the patient in the supine position and tilt the table 15° head down. Keep the arm straight and move it about 45° away from the patient's side (this manoeuvre straightens out the axillary vein).

Position of operator
Stand on the same side as the puncture site.

Equipment used in original description
Seldinger guide wire technique (Leader-Cath-Vygon). Size 14–16 gauge catheter.

Advice on current equipment
18 gauge O.D. needle, length 60 mm (minimum). Guide wire length 400 mm (minimum). Catheter length 200 mm (minimum).

Anatomical landmarks (Figure 4.13c)
Mark position A–3 fingers breadth (about 5 cm) below the lower border of the coracoid process. In children, the child's own fingers may be used to estimate this landmark.[21] Mark position B – where the space between the clavicle and the thorax just becomes palpable. This corresponds to a point immediately below the lower border of the clavicle at the junction of its medial quarter and its lateral three-quarters. Outline the medial border of pectoralis minor by drawing a line starting at the coracoid process and swinging towards the mid-line and mark the point at which it crosses the line A–B.

Preparation
Perform the puncture under sterile conditions using local anaesthetic if indicated.

Point of insertion of the needle (Figure 4.13b and c)
This is lateral to the medial border of pectoralis minor and on the line A–B.

Initial location of vein with small-gauge needle
Recommended (21 or 22 gauge). If an ordinary needle is too short a similar gauge spinal needle may be used.

Direction of the needle and procedure (Figure 4.13b and d)
Place the point of the needle at the entry site and the syringe on the skin. Elevate the attached syringe about 20° with the needle pointing medially along the line A–B. Whilst palpating the axillary artery (ideal, but not always possible) advance the needle slowly, aspirating continuously and aim to enter the vein half way between the medial border of pectoralis minor and point B. If resistance is met, withdraw the needle and redirect in an anteroposterior plane parallel to the line A–B. At all times keep the tip of the needle below the lower border of the clavicle to prevent inadvertent puncture of the lung.

After insertion of the catheter take a chest x-ray to confirm the position of the catheter tip and to exclude pneumothorax.

Success rate
Nickalls[20] 92% (n = 14). Taylor and Yellowlees[21] 97% (n = 95).

Complications
Nickalls.[20] None in this series but the risk of inadvertent puncture of the axillary artery is noted.

Taylor and Yellowlees.[21] In 92 successful cannulations, the complications were arterial puncture (5 cases) and paraesthesia (2 cases).

(a)

(b)

45°

(c)

Artery

Coracoid
process

B

Axillary
vein

A

Medial border of
pectoralis minor

Line of medial
border of
pectoralis minor

(d)

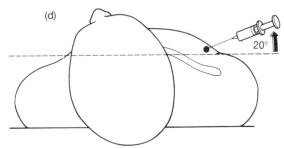

20°

Figure 4.13 Axillary vein: infraclavicular
approach (Nickalls, 1987[20]).

Table 4.1. Arm vein – results and complications.

Author and year	Classification of technique (vein used)	Success rate	No. cases	Complications	No. complications (%)	Personnel	Comments
Holt (1967)[1]	Basilic Cephalic	71% 44%	56 78	Local phlebitis, cellulitis of upper arm	11 (8·2) 2 (1·5)	Authors	Duration of catheterisation 3 days (mean), 0–9 days (range)
Gilday and Downs (1969)[2]	Mainly basilic	66·5%	200	Not stated			Cephalic vein found to be unsatisfactory
Deitel and McIntyre (1971)[3]	Basilic Cephalic	75·3% 14%	130 7	Not stated			Duration of catheterisation up to 25 days
Langston (1971)[4]	Basilic (207) Cephalic (93)	62% (75·3% if catheter in right atrium or right ventricle withdrawn)	300	Not stated		Various residents	
Johnston and Clark (1972)[5]	Basilic and cephalic	64% (77·5% if catheters in right atrium or right ventricle withdrawn)	73	Thrombophlebitis at puncture site	2 (2·7)	One operator	Arm abducted 90° Strict aseptic technique
Ng and Rosen (1973)[6]	Basilic (I-Catheters and Drum Cartridge Catheters)	52·8% 77·7%	106 94	Not stated		Mainly authors but some supervised residents	
Webre and Arens (1973)[7]	Basilic Cephalic	65% 45%	71 29	Not stated			Most of the unsatisfactory catheters were in the internal jugular vein
Lumley and Ressell (1975)[9]	Basilic Cephalic	75·6% 73·9%	82 23	Not stated		Various	
Sorensen and Sonne-Holm (1975)[8]	Basilic (left)	69%	55	None initially. Later: swelling of arm; inflammation at site of insertion; septicaemia	5 (9·1) 3 (5·4) 1 (1·8)		
Burgess et al. (1977)[29]	Basilic (head in mid position, turned towards arm of insertion)	58–80%	50 50	Not stated			

Authors	Vein/technique	Success rate	No. of patients	Complication	n (%)	Comments
Bridges et al. (1979)[33]	Basilic	72·5%	51	Not stated		
	Cephalic	76%	25			
Smith (1984)[36]	Basilic vein, sitting position, special technique, 'soft' catheter	98%	50	Unable to cannulate	4 (5)	No serious complications
	Basilic	70%		Unable to advance wire	3 (3.8)	
	Cephalic	30%		Malposition but intrathoracic	3 (3.8)	
	J-tipped guide wire used	91%	77	Premature Ventric. beat	3 (3.8)	
Spracklen et al. (1976)[16]	Proximal basilic or axillary vein	90%	50	Transient pain or paraesthesiae during venepuncture. No cases of local infection or thrombophlebitis	10 (20)	Duration of catheterisation not stated
Ayim (1977)[17]	Axillary vein	95·9%	73 (4–80 years)	? Venous thrombosis	1 (1·4)	Duration of catheterisation 7·8 days (mean)
	Proximal basilic	93·1%	54 (1–75 years)	Venous haematoma	3 (5·5)	Duration of catheterisation 4·3 days (mean)
				? Thrombosis	1 (1·8)	
Gouin et al. (1985)[18]	Axillary vein	87%	323	Malposition	22 (9)	
Martin et al. (1986)[19]	Axillary vein	87·5%	63	Arterial puncture (no sequelae)	(11)	
				Thrombosis of axillary and subclavian veins Used for PA catheters in all patients	1 (1·8)	
Nickalls (1987)[20]	Axillary vein	92%	14			
Taylor (1990)[21]	Axillary vein	Not stated	95	Arterial puncture	5 (5%)	
				Parasthesiae	2 (2)	
Saissy et al. (1985)[13]	Deep brachial vein	60%	50	Arterial puncture (minor)	6 (12)	

REFERENCES

1. Holt, H. M. (1967). Central venous pressure via peripheral veins. *Anesthesiology*, **28**, 1093.
2. Gilday, D. L. and Downs, A. R. (1969). The value of chest radiography in the localization of central venous pressure catheters. *Canadian Medical Association Journal*, **101**, 363.
3. Deitel, M. and McIntyre, J. A. (1971). Radiographic confirmation of site of central venous pressure catheters. *Canadian Journal of Surgery*, **14**, 42.
4. Langston, C. S. (1971). The aberrant central venous catheter and its complications. *Radiology*, **100**, 55.
5. Johnston, A. O. B. and Clark, R. G. (1972). Malpositioning of central venous catheters. *Lancet*, **2**, 1395.
6. Ng, W. Shang and Rosen, M. (1973). Positioning central venous catheters through the basilic vein. A comparison of catheters. *British Journal of Anaesthesia*, **45**, 1211.
7. Webre, D. R. and Arens, J. F. (1973). Use of cephalic and basilic veins for introduction of central venous catheters. *Anesthesiology*, **38**, 389.
8. Sorensen, T. I. A. and Sonne-Holm, S. (1975). Central venous catheterization through the basilic vein or by infraclavicular puncture. *Acta Chirurgica Scandinavica*, **141**, 323.
9. Lumley, J. and Russell, W. J. (1975). Insertion of central venous catheters through arm veins. *Anaesthesia and Intensive Care*, **3**, 101.
10. Christensen, K. H., Nerstrom, B. and Baden, H. (1967). Complications of percutaneous catheterization of the subclavian vein in 129 cases. *Acta Chirurgica Scandinavica*, **133**, 615.
11. Colvin, M. P., Blogg, C. E., Savege, T. M., Jarvis, J. D. and Strunin, L. (1972). A safe long term infusion technique? *Lancet*, **2**, 317.
12. Roseman, J. M. (1983). Deep, percutaneous antecubital venipuncture: an alternative to surgical cutdown. *American Journal of Surgery* **146**, 285.
13. Saissy, J. M., Driss-Kamili, N., Berdouz, S., Atmani, M. and Dimou, M. (1985). Percutaneous catheterization of the deep brachial vein. *Annales Francais D Anesthesie et de Reanimation* **4**, 316.
14. Gilette, J. F. and Susini, J. (1984). Deep brachial vein catheterization for total parenteral nutrition – an alternate approach: review of 154 cases. *Journal of Parenteral and Enteral Nutrition*, **8**, 49.
15. Koing-Bo, K., Gorfine, S., Berman, M. *et al.* (1984). Percutaneous catheterization of the brachial vein for central venous access. *Surgery, Gynaecology and Obstetrics* **159**, 287.
16. Spracklen, F. H. N., Niesche, F., Lord, P. W. and Beterman, E. M. M. (1967). Percutaneous catheterisation of the axillary vein. *Cardiovascular Research*, **1**, 297.
17. Ayim, E. N. (1977). Percutaneous catheterisation of the axillary vein and proximal basilic vein. *Anaesthesia*, **32**, 753.

18. Gouin, F., Martin, C. and Saux, P. (1985). Central venous and pulmonary artery catheterizations via the axillary vein. *Acta Anaesthesiologica Scandinavica, Suppl.* **81**, 27.
19. Martin, C., Auffray, J. P., Albanese, J. *et al.* (1986). Pulmonary artery catheterization via the axillary vein. *Annales Francais D Anesthesie et de Reanimation* **5**, 64.
20. Nickalls, R. W. D. (1987). A new percutaneous infra-clavicular approach to the axillary vein. *Anaesthesia* **42**, 151.
21. Taylor, B. L. and Yellowlees, I. (1990). Central venous cannulation using the infraclavicular axillary vein. *Anesthesiology* **72**, 55.
22. Gustavsson, B., Linder, L. E., Hultman, E. and Curelaru, I. (1985). 'Half-Way' venous catheters. 1. Theoretical premises and aims. *Acta Anaesthesiologica Scandinavica, Suppl.* **81**, 30.
23. Curelaru, I., Gustavsson, B., Wojciechowski, J. *et al.* (1985). 'Half-Way' venous catheters. 2. Anatomoradiological basis. *Acta Anaesthesiologica Scandinavica, Suppl.* **81**, 32.
24. Linder, L. E., Wojciechowski, J., Zachrisson, B. F. *et al.* (1985). 'Half-Way' venous catheters. 4. Clinical experience and thrombogenicity. *Acta Anaesthesiologica Scandinavica, Suppl.* **81**, 40.
25. Ricksten, S.-E., Medegard, A., Curelaru, I. *et al.* (1986). Estimation of central venous pressure by measurement of proximal axillary venous pressure using a 'half-way' catheter. *Acta Anaesthesiologica Scandinavica, Suppl.* **30**, 13.
26. Zohman, L. R. and Williams, M. H. (1959). Percutaneous right heart catheterization using polyethylene tubing. *American Journal of Cardiology*, **4**, 373.
27. Jaikaran, S. M. N. and Sagay, E. (1968). Normal central venous pressure. *British Journal of Surgery*, **55**, 609.
28. Kellner, G. A. and Smart, J. F. (1972). Percutaneous placement of catheters to monitor 'central venous pressure'. *Anesthesiology*, **36**, 515.
29. Burgess, G. E., Marino, R. J. and Peuler, M. J. (1977). Effect of head position in the location of venous catheters inserted via basilic veins. *Anesthesiology*, **46**, 212.
30. Woods, D. G., Lumley, J., Russell, W. J. and Jacks, R. D. (1974). The position of central venous catheters inserted through arm veins: a preliminary report. *Anaesthesia and Intensive Care*, **2**, 43.
31. Ragasa, J., Shah, N., Watson, R. and Bedford, M. D. (1988). Where antecubital CVP catheters go: a study under fluoroscopic control. *Anesthesiology* **69** (Suppl. 3A), A231.
32. Kuramoto, T. and Sakabe, T. (1975). Comparison of success in jugular versus basilic vein technics for central venous pressure catheter positioning. *Anesthesia and Analgesia: Current Researches*, **54**, 696.
33. Bridges, B. B., Carden, E. and Takacs, F. A. (1979). Introduction of central venous pressure catheters through arm veins with a high success rate. *Canadian Anaesthetists' Society Journal*, **26**, 128.

34. Wright, P. J. and Walker, D. A. J. (1989). Central venous cannulation in neurosurgical patients. *Intensive Therapy and Clinical Monitoring* **82**, 84.

35. Blitt, C. D., Wright, W. A., Petty, W. C. and Webster, T. A. (1974). Central venous catheterisation via the external jugular vein. A technique employing the J-wire. *Journal of the American Medical Association* **229**, 817.

36. Smith, S. L., Albin, M. S., Ritter, R. D. and Bunegin, L. (1984). CVP catheter placement from the antecubital veins using a J-wire catheter guide. *Anesthesiology* **60**, 238.

37. Colley, P. S. and Artru, A. A. (1984). ECG-guided placement of Sorensen CVP catheters via arm veins. *Anesthesia and Analgesia* **63**, 953.

38. *Lancet* (1986). Central venous catheterisation. Editorial. **2**, 669.

39. Kalso, E., Rosenberg, P. H., Vuorialho, M. and Pietila, K. (1982). How much do arm movements displace cubital venous catheters? *Acta Anaesthesiologica Scandinavica* **26**, 354.

5

The Subclavian Vein

Aubaniac[1] first described the technique of infraclavicular subclavian venepuncture in 1952. He pointed out that the vein was large and was prevented from collapsing by the surrounding tissue. Wilson and his colleagues,[2] in 1962, used the infraclavicular route to introduce a catheter into the superior vena cava. Since then catheterisation of the subclavian vein has been widely used for a large range of diagnostic and therapeutic procedures. In addition to its widespread use in central venous pressure monitoring, the technique has been used in cardiac pacing[3,4] and pulmonary artery angiography.[5] Equally the technique has gained a recognised and important place in rapid fluid and blood replacement therapy[2,6] and especially in long-term parenteral nutrition.[7] The administration of potent cardiovascular drugs and agents which are irritant to veins such as those used in chemo-therapy are now invariably administered through central veins and the subclavian route is often favoured especially when longer-term administration is envisaged.

Yoffa[8] introduced the technique of supraclavicular subclavian venepuncture for central venous catheterisation and parenteral nutrition in 1965. Subsequently, several modifications to both infraclavicular and supraclavicular techniques as originally described have been put forward to improve the success rate and to reduce the risks. The subclavian vein therefore established itself as a route applicable when peripheral veins are either unavailable or unsuitable. The subclavian route was especially indicated in shock conditions because of the vein's large diameter and because it remained patent even in such poor haemodynamic states.

Many occasional users of the subclavian technique have probably been encouraged to use this method because of the relatively low rate of complications reported by authors who have become skilled in the technique. Not surprisingly, when subclavian cannulation is carried out by a wide range of physicians of varied levels of experience a much higher incidence of complications is manifest. Pneumothorax reached an incidence of 12·4% in one such group.[9] The popularity of the subclavian route in adults was maintained for many years in spite of numerous reports of a significant incidence of serious complications and death (Tables 5.1, 5.2, and 5.3). The same popularity has never been achieved for subclavian vein catheterisation in infants and small children. Although some workers have used the infraclavicular subclavian approach with good success and few complications, it is generally accepted that with infants and small children there is a much greater potential for serious harm, so the newcomer to the technique should carry out the procedure in these patients only under the strictest supervision by an experienced operator.[7,10,11] In the last decade or so the place of the subclavian route has been overtaken in popularity by the internal jugular approach because it has been perceived as a safer method and no more technically demanding than subclavian vein catheterisation. Indeed, in the anaesthetic field most other techniques appear to have been abandoned in favour of the internal jugular approach. However, in intensive care and other critical care areas the subclavian vein remains the route for many of the longer-term uses of central lines, notably for prolonged parenteral nutrition.

ANATOMY (Figure 5.1)

The subclavian vein lies in the lower part of the supraclavicular triangle (Figure 5.1). This triangle is bounded medially by the posterior border of the sternomastoid muscle, caudally by the middle third of the clavicle, and laterally by the anterior border of the trapezius muscle.

The subclavian vein is the continuation of the axillary vein and begins at the lower border of the first rib. Initially the vein arches upwards across the first rib and then inclines medially, downwards, and slightly forwards across the insertion of the scalenus anterior muscle in the first rib to enter the thorax, where it unites with the internal jugular vein behind the sternoclavicular joint. From here, as the innominate vein, it turns towards the mediastinum and unites with its counterpart from the other side to form the superior vena cava.

Anteriorly, the vein is separated from the skin throughout its entire course by the clavicle. It attains its highest point just medial to the midpoint of the clavicle, where it rises to the upper border of the bone. The lateral portion of the vein lies anterior to and below the subclavian artery as both these structures cross the upper surface of the first rib. Medially the fibres of the scalenus anterior muscle separate the vein in front from the artery behind. Behind the artery is the cervical pleura. The cervical pleura rises above the sternal end of the clavicle. The subclavian vein crosses in front of the phrenic nerve. The thoracic duct arches over the apex of the pleura on the left side to enter the angle made by the junction of the internal jugular and subclavian veins.

CHOICE OF TECHNIQUE (Figure 5.2)

No clear choice between supraclavicular and infra-clavicular approaches can be recommended from a comparison of their success and complication rates (Tables 5.1 and 5.2). The few trials that have been undertaken show no difference in success and complication rates.[12] However, several reports suggest that the supraclavicular approach leads to a much higher success rate in satisfactory positioning of the catheter tip.[12,13] This is particularly apparent when central venous catheterisation is being performed during the rather special circumstances of cardiopulmonary resuscitation.[14] Nevertheless, the infraclavicular approach is much more popular judging by the far greater volume of reports in the literature; this may, however, be due to its earlier introduction into medical practice. For central venous catheterisation in infants and small children, only the infraclavicular approach (see Figure 5.2 – Morgan and Harkins (1972)[10]) has been used[2,7,10,11,15] and all authors urge great caution on the operator.

Consideration of some practical points will assist in making a choice. With either approach, accurate identification of the landmarks may be difficult in obese patients and the choice may then be influenced by which landmarks can be determined.

The supraclavicular approach offers some practical advantages. The distance from skin to vein is shorter and the needle has only to pierce skin and fascia,[8] the catheter is also more likely to reach a satisfactory central position.[14,16] During operations the supraclavicular area is usually accessible to the anaesthetist at the head of the patient. Many would advocate using the internal jugular vein under these circumstances. Nevertheless, in some cases the subclavian vein may be chosen. Certainly, there is less interruption of cardiopulmonary resuscitation manouevres when the supraclavicular approach to cannulating the subclavian vein is chosen since the operator stands at the head of the patient away from those carrying out airway management and chest compression.[14] However, because of the hollow contour of the supraclavicular fossa, securely fixing catheter and surgical dressing may be difficult. Furthermore, it is not easy to keep the site dry and free from infection, since perspiration tends to collect in the hollow.

With the infraclavicular approach, a longer needle may be necessary since it has to pass through a muscle layer as well as skin and fascia before reaching the vein. However, the method is preferable

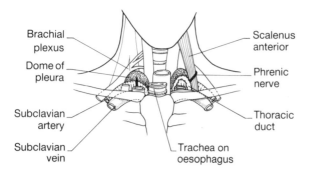

Brachial plexus — Scalenus anterior — Dome of pleura — Phrenic nerve — Subclavian artery — Thoracic duct — Subclavian vein — Trachea on oesophagus

Figure 5.1. Anatomy of the subclavian vein.

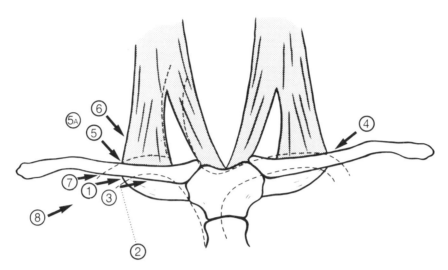

Figure 5.2. Approaches to the catheterisation of the subclavian vein. 1 = Aubaniac (1952),[1] Wilson *et al.* (1962);[2] 2 = Mogil *et al.* (1967);[32] 3 = Morgan and Harkins (1972);[10] 4 = Yoffa (1965);[8] 5 = James and Myers (1973);[33] 5A = Brahos (1977);[18] 6 = Haapaniemi and Slatis (1974);[16] 7 = Tofield (1969);[17] 8 = Untracht (1988).[19] Adults: methods 1, 2, 3, 4, 5, 6 or 7. Infants: method 3.
Methods preferred by authors: Aubaniac (1952),[1] Wilson *et al.* (1962)[2] for adults.
Although the only approach described by the authors as performed on children is that of Morgan and Harkins (1972)[10] this does not necessarily imply that the others are unsuitable.

for long-term catheterisation because the catheter and surgical dressing can be more easily and securely fixed. There is also less chance of infection.

There are differences in technique with both approaches. Accounts of the supraclavicular route usually describe the same point for insertion of the needle, but the landmarks used to guide the direction of the needle are varied. However, Haapaniemi and Slatis[16] advocate a point of insertion somewhat higher up in the neck so that the venepuncture is made into the junction of the internal jugular and subclavian veins. They claim that the catheter passes more easily, but their results are no different from those of other techniques (Table 5.2).

Five techniques have been described for the infraclavicular approach. They differ on the point of insertion of the needle in relation to the midpoint of the clavicle. Most authors use the midpoint or a position slightly lateral to this. A much more lateral point of insertion was advocated by Tofield[17] to reduce the risk of producing a pneumothorax, but no results were given. A recent modification to the infraclavicular route[19] recommends a point of insertion more laterally and using the palpable axillary artery as a definite and reliable landmark. The method appears to warrant more study. Other authors[15,20,21] claim that a more medial point (at the junction of the medial and middle thirds of the clavicle) is safer in avoiding trauma to the subclavian artery, brachial plexus, and pleura. The results again do not appear to be markedly different (Table 5.1). There are many anatomical differences between left- and right-sided approaches to the central veins through the subclavian vein but the choice of which side to use remains uncertain since success rates and complication rates are not related to the side of puncture in most reported series. Most authors recommend the right side whether through a supraclavicular or infraclavicular approach as this gives a more direct route to the superior vena cava, avoids trauma to the thoracic duct and facilitates the procedure for a right handed operator.

Some authors have found no difference in failure and complication rates when left and right side infraclavicular catheterisations were compared[22] but others[23–25] have shown a significantly higher rate of misplacement of the catheter tip in right-sided catheterisations – 15% compared to 2% in one report.[26] Catheter tips which were considered unsatisfactory lay in the ipsilateral internal jugular vein and the innominate vein (right-sided) or contralateral subclavian vein. Much the same finding over 13 000 cannulations of which 98%

were through the infraclavicular route.[27]

Retracting the shoulders and turning the head away from the side of puncture are often recommended to improve successful cannulation but such manoeuvres are probably inconsequential.[25] Indeed, distortion of the anatomy may lead to more difficult catheterisation.[22]

Method preferred by authors

We favour the infraclavicular approach to the subclavian vein as described below (Aubaniac,[1] Wilson *et al.*[2]). The technique for infants, described later (Morgan and Harkins[10]), is essentially the same. The infraclavicular technique employs more definite landmarks and has been safer in our hands. Subclavian vein catheters are popular for long-term use and catheters inserted into the infraclavicular site are more readily kept free from infection than those inserted into the supraclavicular fossa.

LOCATING THE VEIN WITH AN ULTRASOUND BLOOD FLOW DETECTOR

The position of the subclavian vein as it passes below the clavicle can be detected with an ultrasound flow probe[28] (e.g. Sonicaid; Sonicaid Ltd, Hook Lane, Nyetimber, Bognor Regis, Sussex). A characteristic venous hum is heard, which is accentuated when the arm on the same side is firmly squeezed. The venous hum ceases abruptly when a sudden Valsalva effect is produced (a co-operative patient is instructed to breathe out sharply against a closed glottis; in a patient connected to a breathing circuit the inspiratory phase is briefly held). The position of the subclavian artery is given by detecting its pulsatile flow sounds.

An ultrasound probe is easy to use and can be recommended as a preliminary step when cannulating the subclavian vein by any approach, especially in obese and heavily built patients. Its use does not guarantee success or eliminate complications, although it is likely to increase the former and diminish the latter.

Modern sophisticated and real time ultrasound technology can make all forms of deep vein catheterisation a more successful and safer procedure. High resolution imaging enables accurate delineation of all the anatomical structures together with visualisation of the needle and catheter. The technique is not appropriate to all clinical situations but is particularly suited for training the inexperienced and in catheterisation where the anatomy is abnormal or distorted.[29–31]

Descriptions of the
techniques follow

INFRACLAVICULAR APPROACH
Aubaniac (1952),[1] *Wilson* et al. *(1962)*[2]

Patient category

Adults and children.

Preferred side

Not stated. Most other authors using this technique prefer the right side.

Position of patient (Figure 5.3a)

Place the table in a 25° head-down position. Place the patient in the supine position with both arms at the side. *Turn the head away from the side of the puncture. Position a pillow under the chest to thrust up the clavicular area above the shoulders.*

Position of operator (Figure 5.3b)

Stand on the same side as the puncture site.

Equipment used in original descriptions

Adults. 14 gauge O.D. introducing needle. Catheter-through-needle.
Infants. 17 gauge O.D. introducing needle. Catheter-through-needle. Catheter length 200 mm.

Advice on current equipment

Adults. Guide wire technique strongly recommended using an 18 or 16 gauge introducer needle. Catheter thro' cannula, 14 or 16 gauge O.D. needle or introducer, length 60 mm (minimum). Catheter length 200 mm (minimum).
Long cannula on long needle, length 130 mm (minimum).
Neonates. 20 gauge O.D. needle or introducer, length 30 mm (minimum). Catheter length 80 mm (minimum).
Long cannula on long needle, length 40 mm (minimum).

Anatomical landmarks (Figure 5.3c)

Midclavicular point. The lower border of the clavicle. The triangle formed by the sternal and clavicular heads of the sternomastoid muscle with the upper border of the clavicle.

Preparation

Perform the puncture under sterile conditions using local anaesthesia if indicated.

Precautions and recommendations

Ensure that syringe can be removed easily from the needle.

Point of insertion of needle (Figure 5.3c)

1 cm below the midpoint of the lower border of the clavicle in adults.
Immediately below the midpoint of the lower border of the clavicle in neonates.

Direction of the needle and procedure (Figure 5.3d, e)

Place the point of the needle at the entry site on the skin and point the needle and syringe towards the head (A). Then swing the syringe laterally so that the needle points medially towards the small triangle formed by the sternal and clavicular attachments of the sternomastoid muscle and the upper border of the clavicle (A to B). *If this landmark is not clearly defined, point the needle towards the suprasternal notch, keeping a finger tip in the notch to act as a target.*
Advance the needle posterior to the clavicle keeping close to its posterior aspect, maintaining the needle and syringe parallel to the coronal plane (Figure 5.3e). Maintain a slight negative pressure in the syringe as the needle is advanced until the vein is entered. Introduce the catheter.

Take a chest x-ray to confirm the position of the catheter tip and to exclude pneumothorax.

Success rate

Rate not stated in a total of 250 catheterisations.

Complications

The authors state that there were no complications in the 250 cases, but that a 'number of pneumothoraces' occurred in subsequent cases performed by residents.

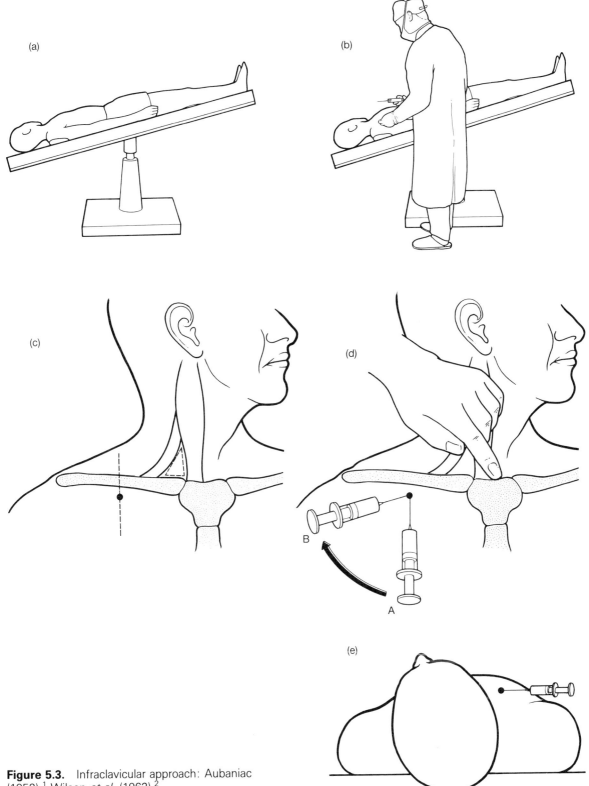

Figure 5.3. Infraclavicular approach: Aubaniac (1952),[1] Wilson *et al.* (1962).[2]

INFRACLAVICULAR APPROACH
Morgan and Harkins (1972)[10]

Patient category
Adults and neonates. This series included neonates.

Preferred side
The left. The right side may, nevertheless, be used.

Position of patient (Figure 5.4a)
Place the table in a 25° head-down position. Place the patient supine with arms at his sides. Turn the head away from the side of puncture. A rolled towel placed beneath the vertebral column thrusts the clavicular area upwards and opens up the small space between the clavicle and first rib.

Position of operator (Figure 5.4b)
Stand on the side of the puncture site.

Equipment used in original description
Neonates. Catheter-through-17 gauge O.D. needle.
Older infants. Catheter-through-14 gauge O.D. needle.

Choice of current equipment
Neonates. 20 gauge O.D. needle or introducer, length 30 mm (minimum). Catheter length 80 mm (minimum). Guide wire technique strongly recommended.
Older infants. Larger size equipment may be appropriate.

Anatomical landmarks (Figure 5.4c)
Midpoint of inferior border of clavicle. Suprasternal notch. (Alternatively the small triangle formed by the sternal and clavicular heads of the sternomastoid muscle.)

Preparation
Perform the puncture under sterile conditions using local anaesthesia if indicated.

Precautions and recommendations
An operator unfamiliar with this technique and proposing to use it in infants should be strictly supervised by an experienced operator. The technique should be performed in an operating room environment. Immobilise infants and take measures to prevent excessive heat loss (for instance, use an overhead radiant heater).

Point of insertion of needle (Figure 5.4c)
Just below the midpoint of the clavicle.

Direction of the needle and procedure (Figure 5.4d, e)
Place the point of the needle at the entry site on the skin and point the needle cephalad (A). Then swing the needle and syringe laterally so that the needle points towards the tip of a finger of the free hand pressed firmly into the suprasternal notch (A to B).

Advance the syringe behind the clavicle keeping the syringe and needle parallel to the coronal plane (Figure 5.4e). Maintain a slight negative pressure in the syringe whilst advancing the needle.
If no 'flashback' is obtained, withdraw the needle slowly to the subcutaneous tissue before attempting venepuncture using a slightly different direction. As the syringe is withdrawn maintain the negative pressure, since the needle tip may enter the lumen of the vein during withdrawal. After inserting the catheter take a chest x-ray to confirm its position and to exclude a pneumothorax.

Success rate
'Almost invariably successful' in over 400 infants and older children. Operators were experienced or closely supervised.

Complications
One hundred consecutive catheterisations were analysed: 74 were performed in patients less than 12 months of age. Of these, 37% were less than 6 weeks old and included 15 premature babies weighing less than 1·5 kg. No complications occurred in the younger infants. In the older infants there were 2 instances of arterial puncture with local bleeding and one case each of the catheter entering the pericardial cavity and the pleural cavity. Both latter cases were detected radiologically before the infusion was started and in both the catheter was withdrawn immediately and produced no clinical problem.

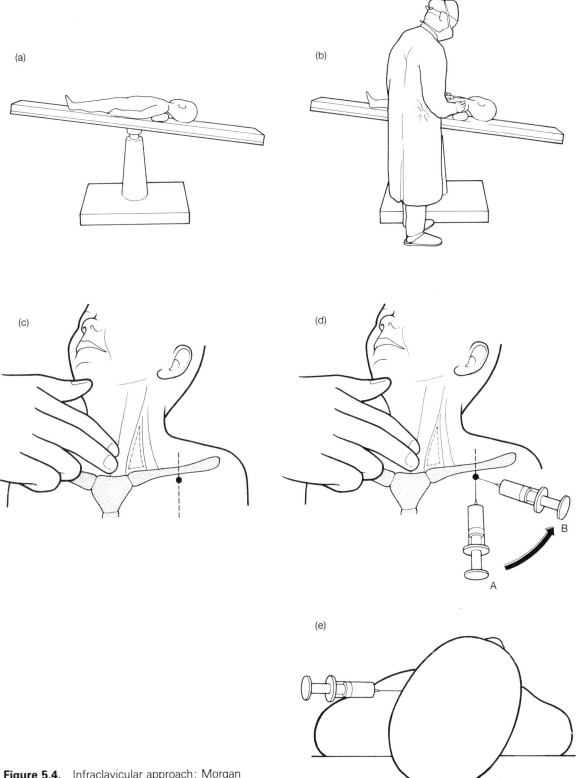

Figure 5.4. Infraclavicular approach: Morgan and Harkins (1972).[10]

INFRACLAVICULAR APPROACH
Mogil et al. (1967)[32]

Patient category

Adults. The description of the technique by the original authors did not include its application in children, but this does not necessarily exclude its use in this age group.

Advantages and disadvantages

The original authors claim that this technique is safer when compared to techniques using a more lateral approach, where the subclavian artery, brachial plexus, and pleura are in danger from the needle.

Preferred side

The right, in order to avoid injury to the thoracic duct: it is also technically easier for a right-handed operator.

Position of patient (Figure 5.5a)

Place the table in a 25° head-down position. Place the patient in the supine position with both arms at his side. Do not place a pillow under the head, but a pillow under the back may be used to let the shoulders fall back so that the head of the humerus is not in the way.

Position of operator (Figure 5.5b)

Stand on the same side as the puncture site.

Equipment used in original description

Adults. 14 or 16 gauge O.D. introducing needle. 200 or 300 mm catheter-through-needle.

Advice on current equipment

Adults. Guide wire technique strongly recommended using an 18 or 16 gauge introducer needle. Catheter thro' cannula, 14 gauge O.D. introducing needle or cannula, length 60 mm (minimum). Catheter length 200 mm (minimum). Long cannula on long needle, 130 mm length (minimum).

Anatomical landmarks (Figure 5.5c)

Junction of the medial and middle thirds of the lower border of the clavicle. Small triangle formed by the two heads of the sternomastoid muscle and the clavicle.

Preparation

Perform the puncture under sterile conditions using local anaesthesia if needed.

Precautions and recommendations

If a syringe is used, ensure that it can easily be detached from the needle.

Point of insertion of needle (Figure 5.5c)

Just below the lower border of the clavicle at the junction of the medial and middle thirds of the clavicle.

Direction of the needle and procedure (Figure 5.5d, e)

Place the point of the needle at the entry site on the skin and point the needle cephalad (A). Then swing the needle and syringe laterally so that the needle points towards the small triangle formed by the two heads of the sternomastoid muscle and the upper border of the clavicle (A to B).

Advance the syringe behind the clavicle, keeping the syringe parallel to the coronal plane (Figure 5.5e). Maintain a slight negative pressure in the syringe whilst advancing the needle, until the vein is entered. A finger placed in the sternal notch is a useful guide to the landmarks, especially in obese patients. Do not alter the direction of the needle without first withdrawing its tip to the subcutaneous tissue. Having inserted the catheter take a chest x-ray to confirm the position of the catheter tip and to exclude a pneumothorax.

Results

95·9% success in 219 attempts at catheterisation made by the authors.

Complications

There were six complications (an incidence of 2·7%): pneumothorax (1); haematoma (3); bleeding at puncture site (2).

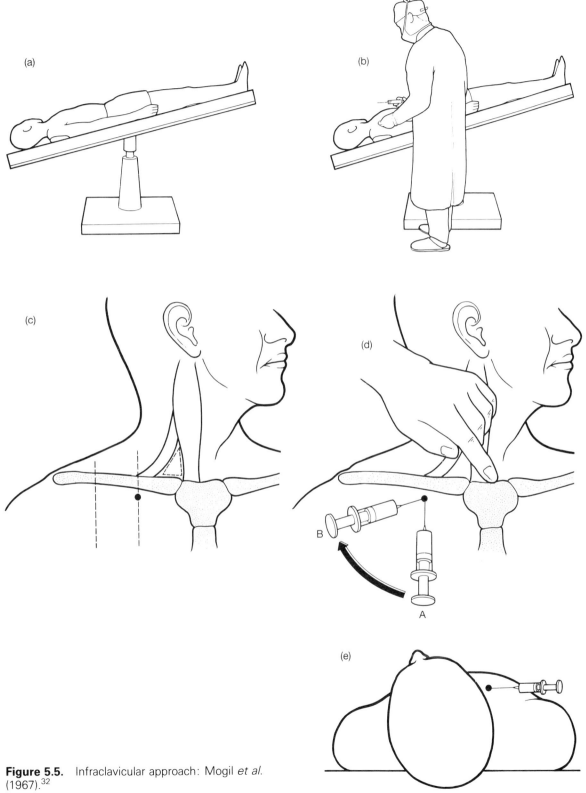

Figure 5.5. Infraclavicular approach: Mogil *et al.* (1967).[32]

INFRACLAVICULAR APPROACH
Tofield (1969)[17]

Patient category

Adults. The description of the technique by the original authors did not include its application in children, but this does not necessarily exclude its use in this age group.

Advantages and disadvantages

The more lateral and oblique approach is claimed to reduce the risk of pneumothorax and puncture of the subclavian artery.

Preferred side

Not stated.

Position of patient (Figure 5.6a)

Place the table in a 25° head-down position. Place the patient in the supine position with both arms at his side. Turn the head away from the side of the puncture.

Position of operator (Figure 5.6b)

Stand on the same side as the puncture site.

Equipment used in original description

Catheter-through-needle. Size not stated.

Advice on current equipment

Adults. Guide wire technique strongly recommended using an 18 or 16 gauge introducer needle. Catheter thro' cannula, 14 or 16 gauge O.D. needle or introducer, length 70 mm (minimum). Catheter length 200 mm (minimum).

Long cannula on long needle, length 130 mm (minimum).

Anatomical landmarks (Figure 5.6c)

Midclavicular point. The lower border of the clavicle. Suprasternal notch.

Preparation

Perform the puncture under sterile conditions using local anaesthesia if indicated.

Precautions and recommendations

Ensure that the syringe can be removed easily from the needle.

Point of insertion of needle (Figure 5.6c)

Lateral (precise distance not stated) to the midclavicular point, *1 cm* below the lower border of the clavicle.

Direction of the needle and procedure (Figure 5.6d, e)

Place the point of the needle at the entry site on the skin and point the needle and syringe towards the head (A). Then swing the needle and syringe laterally so that the needle points medially towards the tip of the index finger of the free hand, firmly pressed into the suprasternal notch.

Advance the needle posterior to the clavicle, keeping close to its posterior aspect and aiming all the time for the tip of the index finger in the suprasternal notch. Maintain a slight negative pressure in the syringe as the needle is advanced until the vein is entered. Insert the catheter.

Take a chest x-ray to confirm the position of the catheter tip and to exclude a pneumothorax.

Success rate

Not stated.

Complications

Not stated.

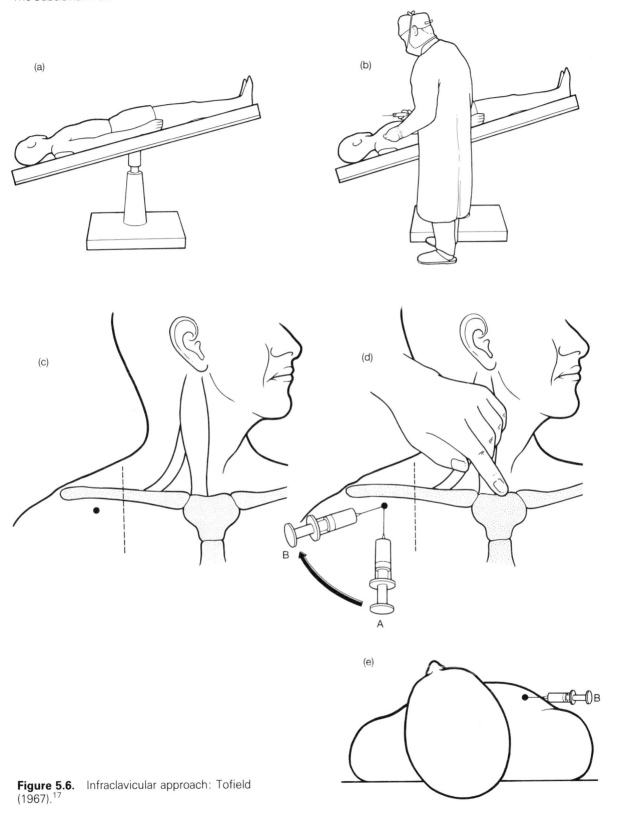

Figure 5.6.   Infraclavicular approach: Tofield
(1967).[17]

INFRACLAVICULAR APPROACH: THE AXILLARY ARTERY AS A LANDMARK
Untracht (1988)[19]

Patient category
Adults.

Advantages and disadvantages
In most other infraclavicular methods there are no clear landmarks. Also, because the needle must be inserted almost directly backwards towards the spine in order to initially pierce the tissues immediately below the clavicle, the pleura is at risk. The axillary artery is a more constant relative landmark and the path of the needle is more parallel to the pleura so reducing the risk of pneumothorax. An added advantage is that after successful catheterisation, a long skin tunnel confers extra security.

Preferred side (Figure 5.7a)
Not stated but a left-sided approach is described.

Position of patient (Figure 5.7a)
Place the patient in the 25° head-down position with arms at the side. Place a rolled towel under the spine at the thoracic level so that the shoulders fall away towards the table. Turn the head away from the side of venepuncture.

Position of operator (Figure 5.7b)
On the same side as the venepuncture.

Equipment used in the original description
Not stated.

Advice on current equipment
Adults. Guide wire technique highly recommended. Small diameter (18 or 16 gauge) needle, length 70 mm minimum, to introduce wire. Catheter length 200 mm minimum.
Long catheter on long needle 130 mm (minimum).

Anatomical landmarks (Figure 5.7c)
Suprasternal notch, lower border of the clavicle, mid-clavicular line. Palpate the axillary artery lateral to the mid-clavicular line.

Preparation
Perform the procedure under sterile conditions using local anaesthetic if indicated.

Point of insertion of needle (Figure 5.7c)
Approximately 2·5 cm below the axillary pulse and lateral to the mid-clavicular line. Point 'a' in Figure 5.7c.

Direction of the needle and procedure (Figure 5.7c, d)
If local anaesthetic is used, it is infiltrated along a line between the skin puncture site and suprasternal notch (line a–b in the figure) up to and including the periosteum of the clavicle. The introducer needle is advanced along the same track as described below.
With the needle at the entry point, aim the needle and syringe towards the head. Then swing the needle laterally so that the needle points medially towards the suprasternal notch, keeping a finger in the notch to act as a target.
Advance the needle parallel to the coronal plane (Figure 5.7e) which keeps the needle parallel to the pleura as it passes under the lower border of the clavicle usually, but not always, between the middle and medial one-thirds. Maintain a slight negative pressure in the syringe to identify entry into the vein, which occurs as the needle point passes under the clavicle. Proceed with the catheterisation procedure.
Take a chest x-ray to confirm position of the catheter tip and to exclude a pneumothorax.

Success rate
80 successful cannulations usually at the first or second pass. No failure rate stated.
Complications: no pneumothorax; one case of axillary artery puncture.

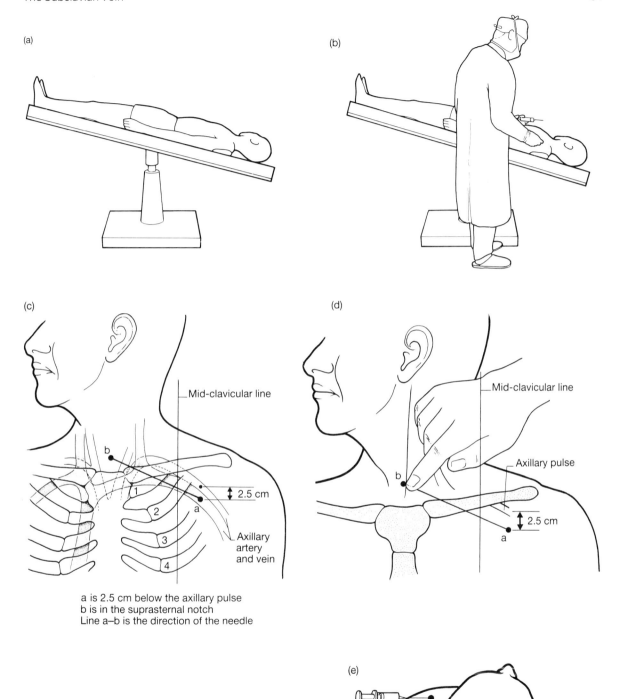

(a)

(b)

(c)

Mid-clavicular line

b

1

2

a

3

4

2.5 cm

Axillary
artery
and vein

a is 2.5 cm below the axillary pulse
b is in the suprasternal notch
Line a–b is the direction of the needle

(d)

Mid-clavicular line

b

Axillary pulse

2.5 cm

a

(e)

Figure 5.7. Infraclavicular approach: Untracht
(1988).[19]

SUPRACLAVICULAR APPROACH
Yoffa (1965)[8]

Patient category
Adults. The description of the technique by the original authors did not include its application in children, but this does not necessarily exclude its use in this age group.

Advantages and disadvantages
Several advantages over the infraclavicular approach are claimed. There is a reduced risk of pneumothorax because the needle points away from the pleura. There is a definite skin landmark. The distance from skin to vein is shorter (0·5–4·0 cm). Only fascial tissue has to be pierced.

Preferred side
The left side for the right-handed operator.

Position of patient (Figure 5.8a)
Place the table in a 25° head-down position. Place the patient in the supine position with no pillow and with both arms at his side. *Turn the head slightly away from the side of the puncture.*

Position of operator (Figure 5.8a)
Stand at the head of patient on the side of the puncture site.

Equipment used in original description
Catheter-through-14 gauge O.D. introducing needle.

Choice of current equipment
Adults. Guide wire technique strongly recommended using an 18 or 16 gauge introducer needle. Catheter thro' cannula, 14 or 16 gauge O.D. needle or introducer. Length 60 mm (minimum). Catheter length 200 mm (minimum).
Long cannula on long needle, length 130 mm (minimum).

Anatomical landmarks (Figure 5.8b)
Lateral border of the clavicular head of the sternomastoid muscle just above the clavicle. If the patient is conscious, ask him to raise his head against the resistance of a hand placed on the forehead to make the muscle stand out.

Preparation
Perform the puncture under sterile conditions using local anaesthetic.

Precautions and recommendations
Ensure that the syringe, if used, can be easily disengaged from the needle.

Point of insertion of needle (Figure 5.8b)
Precisely into the angle between the clavicular head of sternomastoid and the upper border of the clavicle.

Direction of the needle and procedure (Figure 5.8c, d, e)
Place the point of the needle at the entry site on the skin and point the needle and syringe caudally (A). Then swing the needle and syringe 45° laterally (A to B). Elevate the needle and syringe 15° above the coronal plane (B to C). Maintain a negative pressure in the syringe as the needle is advanced. The vein is entered usually 1·0–1·5 cm from the skin (perhaps as little as 0·5 cm). If the catheter does not pass freely, its passage may be assisted by rotating the needle or introducer slightly whilst advancing the catheter. Take a chest x-ray to confirm the position of the catheter tip and to exclude a pneumothorax.

Success rate
97% (130 cases).

Complications
None, although there was one pneumothorax in a later series.

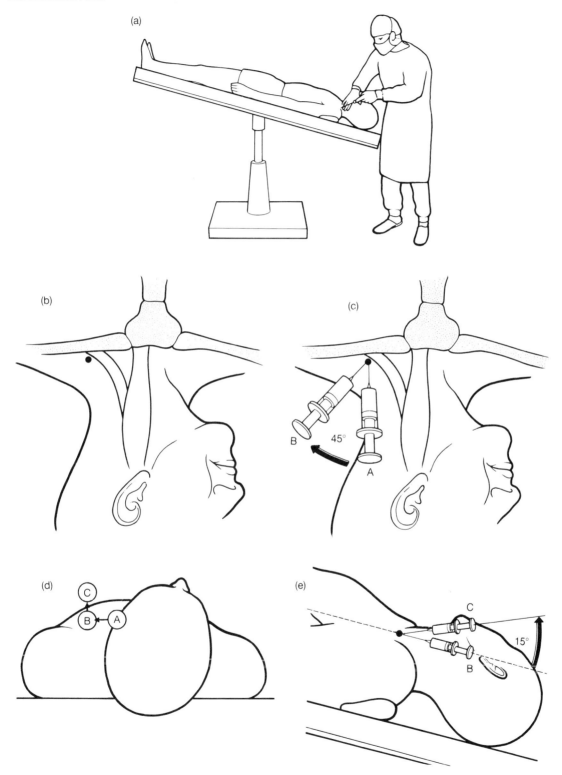

Figure 5.8. Supraclavicular approach: Yoffa (1965).[8]

SUPRACLAVICULAR APPROACH
James and Myers (1973)[33]

Patient category

Adults. The description of the technique by the original authors did not include its application in children, but this does not necessarily exclude its use in this age group.

Preferred side

Not stated.

Position of patient (Figure 5.9a)

Position the table in a 25° head-down tilt position. Place the patient in the supine position, with both arms at his sides. Turn the head away from the side of the puncture.

Position of operator (Figure 5.9a)

Stand at the head of the patient.

Equipment used in original description

14 gauge O.D. introducing needle. Catheter-through-needle.

Choice of current equipment

Adults. Guide wire technique strongly recommended using an 18 or 16 gauge introducer needle. Catheter thro' cannula, 14 gauge O.D. needle or introducing cannula, length 60 mm (minimum). Catheter length 200 mm (minimum).
Long cannula with long needle, length 130 mm (minimum).

Anatomical landmarks (Figure 5.9b)

Posterior border of the sternomastoid muscle and superior border of the clavicle.

Preparation

Perform the puncture under sterile conditions using local anaesthetic if indicated.

Precautions and recommendations

The borders of the sternomastoid can be made more prominent by asking the patient, if conscious, to tense the muscle by raising his head against resistance.
    Fill the syringe with saline to eject small plugs of fat and tissue to keep the needle patent. Ensure that the syringe can be easily detached.

Point of insertion of the needle (Figure 5.9b)

Into the angle made by the posterior border of the clavicular head of the sternomastoid muscle and the clavicle.

Direction of needle and procedure (Figure 5.9c, d, e)

Place the point of the needle at the entry site on the skin and point the needle caudally (A). Then swing the needle and syringe laterally so that the needle lies along the line bisecting the angle between the clavicle and the clavicular head of the sterno-mastoid muscle (A to B). Elevate the syringe 10° above the coronal plane (B to C). Advance the needle – its direction will be towards the retro-manubrial area at the level of the sternal angle – until the vein is entered. Keep the needle clear by injecting a small volume of saline; otherwise maintain a slight negative pressure in the syringe as the needle is advanced. Insert the catheter if venepuncture is successful. If venepuncture and catheterisation are unsuccessful, delay any attempt on the other side if possible.
A chest x-ray should be performed to exclude a pneumothorax in all cases.

Success rate

A 95% success rate was achieved in 3000 attempted catheterisations. The operators were experienced or closely supervised.

Complications

In the 3000 cases the overall complication rate was 11·2%: 1·2% major and 10% minor. The major complications included pneumothorax (0·4%), hydrothorax (0·09%), subclavian thrombophlebitis (0·06%), haemorrhage (0·06%), air embolus (0·03%), and arteriovenous fistula (0·03%).
Minor complications included failure to puncture the vein or to thread the catheter.

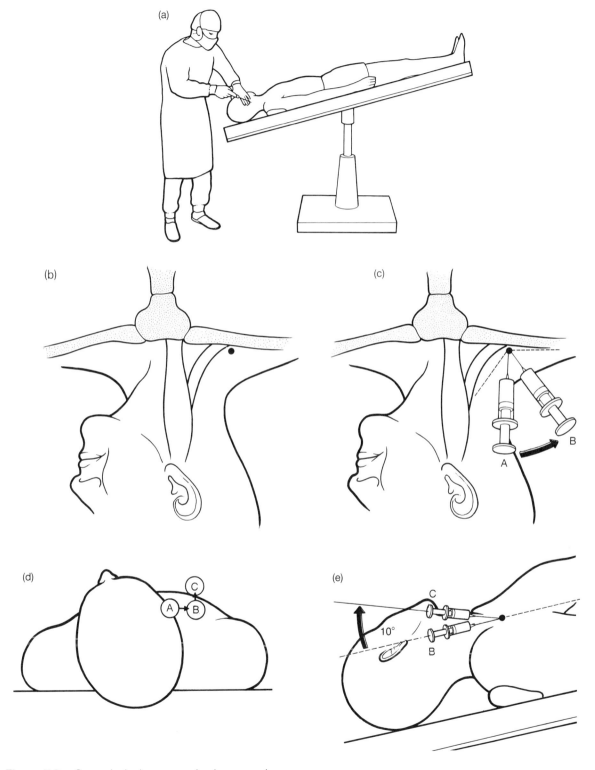

Figure 5.9. Supraclavicular approach: James and Myers (1973).[33]

SUPRACLAVICULAR APPROACH
Brahos (1977)[18]

Similar to James and Myers (see p. 66) but with small detail differences.

Patient category
Adults and children down to 8 years of age described.

Preferred side
Either side may be attempted but the right is preferable because the vein on this side is usually larger and has a more direct route to the superior vena cava (SVC). Avoids the thoracic duct.

Position of patient (Figure 5.10a)
Tilt the patient in the 20–25° head position. Turn the patient's head to the opposite side.

Position of operator (Figure 5.10a)
Stand at the head.

Equipment used in original description
Introducer needle 14 gauge, length 2 inches. Catheter 16 gauge, length 8–9 inches for the right side, 10 inches for the longer path of the left side.

Advice on current equipment
The use of a guide wire technique is strongly recommended.
Long cannula on long needle, length 130 mm minimum.

Anatomical landmarks (Figure 5.10b)
Identify the angle between the clavicle and the lateral border of the sternomastoid muscle – usually just medial to the external jugular vein. In a conscious patient the landmarks are more easily seen in the obese if the patient actively lifts his head.

Preparation
Perform the procedure under sterile conditions using local anaesthesia if indicated.

Point of insertion of needle (Figure 5.10b)
In the angle of between the lateral border of the sternomastoid muscle and the upper border of the clavicle.

Direction of the needle and procedure (Figure 5.10c)
Place the needle point at the entry site and point the needle and syringe towards the feet. Then swing the needle and syringe laterally so that it lies along a line which bisects the clavisternomastoid angle. The line points just caudad to the opposite nipple. Elevate the needle about 10° above the horizontal plane and advance along the line described, just beneath the sternomastoid muscle. If no flashback occurs when about 5 cm of needle has been inserted, withdraw and elevate the needle a little more and repeat the insertion. Increase the angle step by step to a maximum of 25° above the coronal plane. Flashback usually occurs when the needle is about 15–20° above the coronal plane with about 3–4 cm needle inserted. Proceed with the rest of the catheterisation procedure.
Take a chest x-ray to confirm that the catheter tip is correctly placed and to exclude pneumothorax.

Success rate
All procedures were carried out by residents supervised by the author. No more than two attempts in any case were allowed.
Right-sided attempts 100% (68 cases).
Left-sided attempts 100% (32 cases).

Complications
Inability to thread catheter or unsatisfactory placement 5%. Arterial puncture 1%. Pneumothorax 1%.

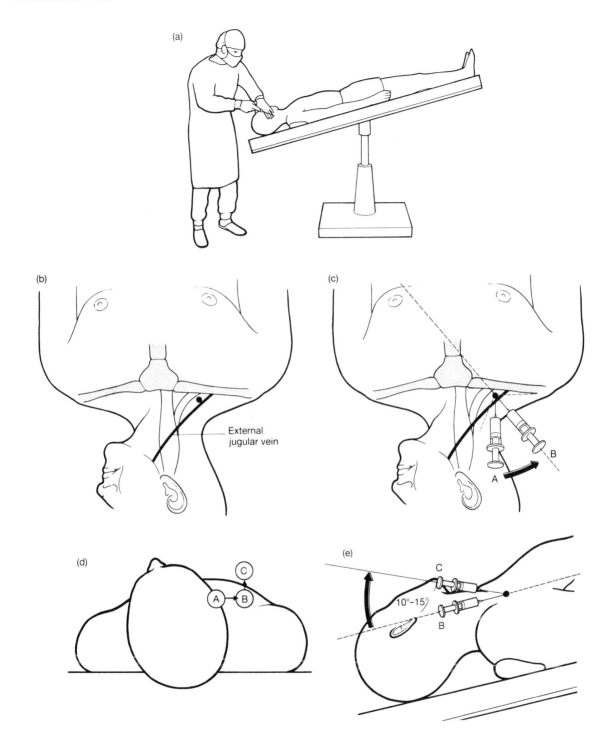

External
jugular vein

Figure 5.10. Supraclavicular approach: Brahos
(1977).[18]

SUPRACLAVICULAR APPROACH
Haapaniemi and Slatis (1974)[16]

Patient category

Adults. The description of the technique by the original authors did not include its application in children, but this does not necessarily exclude its use in this age group.

Advantages and disadvantages

The authors claim that advancing the catheter is easier because there is a less obtuse angle between the needle and the vessel wall than in other supraclavicular and infraclavicular techniques. Furthermore, they claim that there is less risk of introducing the catheter into neck veins compared to the infraclavicular route.

Preferred side

The right. The left side may be used, however.

Position of patient (Figure 5.11a)

Place the table in a 10° head-down position. Place the patient supine with both arms at his sides and with shoulders depressed. Turn the head slightly away from the side of the puncture.

Position of operator (Figure 5.11a)

Stand at the head of the patient or on the opposite side to the puncture site.

Equipment used in original description

Polypropylene catheter-through-14 gauge O.D. needle.

Advice on current equipment

Adults. Guide wire technique strongly recommended using an 18 or 16 gauge introducer needle. 14 or 16 gauge O.D. needle or introducer. Length 60 mm (minimum). Catheter length 200 mm (minimum). Long cannula with long needle, length 130 mm (minimum).

Anatomical landmarks (Figure 5.11b)

The posterior border of the sternomastoid muscle.

Preparation

Perform puncture under sterile conditions using local anaesthetic if indicated.

Precautions and recommendations

Maintain positive intrathoracic pressure during venous cannulation to distend the vein.

Point of insertion of needle (Figure 5.11b)

2–3 cm above the clavicle close to the posterior border of the sternomastoid muscle.

Initial location of vein with small-gauge needle

Locate the vein with a fine needle (21 or 22 gauge) using the directions given below. Then remove the fine needle and insert the large needle attached to a saline-filled syringe along the same path.

Direction of the needle and procedure (Figure 5.11c, d, e)

Place the point of the needle at the entry site on the skin and point the needle caudally (A). Then swing the needle and syringe laterally 35° (A to B). Elevate the syringe slightly above the coronal plane (B to C). Maintain a slight negative pressure in the syringe as the needle is advanced. The vein is entered 2–3 cm (occasionally up to 5 cm) from the puncture site. The needle enters the vein behind the medial portion of the clavicle 1–2 cm lateral to the sternoclavicular joint. The point of entry into the vein corresponds to the junction of the subclavian and internal jugular veins. Advance the needle 3–4 mm into the vein and then introduce the catheter. Take a chest x-ray to confirm the position of the catheter and to exclude a pneumothorax.

Success rate

85·4% successful in the first 171 cases.
97% successful in the subsequent 429 cases.

Complications

Overall complication rate: 5%. There was a 0·6–1·0% incidence each of arterial puncture, haematoma, local infection, and puncture of the thoracic duct. The incidence of pneumothorax, air embolus, sepsis, and thrombophlebitis was 0·1–0·5% each.

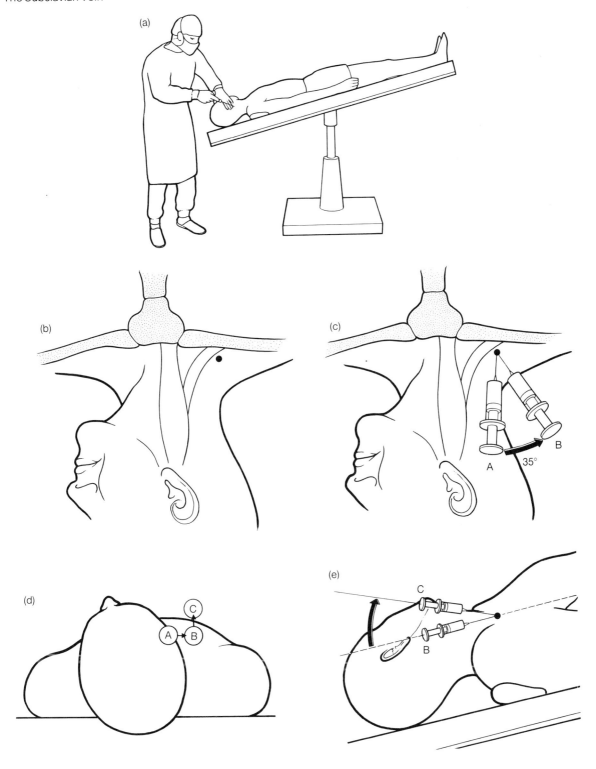

Figure 5.11. Supraclavicular approach: Haapaniemi and Slatis (1974).[16]

CASE REPORTS OF COMPLICATIONS RELATED TO THE SUBCLAVIAN VEIN ROUTE (TABLE 5.3)

The commonly occurring hazards of central venous catheterisation through the subclavian vein are now well known. The case reports from the literature set out below illustrate some unusual presentations of common complications as well as descriptions of some rare problems. Some cases include instructive as well as salutary lessons in diagnosis and management.

Pleural space and lung

The hazard of pneumothorax complicating subclavian venepuncture is the most well-known and obvious risk and is well documented in numerous series (see Table 5.1, pp. 107–109). The incidence ranges from 0% to 4·7% and up to 12·4% in certain physician groups.[9] Several case reports have warned of the apparent onset of a pneumothorax after some delay, sometimes days later. The chest x-ray taken immediately after the venepuncture has been clear.

Other types of respiratory tract complications appear to be rare.

Delayed pneumothorax[100]

The significance of 'difficult' subclavian catheterisation is illustrated in three cases where pneumothorax from a slow pleural air leak only became manifest later. A repeat chest x-ray is worth considering in such cases. The diagnosis may be anticipated if air was aspirated at the time of venepuncture or if subcutaneous emphysema develops. Pleuritic or any persistent chest pain should alert to the possibility. Chest x-ray in such patients about to undergo surgery is advised.

Late appearance of pneumothorax[43]

An immediate chest x-ray taken after a difficult catheterisation showed a correctly placed tip and no pneumothorax. Five days later, because of persistent shoulder tip pain and proposed surgery requiring positive pressure ventilation, a repeat x-ray revealed a pneumothorax. The value of a preoperative film in such patients is obvious.

Bilateral pneumothorax[44]

A common pleural space was produced by inadvertent entry of both pleural cavities at median sternotomy. Subsequently pneumothorax complicated a subclavian venepuncture. The air leak was able to spread bilaterally with life threatening effect.

Hydrothorax[45]

Perforation of the central vein wall occurred after apparently successful subclavian catheterisation in two patients (children). In both patients the line was used to administer fluid therapy which was followed by deterioration of the patients' general condition instead of the expected improvement. Progressive respiratory distress accompanied by dullness to percussion and diminished breath sounds led to the diagnosis, which was confirmed radiologically. Pleurocentesis produced clear (i.e. the infused) fluid.

Perforation of the central vein is of course more likely to be related to the catheter material and the design of its tip and its position in the central veins rather than the route of insertion.

Bilateral hydrothorax and hydromediastinum[46]

A patient developed bilateral hydrothorax. However, injection of radio-opaque medium through the catheter demonstrated only a leak into the mediastinum. It was thought that the hydrothorax resulted from a shift of fluid from the mediastinum due to pressure differences in the two compartments.

Contralateral haemothorax[47]

The case demonstrates the difficulty in diagnosis when late and especially contralateral manifestations follow central venous catheterisation. In this case two subclavian catheters had been inserted, the right-sided one several days later than the left catheter. Haemorrhage into the right chest was interpreted as a complication of the right-sided catheterisation. However, chyle-like fluid continued to flow from the right chest drain and anaesthetic drugs (methohexitone and suxamethonium) injected through the left catheter failed to be effective. Eventually, contrast studies established that perforation of the left-sided catheter into the right pleural cavity had occurred. The erosion of the superior vena caval wall was attributed to the stiff material of the catheter and the use of a left-sided approach. Cannulation from the left side allows the catheter to take an approximately horizontal course, its tip coming to abut at about 90° to the wall of the superior vena cava.

Contralateral effusions[48]

Two cases are presented. Radiological studies were performed to elucidate the mechanisms.

Contralateral hydrothorax following guide wire catheter replacement[49]

Fatal contralateral hydrothorax followed replacement of a central venous catheter using the guide wire technique.

Venopulmonary fistula[50]

Two weeks after insertion of a silicone parenteral nutrition catheter into a 13-year-old child through the subclavian vein, pneumonitis and life-threatening respiratory failure developed. Removal of the catheter was followed by complete resolution.

Puncture of the trachea[51]

This occurred during infraclavicular subclavian catheterisation using a 14 gauge diameter needle of 7 cm length. The injury was revealed by leakage of inflated gases from around the tracheostomy tube through which the patient was receiving positive pressure ventilation. Changing the tube solved the problem; the original tube had a puncture of 1 mm diameter. The trachea lies in close relation to subclavian venepuncture, but in this case the puncture was made more likely by the tracheal wall reaching much more laterally. This resulted from dilatation of the trachea after prolonged tracheal intubation.

Acute airway obstruction[52]

During an emergency resuscitation of a shocked patient in pulmonary oedema, attempts were made at infraclavicular venepuncture with a large bore 14 gauge (1·9 mm) needle. At the fourth attempt arterial blood was aspirated. Twenty minutes later a swelling appeared in the suprasternal notch and the neck also became swollen. Intense cyanosis appeared and total airway obstruction supervened only relieved by tracheal intubation. This proved extremely difficult because of the stiffness of the tissues which were distended with blood together

with obstruction to passage of the tube. Radiological studies performed later showed a marked widening of the retropharyngeal space (by haematoma) and tracheal deviation. The subclavian artery was almost certainly lacerated because of its proximity to the venepuncture site.

Once again the danger inherent in needling of deep veins with a large bore device is illustrated.

Vascular

Puncture of the ascending aorta[53]

In this case of attempted left infravlavicular subclavian venepuncture, an 80 mm needle was of sufficient length and size (12 gauge) to puncture the ascending aorta within 2 cm of the aortic valve route causing a fatal haemopericardium. It was thought that gross abdominal distension together with the head-down tilt position adopted during cannulation resulted in the mediastinum being distorted upwards. This was supported at postmortem examination. A Seldinger guide wire technique using a small short introducer needle is advised in cases of marked abdominal distension.

Pulmonary artery puncture[54]

Infraclavicular subclavian venepuncture was performed with a long cannula-over-needle (140 mm) and illustrates the danger of this type of device. Although the vein can be reached by a needle of 60–70 mm length, the extra length of the long cannula-over-needle type of device means that it can reach and injure mediastinal structures if it is inserted too deeply. In this patient, at emergency sternotomy, the apex of the pulmonary artery was found to be punctured together with holes in the anterior pericardium and a large haemopericardium. The author stressed the need to consider cardiac tamponade in a patient presenting with cardiovascular collapse after central venous catheterisation.

Intercostal artery laceration[55]

Severe pneumothorax followed subclavian venepuncture with injury to the first intercostal artery. Emergency thoracotomy and intensive care saved the patient.

Subclavian arteriovenous fistula[56]

Inadvertent puncture of the subclavian artery was noted when infraclavicular venepuncture was carried out using a 14 gauge needle. Ten days after discharge the patient became aware of a loud murmur over the subclavian area. At operation a fistula was found encased in a 3 cm fibrous mass; a vein graft was used to bypass the fistula. The danger of using wide bore venepuncture needles is commented upon.

Vertebral artery pseudoaneurysm[57]

Stridor and dysphagia followed 5 days after a difficult attempt at subclavian catheterisation. A CT scan showed a superior mediastinal, contrast enhancing mass in the region of the right subclavian artery with the 'bull's eye' sign suggestive of a pseudo-aneurysm. Arteriography proved the aneurysm to originate from the vertebral artery which had presumably been lacerated at the time of venepuncture. The aneurysm was successfully ligated.

Benign intracranial hypertension[58]

This resulted from an arteriovenous fistula complicating subclavian catheterisation.

Spurious central venous pressure[59]

During an operation in a very ill patient, two markedly different central venous pressure measurements were obtained from two different sites of cannulation. A falsely elevated pressure (30 cm water pressure versus only 15 cm in the other catheter) recorded from one catheter inserted through the subclavian vein was related to the increased blood flow and pressure in a patent arteriovenous shunt which had been previously inserted for haemodialysis. There could have been errors in fluid management if the higher figure had been accepted. In addition the high and fluctuating pressure in the catheter which was in communication with the A–V fistula produced dangerous fluctuations in vasoactive drugs being administered through the same line.

A–V fistula of the internal mammary artery and innominate vein[60]

Some days following a difficult subclavian vein catheterisation a machinery-like murmur was heard over the right clavicle. Further studies demonstrated an arteriovenous fistula. To avoid surgical exploration in an ill patient, transcatheter intravascular coil occlusion was successfully attempted. The steel coil prevents arterial blood from entering the arterial to venous fistula.

Innominate vein stenosis[61]

The patient presented with left upper arm swelling which was related to acute exercise. The patient had undergone repeated and prolonged central venous catheterisation 10 months previously. Phlebography revealed left innominate vein stenosis. There was no subclavian vein thrombosis.

Heart and mediastinum

Cardiac tamponade[62]

This early case report is a classic example of the ease with which the correct diagnosis of perforation of a central venous catheter into the mediastinum is overlooked. The patient was in the post-cardiac surgery phase and although the clinical features were rightly interpreted as those of cardiac tamponade this was never attributed to inadvertent pericardial infusion through a central venous line that had perforated into the mediastinum. This was only too apparent at emergency thoracotomy. Interestingly, the anaesthetist noted that drugs injected through the line had no effect. The authors point out that if perforation had been considered, injection of radio-opaque dye would have easily confirmed the diagnosis and the patient spared exploratory thoracotomy.

Other cases, see Adar and Mozes[63] and Defalque.[64]

Radiological demonstration of cardiac tamponade[65]

Radiological demonstration of a central venous catheter which had perforated into the pericardial sac explained why a patient developed a shocked state some hours after commencement of intravenous alimentation administered through the same line. A post-insertion chest x-ray had not permitted a clear view of the terminal portion of the catheter which was 'lost' amongst the equally radio-opaque mediastinal structures. The true position of the tip only became apparent after the injection of radio-opaque dye. When the correct diagnosis is made, the authors recommend aspiration of tamponade fluid through the line before its withdrawal.

Perforation of heart by a guide wire[66]

A straight soft-tipped guide wire used to insert a subclavian dialysis catheter perforated the heart. The use of a J-tipped wire is advised to avoid this life-threatening complication.

Massive mediastinal haematoma caused by a double lumen catheter[67]

This was a special subclavian double lumen catheter inserted for gaining temporary access for extracorporeal circulation. This worked perfectly well on the first occasion. At the start of the second treatment, the patient experienced excruciating pain and was found to have developed a massive mediastinal haematoma. Whilst the proximal orifice remained inside the vein so that blood could still move freely into the circuit, blood was forcibly pumped through the distal orifice of the catheter tip, which had perforated the vein wall, into the mediastinum.

Cardiac tamponade with a multilumen catheter[68]

In two cases the possibility of perforation of the central vein by the catheter and subsequent infusion through the line causing a pericardial collection was not considered as the cause of acute hypotension and cardiac arrest. However, at emergency thoracotomy the catheter tip was found to have penetrated the posterior aspect of the heart and was lying in a fluid-filled pericardium. The position of the catheter tip is all important and in these cases the catheters were inserted well beyond the 20 cm mark recommended by the manufacturers. The check x-ray should confirm that the catheter tip should lie no further than 2 cm below a line joining the inferior borders of the clavicles. The temptation to insert excess catheter to be sure that the most proximal orifice of the multilumen catheter is within the central vein should be guarded against.

'Ring around the artery' sign in pneumomediastinum[69]

Following subclavian catheterisation, a small pneumomediastinum resulted in the collection of a thin layer of gas around the right pulmonary artery, which on lateral chest x-ray produced a distinctive oval shadow at the right hilum.

Hydromediastinum from perforation of the innominate vein[63,64,70]

These early reports of fatal hydromediastinum following subclavian catheterisation warned of the delay in onset of symptoms and signs for over 24 hours. The possibility of the catheters advancing spontaneously was suggested so emphasising the need for secure fixing of the catheter at the time of insertion. Any sudden unexpected deterioration in a patient's condition should throw suspicion on the central venous catheter. X-ray and ECG changes may be absent. Timely aspiration of the mediastinum or pericardium can be life saving.

Lymphatic system

Laceration of the thoracic duct[4]

Trauma to the thoracic duct occurred at an attempt to insert a pacing electrode through the track previously occupied by an electrode wire (which had failed and been removed) into the left subclavian vein. Lymph drainage stopped spontaneously after four days.

Lymphatic fistula[71]

The thoracic duct or one of its branches must have been inadvertently punctured at left subclavian venepuncture. Chylous fluid (confirmed by its high fat content and lymphocyte content) was leaking from the skin entry site one week later. The fistula healed spontaneously in 36 hours. The authors correctly point out that injury to the thoracic duct cannot occur with right subclavian puncture but this does not eliminate the danger of damage to the lymphatic system as shown in the next report.

Lymph leakage after right-sided catheterisation[72]

Two days after easy right-sided infraclavicular subclavian venepuncture to insert a pacing electrode in a 6-year-old child, milky fluid (confirmed to be lymph) leaked out from around the catheter. No chylothorax developed and after four days the leak stopped spontaneously. Right-sided subclavian venepuncture is often recommended in order to avoid thoracic duct injury. However, the right lymphatic duct enters the superior margin of the subclavian vein near its junction with the internal jugular vein so the lymphatic system is still vulnerable although to a far lesser degree.

Neurological

Neurological sequelae of subclavian cannulation are uncommon. Unless the possibility of the clinical features being related to injury from venepuncture is borne in mind, the correct diagnosis must be difficult to arrive at.

Phrenic nerve paralysis due to local anaesthetic[73]

Left-sided infraclavicular puncture preceded by 5 ml 2% lignocaine infiltration was performed with a guide wire technique. Respiratory distress and cyanosis developed immediately. Radiological studies revealed elevation of the left hemidiaphragm, deviation of the trachea to the right and paradoxical movement of the left hemidiaphragm. The paralysis lasted for 3 hours and was attributed to block of the phrenic nerve by the local anaesthetic used. The authors comment that such cases appear to be rare although the phrenic nerve lies so closely related, behind the subclavian vein, to the site of venepuncture.

Diaphragmatic paralysis[74]

Two cases of hemidiaphragmatic paralysis following right-sided supraclavicular subclavian puncture are described after apparently easy catheterisations. In both cases there were no symptoms and diaphragmatic paralysis was only seen on routine chest x-rays some days later. Extensive investigations were performed to determine the cause of this finding but were negative. The abnormal hemidiaphragm remained in both cases up to 3 years later. It was concluded that the phrenic nerve which lies in close proximity at subclavian venepuncture had been damaged at the time of catheterisation.

Recurrent laryngeal nerve paralysis[75]

This followed pacemaker insertion through the subclavian vein.

Brown–Sequard syndrome[76]

This followed spinal cord infarction following subclavian vein catheterisation.

Pain in the left arm and leg was experienced immediately at the time of attempted infraclavicular venepuncture. No flashback of blood was obtained. Left hemiplegia was severe and accompanied by a partial left Horner's syndrome. There was diminished sensation on the right corresponding to a lesion between C8 and T4 spinal segments. These signs persisted over 3 months.

It was thought that needling at the time of attempted subclavian venepuncture induced severe spasm of one of the arteries of the costocervical plexus and consequent ischaemia to the left anterior part of the lower spinal cord leading to infarction of the cervicothoracic spinal cord. Apparently spasm of arteries in this area due to the mechanical irritation of needling is sometimes seen during angiographic studies.

Transient paralysis of the upper arm[77]

In two elderly patients transient motor and sensory paralysis of the upper limb was attributed to excessive amounts of lignocaine infiltrated too deeply and too laterally. The amounts of lignocaine 2% used were 16 ml and 25 ml respectively and had in fact produced a brachial plexus block.

Injury to the lower cord of the brachial plexus[78]

Clinical evidence supported by electrophysiological tests confirmed injury to the brachial plexus after cannulation through the infraclavicular route. The rarity of brachial plexus injuries with infraclavicular catheterisation can be attributed to the anatomical distance between the plexus and the point of insertion of the catheter. Of course, minor neurological deficits may easily miss detection.

Unsuspected cerebral perfusion[79]

During an emergency, drugs were infused into a line the position of which had not been confirmed radiologically. The tip, in fact, lay deep in the internal jugular vein so that the drugs administered produced cerebral effects by retrograde perfusion of the intracranial venous sinuses. Adrenaline produced very severe headache; lignocaine led to an increased clouding of consciousness. Yet there was virtually no therapeutic effect on the heart from either of these drugs.

Cortical blindness[80]

After subclavian venepuncture, the patient became acutely confused and developed a transient left hemiplegia. Loss of vision followed. Pupillary reflexes and examination of the optic fundi were normal so the pathology was attributed to an acute cortical lesion produced by an air embolus.

Air embolus

Air embolism: a lethal but preventable complication[81]

Fourteen cases of air embolism related to sub-clavian vein catheterisation are reported. In 13 of these, a sudden catastrophe was associated with inadvertent disconnection of the catheter. Four (29%) died; nine (65%) had profound neurological impairment of whom five recovered. Five others had severe cardiorespiratory complications. Lack of integrity of catheter connections was the over-whelming cause of this serious but preventable hazard and the authors stress the need to ensure secure connection between the catheter and intravenous tubing.

Air embolism in the sitting position[82]

With the patient in the sitting position during neurosurgery, downward traction of the cannula enlarged the opening around the puncture site of the subclavian catheter, so allowing air to enter. Air embolism was diagnosed by the appearance of typical precordial Doppler sounds, fall of end-tidal PCO_2 and acute hypotension. Packing and pressure over the puncture site effected a temporary cure. A through-needle catheter had been used which means that the puncture would have been larger than the catheter. A guide wire technique would have been safer, because the puncture would have been smaller than the catheter.

Air embolism causing acute pulmonary oedema[83]

Immediately after the removal of a triple lumen subclavian catheter, whilst in the sitting position, the patient suddenly developed a sense of retro-sternal oppression and became acutely dyspnoeic. Consciousness was lost for 5 minutes. An hour later symptoms and signs developed and chest x-ray confirmed the clinical diagnosis of bilateral pul-monary oedema. All these features were attributed to venous air embolism which must have entered along the large (2·3 mm diameter) catheter track aided by the patient being in the sitting position.

Other reports, Flanagan et al.,[84] Aulenbacher,[85] Johnson et al.[86] and Levinsky.[87]

Infection

Catheter-related infections and septicaemia are common and important sequelae to central venous catheterisation especially in relation to long-term use. These problems have received extensive atten-tion. However, some rare and unusual infective conditions have also been reported.

Osteomyelitis of the first rib[88]

This presented as a cold chest wall mass 9 months after subclavian catheterisation for insertion of temporary pacing wires. Further investigation re-vealed a Staphylococcus osteomyelitis of the first rib.

Breast 'abscess'[89]

Eight days after successful insertion of an infra-clavicular subclavian catheter, the patient devel-oped severe pleuritic pain in the right chest. Injection of drugs into the catheter induced severe right-sided chest pain. Simultaneously a fluctuant right 'breast abscess' was drained. Fluid emerged from the drain in this lesion at the same rate as infusion into the venous line. Contrast studies showed inadvertent catheterisation of the right internal mammary vein from which a track had formed leaking into the right breast tissues.

Clavicular periostitis[90]

Three children developed this benign condition following percutaneous subclavian catheterisation.

Osteomyelitis of both clavicles[91]

In this case there was no systemic signs of infection, but simply local pain and tenderness over the affected area.

Miscellaneous complications

Intravascular knot formation[92]

Suspicion was aroused when after several attempts, resistance to withdrawal was noted and the cathe-ter appeared kinked. If knotting is suspected further pulling should be avoided as this may tighten the knot and make attempts to remove the catheter by unravelling the knot with a pig-tail catheter impossible, in which case surgical exploration is necessary.

Extravascular knotting of a guide wire[93]

Although the Seldinger technique is usually recom-mended for catheterisation of deep veins, the technique itself can lead to problems. In this case although the wire was advanced with ease, the catheter could not be. Attempts to withdraw the wire were unsuccessful. Surgical exploration revealed that the wire had perforated the posterior wall of the subclavian vein and knotted itself outside the vein. Undoubtedly, the vein was abnormal from many previous catheterisations for chemotherapy. Although no resistance was encountered when the wire was introduced in this case, when resistance is felt, it should always be a signal to withdraw or to proceed with extreme caution. This especially applies when there is a history of previous central venous catheterisations. Almost certainly, a J-tipped wire should be used in these cases.

Other report, Nicholas *et al.*[94]

Catheter embolism[95,96]

Intravascular foreign body[97]

Infraclavicular subclavian catheterisation was being attempted by an experienced operator using a Seldinger technique. Difficulty was encountered advancing the straight guide wire which was used. When the wire was retracted it broke. Immediate chest x-ray showed the wire. At exploration under local anaesthesia the tip of the fractured wire was found under the clavicle where it had become caught in the clavicular periosteum. Perhaps use of a J-tipped guide wire would have avoided this problem.

Misplacement of guide wire and loop formation[98]

During attempted insertion of a catheter using the guide wire technique, resistance was felt in trying to advance the wire. Catheterisation was impossible, but attempts to remove the wire failed. Chest x-ray demonstrated loop and knot formation. At surgical exploration, the wire was seen to have perforated the wall of an almost occluded subclavian vein and buried itself in the scalenus anterior muscle. In this case the patient had received numerous previous catheterisations for chemotherapy which no doubt had led to a partially thrombosed and softened vein wall.

Contact dermatitis[99]

From a subclavian catheter.

Table 5.1. Subclavian vein: infraclavicular approach – results and complications.

Author and year	Classification of technique (point of insertion)	Success rate	No. cases	Complications	No. complications (%)	Personnel	Comments
Wilson et al. (1962)[2]	Mid-clavicular point	Not stated	250	None (pneumothorax in some later cases performed by residents)	0	Authors	Series included infants
Davidson et al. (1963)[15]	Junction of middle and medial thirds of clavicle	94%	100	Pneumothorax Haematoma	1 (1) 3 (3)		Adults and children; youngest patient $3\frac{1}{2}$ years
Smith et al. (1965)[35]	Mid-clavicular point	Not stated	200	Lacerated subclavian vein communicating with pleura (both patients died) Severe subcutaneous emphysema – tracheostomy needed Brachial plexus palsy Haemothorax Septicaemia	2 (1) 2 (1) 1 (0·5) 1 (0·5) 1 (0·5)		
Mogil et al. (1967)[32]	Just lateral to the junction of middle and medial thirds of clavicle	95·9%	219	Overall Pneumothorax Haematoma Bleeding at puncture site	6 (2·7) 1 (0·4) 3 (1·3) 2 (0·9)	Main author only	
Christensen et al. (1967)[20]	Medial to mid-clavicular point	80%	90	Tension pneumothorax	1 (1.1)		
Defalque (1968)[34]	Slightly medial to mid-clavicular point	98·8%	1000	Arterial puncture Pneumothorax	1 (0·1) 3 (0·3)		Some catheterisations performed by supraclavicular approach
Morgan and Harkins (1972)[10]	Mid-clavicular point	Not stated	100	Infants (< 12 months): None Older children: Arterial puncture with local bleeding Catheter in pericardium Catheter in pleural cavity	0 2 (2) 1 (1) 1 (1)	Probably closely supervised personnel	74 catheterisations in children aged < 12 months; 37% of these were < 6 weeks old

Table 5.1. Continued.

Author and year	Classification of technique (point of insertion)	Success rate	No. cases	Complications	No. complications (%)	Personnel	Comments
James and Myers (1973)[33]	Mid-clavicular point	94%	511	Overall Major Pneumothorax Hydrothorax Sepsis	85 (16·6) 38 (7·44) 15 (2·93) 6 (1·17) 8 (1·56)		
Ryan et al. (1974)[39]	Not stated	Not stated	355	Pneumothorax Brachial plexus injury Pleural effusion Carotid artery laceration Mediastinal haemorrhage from innominate vein laceration Death (catheter sepsis)	6 (1·7) 2 (0·6) 1 (0·3) 1 (0·3) 1 (0·3) 1 (0·3)		Some catheters not inserted by the subclavian route
Groff and Ahmed (1974)[11]	Mid-clavicular point		< 1 year, 67 < 2 years, 36	Hydrothorax Haemothorax Pneumothorax Catheter sepsis Death (haemorrhage)	2 (1·9) 1 (0·9) 1 (0·9) 1 (0·9) 1 (0·9)	Experienced	
Blackett et al. (1978)[40]	Mid-clavicular point	84·3%	211	Overall Subclavian artery puncture Bilateral pneumothorax	5 (2·3) 3 (1·4) 1 (0·4)		All patients catheterised for intravenous feeding
Craig et al. (1969)[36]		Not stated	453	Pneumothorax Subcutaneous haematoma Subcutaneous infiltration with fluids	3 (0·6) 14 (3) 6 (1·3)		
Dudrick et al. (1969)[7]	Mid-clavicular point	Not stated	400	None (pneumothorax in later cases performed by residents)	0	Author	Series included infants

Author (year)	Approach/landmark	Success rate	Number	Complications	Number (%)	Operator experience	Comments
Feiler and de Alva (1969)[37]		Not stated	704	Pneumothorax Subclavian vein thrombosis	2 (0·3) 1 (0·1)		This series covered 4½ years. Complications occurred in the first 1½ years only
Tofield (1969)[17]	Lateral to mid-clavicular point	Not stated	Not stated	Not stated			More lateral approach said to avoid the risk of pneumothorax
Borja and Hinshaw (1970)[21]	Junction of medial and middle thirds of clavicle	Not stated	Not stated	Not stated			More medial approach said to be safer than lateral approach to avoid subclavian artery, brachial plexus, and pleural damage
Williams and McDonald (1971)[38]		93·3%	75	Haematoma Pneumothorax Septicaemia	2 (2·6) 1 (1·3) 6 (8)	Included medical students and residents	Average age 64 years (range 20–87 years)
Matthews (1982)[26]		88%	Right side 126	Malposition Pneumothorax Subclavicular artery puncture	16 (12·6) 5 (3·9) 3 (2·3)	Experienced	Choice of side left to operator
		88%	Left side 111	Malposition Pneumothorax Artery puncture Haemothorax	3 (2·3) 4 (3·1) 2 (1·5) 1 (0·8) Died		Malposition greater on right side
Eerola (1985)[27]		88%	13 857 (98% infra-clavicular) 76% Right sided 24% Left sided	Malposition into Internal jugular vein Other malposition Pneumothorax	(10) (0·5) (0·1)	Mainly experienced physicians	
Untracht (1988)[19]		100%	80	Axillary artery puncture	1 (1·2)		

Table 5.2.   Subclavian vein: supraclavicular approach – results and complications.

Author and year	Success rate	No. of cases	Complications	No. of complications (%)	Personnel	Comments
Yoffa (1965)[8]	97·6%	130	None		Author only	Successful venepuncture at first attempt in 80% of cases
Christensen et al. (1967)[20]	38%	21	Subclavian artery puncture Pneumothorax Subcutaneous emphysema	1 (4·7) 1 (4·7) 1 (4·7)	Experienced surgeons	Supraclavicular route attempted only after failure by infraclavicular route
Freeman (1968)[41]	99%	300	Arterial puncture Pneumothorax	2 (0·6) 3 (1·0)		
Defalque and Nord (1970)[42]	98·9%	1500	Pneumothorax Haematoma	4 (0·26) 1 (0·06)		
James and Myers (1973)[33]	95%	3000	Overall Major complication Subclavian thrombophlebitis Haemorrhage Air embolus Pneumothorax Hydrothorax Arteriovenous fistula	337 (11·2) 36 (1·2) 2 (0·06) 2 (0·06) 1 (0·03) 12 (0·4) 3 (0·09) 1 (0·03)	Experienced or supervised	
Brahos (1977)[18]	95	Right side 68 Left side 32	Unable to thread catheter Malposition of catheter Arterial puncture Pneumothorax	4 (4) 1 (1) 1 (1) 1 (1)	Residents supervised by author	
Haapaniemi and Slatis (1974)[16]	85·4% 97%	First 171 Later 429	Overall Malposition Arterial puncture Pneumothorax Haematoma Local infection Sepsis Thrombophlebitis Puncture of thoracic duct Air embolism	30 (5) 10 (1·7) 4 (0·6) 2 (0·3) 4 (0·6) 6 (0·9) 3 (0·5) 3 (0·5) 6 (0·9) 1 (0·2)		

Table 5.3. Complications of subclavian venous catheterisation: case reports.

Pleural space and lung

Delayed pneumothorax
Bilateral pneumothorax
Hydrothorax
Bilateral hydrothorax
Contralateral haemothorax
Contralateral effusion,
    venopulmonary fistula
Puncture of trachea
Airway obstruction

Vascular

Puncture of aorta
Puncture of pulmonary artery
Puncture of intercostal artery
Arteriovenous fistula
Benign intracranial
    hypertension
Spurious central venous
    pressure (CVP)
    measurement

Heart and mediastinum

Cardiac tamponade
Perforation of heart by guide
    wire
Pneumomediastinum
Arrhythmia

Lymphatic system

Laceration of thoracic duct
Lymphatic fistula
Lymph leak after
    venepuncture on right

Neurological

Phrenic nerve paralysis
Diaphragmatic paralysis
Recurrent laryngeal nerve
    paralysis
Brown–Sequard syndrome
Brachial plexus injury
Unsuspected cerebral
    perfusion
Blindness

Air embolus
Infection

Osteomyelitis of ribs
Osteomyelitis of clavicle
Breast 'abscess'

Miscellaneous

Intravascular foreign body
Intravascular knot formation
Catheter embolus
Contact dermatitis

REFERENCES

1. Aubaniac, R. (1952). L'injection intraveineuse sous-claviculaire; advantages et technique. *Presse Médicale* **60**, 1456.
2. Wilson, J. N., Grow, J. B., Demong, C. V., Prevedel, A. E. and Owens, J. C. (1962). Central venous pressure in optimal blood volume maintenance. *Archives of Surgery* **85**, 563.
3. Mobin-Uddin, K., Smith, P. E., Lombardo, C. and Jude, J. (1967). Percutaneous intracardiac pacing through the subclavian vein. *Journal of Thoracic and Cardiovascular Surgery* **54**, 545.
4. Vellani, C. W., Tildesley, G. and Davies, L. G. (1969). Endocardial pacing: a percutaneous method using the subclavian vein. *British Heart Journal* **31**, 106.
5. Lemole, G. M., Soulen, R. L. and Swartz, B. E. (1971). Technique of rapid pulmonary angiography by percutaneous subclavian vein catheterization. *Radiology* **100**, 179.
6. Defalque, R. J. (1972). The subclavian route. A critical review of the literature up to 1970. *Anaesthesist* **21**, 325.
7. Dudrick, S. J. D., Wilmore, D. W., Vars, H. M. and Rhoads, J. E. (1969). Can intravenous feeding as the sole means of nutrition support growth in the child and restore weight loss in an adult. *Annals of Surgery* **169**, 974.
8. Yoffa, D. (1965). Supraclavicular subclavian venepuncture and catheterisation. *Lancet* **2**, 614.
9. Lockwood, A. H. (1984). Percutaneous subclavian vein catheterisation: Too much of a good thing? *Archives of Internal Medicine* **144**, 1407.
10. Morgan, W. W. and Harkins, G. A. (1972). Percutaneous introduction of long-term indwelling venous catheters in infants. *Journal of Pediatric Surgery* **7**, 538.
11. Groff, D. B. and Ahmed, N. (1974). Subclavian vein catheterization in the infant. *Journal of Pediatric Surgery* **9**, 171.
12. Sterner, S., Plummer, D. W., Clinton, J. and Ruiz, E. (1986). A comparison of the supraclavicular approach and the infraclavicular approach for subclavian vein catheterization. *Annals of Emergency Medicine* **15**, 421.
13. Malatinsky, J., Faybik, M., Griffith, M., Majek, M. and Samel, M. (1983). Venepuncture, catheterization and failure to position correctly during central venous cannulation. *Resuscitation* **10**, 259.
14. Dronen, S., Thompson, B., Nowak, R. and Tomlanovich, M. (1982). Subclavian vein catheterization during cardiopulmonary resuscitation. *Journal of the American Medical Association* **247**, 3227.
15. Davidson, J. T., Ben-Hur, N. and Nathen, H. (1963). Subclavian venepuncture. *Lancet* **2**, 1139.
16. Haapaniemi, L. and Slatis, P. (1974). Supraclavicular catheterisation of the superior vena cava. *Acta Anaesthesiologica Scandinavica* **18**, 12.
17. Tofield, J. J. (1969). A safer technique of percutaneous catheterisation of the subclavian vein. *Surgery, Gynecology and Obstetrics* **128**, 1069.

18. Brahos, G. J. (1977). Central venous catheterization via the supraclavicular approach. *Journal of Trauma* **17**, 872.

19. Untracht, S. H. (1988). Axillary artery as a landmark in cannulating the subclavian vein. *Surgery, Gynecology and Obstetrics* **166**, 565.

20. Christensen, K. H., Nerstrom, B. and Baden, H. (1967). Complications of percutaneous catheterisation of the subclavian vein in 129 cases. *Acta Chirurgica Scandinavica* **133**, 615.

21. Borja, A. R. and Hinshaw, J. R. (1970). A safe way to perform infraclavicular subclavian vein catheterisation. *Surgery, Gynecology and Obstetrics* **130**, 673.

22. Jesseph, J. M., Conces, D. J. and Augustyn, G. T. (1987). Patient positioning for subclavian vein catheterization. *Archives of Surgery* **122**, 1207.

23. Malatinsky, J., Kadlic, T., Majek, M. and Samel, M. (1976). Misplacement and loop formation of central venous catheters. *Acta Anaesthesiologica Scandinavica* **20**, 237.

24. Padberg, F. T., Ruggiero, J., Blackburn, G. L. and Bistrian, B. R. (1981). Central venous catheterization for parenteral nutrition. *Annals of Surgery* **193**, 264.

25. Sanchez, R., Halck, S., Walther-Larsen, S. and Heslet, L. (1990). Misplacement of subclavian venous catheters: importance of head position and choice of puncture site. *British Journal of Anaesthesia* **64**, 632.

26. Matthews, N. T. and Worthley, L. I. G. (1982). Immediate problems associated with infraclavicular subclavian catheterisation; a comparison between left and right sides. *Anaesthesia and Intensive Care* **10**, 113.

27. Eerola, R., Kaukinen, L. and Kaukinen, S. (1985). Analysis of 13 800 subclavian vein catheterizations. *Acta Anaesthesiologica Scandinavica* **29**, 193.

28. Peters, J. L., Kenning, B. R., Garrett, C. P. O. and Kurzer, M. (1980). Percutaneous central venous cannulation. *British Medical Journal* **281**, 618.

29. Machi, J., Takeda, J. and Kakegawa, T. (1987). Safe jugular and subclavian venipuncture under ultrasonographic guidance. *American Journal of Surgery* **153**, 321.

30. Kawamura, R., Okabe, M. and Namikawa, K. (1987). Subclavian vein puncture under ultrasonic guidance. *Journal of Parenteral and Enteral Nutrition* **11**, 505.

31. Nolse, C., Nielsen, L., Karstrup, S. and Lauritsen, K. (1989). Ultrasonically guided subclavian vein catheterization. *Acta Radiologica* **30**, 108.

32. Mogil, R. A., Delaurentis, D. A. and Rosemond, G. P. (1967). The infraclavicular venepuncture. *Archives of Surgery* **95**, 320.

33. James, P. M. and Myers, R. T. (1973). Central venous pressure monitoring: complications and a new technic. *American Surgeon* **39**, 75.

34. Defalque, R. J. (1968). Subclavian venipuncture a review. *Anesthesia and Analgesia: Current Researches* **47**, 677.

35. Smith, B. E., Modell, J. H., Gaub, M. L. and Moya F. (1965). Complications of subclavian vein catheterisation. *Archives of Surgery* **90**, 228.

36. Craig, R. G., Jones, R. A., Sproul, G. J. and Kinyot, G. E. (1968). Alternate methods of central venous system catheterisation. *American Surgeon* **34**, 131.

37. Feiler, E. M. and deAlva, W. E. (1969). Infraclavicular percutaneous subclavian vein puncture: a safe technic. *American Journal of Surgery* **118**, 906.

38. Williams, R. W. and McDonald, J. C. (1971). A prospective study of the dangers of central venous pressure monitoring. *American Surgeon* **37**, 719.

39. Ryan, J. A., Abel, R. M., Abbott, W. M., Hopkins, C. C., Chesney, T. McC., Colley, R., Phillips, K. and Fischer, J. (1974). Catheter complications in total parenteral nutrition. *New England Journal of Medicine* **290**, 757.

40. Blackett, R. J., Bakran, A., Bradley, J. A., Halsall, A., Hill, G. L. and McMahon, M. J. (1978). A prospective study of subclavian vein catheters used exclusively for the purpose of intravenous feeding. *British Journal of Surgery* **65**, 393.

41. Freeman, J. (1968). Subclavian vein catheterisation. *Medical Journal of Australia* **2**, 979.

42. Defalque, R. J. and Nord, H. J. (1970). Supraclaviculare Technik der V. subclaviaPunktion fur den Anaesthesisten. *Anaesthesist* **19**, 197.

43. Mitchell, A. and Steer, H. (1980). Late appearance of pneumothorax after subclavian vein catheterisation: an anaesthetic hazard. *British Medical Journal* **281**, 1339.

44. Schorlemmer, G. R., Khouri, R. K., Murray, G. F. and Johnson, G. (1984). Bilateral pneumothoraces secondary to iatrogenic buffalo chest. An unusual complication of median sternotomy and subclavian vein catheterization. *Annals of Surgery* **199**, 372.

45. Rudge, C. J., Bewick, M. and McColl, I. (1973). Hydrothorax after central venous catheterization. *British Medical Journal* **3**, 23.

46. Naguib, M., Farag, N. and Joshi, R. N. (1985). Bilateral hydrothorax and hydromediastinum after a subclavian line insertion. *Canadian Anaesthetists' Society Journal* **32**, 412.

47. Bardosi, L., Mostafa, S. M., Wilkes, R. G. and Wenstone, R. (1988). Contralateral haemothorax: a late complication of subclavian vein cannulation. *British Journal of Anaesthesia* **60**, 463.

48. Ciment, L. M., Rotbart, A. and Galbut, R. N. (1988). Contralateral effusions secondary to subclavian venous catheters. Report of two cases. *Chest* **93**, 926.

49. Armstrong, C. W. and Mayhall, C. G. (1988). Contralateral hydrothorax following subclavian catheter replacement using a guidewire. *Chest* **94**, 231.

50. Demey, H. E., Colemont, L. J., Hartoko, T. J. *et al.* (1982). Venopulmonary fistula: a rare complication of central venous catheterization. *Journal of Parenteral and Enteral Nutrition* **11**, 580.

51. Breen, M. T. and Kageler, W. V. (1989). Puncture of the trachea during catheterization of the subclavian vein. *New England Journal of Medicine* **320**, 1148.

52. O'Leary, A. M. (1990). Acute airway obstruction due to arterial puncture during percutaneous central venous cannulation of the subclavian vein. *Anesthesiology* **75**, 780.

53. Childs, D. and Wilkes, R. G. (1986). Puncture of the ascending aorta-a complication of subclavian venous cannulation. *Anaesthesia* **41**, 331.

54. Hirsch, N. P. and Robinson, P. N. (1984). Pulmonary

artery puncture following subclavian venous cannulation. *Anaesthesia* 39, 727.

55. Bergmann, J., Gok, Y. and Smague, E. (1984). Haemothorax caused by an injury of the first intercostal artery after the trial of a vena subclavian aspiration. *Der Anaesthetist* 33, 592.

56. Hagley, S. R. (1985). Subclavian arteriovenous fistula from central venous catheterisation. *Anaesthesia and Intensive Care* 13, 103.

57. Amaral, J. F., Grigoriev, V. E., Dorfman, G. S. and Carney, W. I. (1990). Vertebral artery pseudoaneurysm. *Archives of Surgery* 125, 546.

58. Rotellar, C. (1987). Benign intracranial hypertension: a complication of subclavian vein catheterization and arteriovenous fistula. *American Journal of Kidney Disease* 9, 242.

59. Barrowcliffe, M. P. (1987). Spurious central venous pressure. *Anaesthesia* 42, 293.

60. Nakamura, T., Nakashima, Y., Yu, K. *et al.* (1985). Iatrogenic arteriovenous fistula of the internal mammary artery. Transcatheter intravascular coil occlusion. *Archives of Internal Medicine* 145, 140.

61. Fourestie, V., Godeau, D., Lejonc, J. L. and Schaeffer, A. (1985). Left innominate stenosis as a late complication of central venous catheterization. *Chest* 88, 636.

62. Dosios, T. J., Magovern, G. J., Gay, T. C. and Joyner, C. R. (1975). Cardiac tamponade complicating percutaneous catheterization of subclavian vein. *Surgery* 78, 261.

63. Adar, R. and Mozes, M. (1971). Fatal complications of central venous catheter. *British Medical Journal* 3, 746.

64. Defalque, R. J. (1971). Fatal complication of subclavian catheter. *Canadian Anaesthetists' Society Journal* 18, 681.

65. James, O. F. and Tredrea, C. R. (1979). Cardiac tamponade caused by caval catheter – a radiological demonstration of an unusual complication. *Anaesthesia and Intensive Care* 7, 174.

66. Blake, P. G. and Uldall, R. (1989). Cardiac perforation by a guide wire during subclavian catheter insertion. *International Journal of Artificial Organs* 12, 111.

67. Vaziri, N. D., Maksy, M., Lewis, M., Martin, D. and Edwards, K. (1984). Massive mediastinal hematoma caused by a double lumen subclavian catheter. *Artificial Organs* 8, 223.

68. Maschke, S. P. and Rogove, H. J. (1984). Cardiac tamponade associated with a multilumen central venous catheter. *Critical Care Medicine* 12, 611.

69. Hammond, D. I. (1984). The 'ring around the artery' sign in pneumomediastinum. *Journal of the Canadian Association of Radiologists* 35, 88.

70. Adar, R. and Mozes, M. (1970). Hydromediastinum. *Journal of the American Medical Association* 214, 372.

71. Ng, Y. C. and Walls, J. (1983). Lymphatic fistula after subclavian vein cannulation. *British Medical Journal* 287, 1264, 1725.

72. Ryan, D. W. (1978). Lymph leakage following catheterization of the right subclavian vein. *Anesthesia and Analgesia* 57, 123.

73. Obel, I. W. P. (1970). Transient phrenic-nerve paralysis following subclavian venipuncture. *Anesthesiology* 33, 369.

74. Epstein, E. J., Quereshi, M. S. A. and Wright, J. S. (1976). Diaphragmatic paralysis after supraclavicular puncture of subclavian vein. *British Medical Journal* 1, 693.

75. Copperman, Y. J., Daiser, M., Samuel, Y. *et al.* (1982). Recurrent laryngeal nerve paralysis following pacemaker introduction. *Pacing and Clinical Electrophysiology* 5, 505.

76. Koehler, P. J. and Wijngaard, P. R. A. (1986). Brown-Sequard Syndrome due to spinal cord infarction after subclavian vein catheterisation. *Lancet* 2, 914.

77. Bastani, B., Bolton, W. K. and Westervelt, F. B. (1987). Transient paralysis of upper extremity after percutaneous cannulation of the subclavian vein for hemodialysis. *American Journal of Kidney Disease* 10, 376.

78. Joyce, D. A. and Stewart Wynne, E. G. (1983). Brachial plexopathy complicating central venous catheter insertion. *Medical Journal Australia* 1, 82.

79. Klein, O. H., Segni, E. D. and Kaplinsky, E. (1978). Unsuspected cerebral perfusion. *Chest* 74, 109.

80. Acalovschi, I., Corbaciu, D. and Paraianu, I. (1988). Cortical blindness after subclavian catheterization. *Journal of Parenteral and Enteral Nutrition* 12, 526.

81. Coppa, G. F., Gouge, T. H. and Hoffstatter, S. R. (1981). Air embolism: a lethal but preventable complication of subclavian vein catheterization. *Journal of Parenteral and Enteral Nutrition* 5, 166.

82. Kloosterboer, T. B., Springman, S. R. and Coursin, D. B. (1986). Subclavian vein catheter as a source of air emboli in the sitting position. *Anesthesiology* 64, 411.

83. Kuhn, M., Fitting, J. W. and Levenberger, Ph. (1987). Acute pulmonary edema caused by venous air embolism after removal of a subclavian catheter. *Chest* 92, 364.

84. Flanagan, J. P., Gradisar, J. A., Gross, R. J. and Kelly, T. R. (1969). Air embolus. A lethal complication of subclavian venipuncture. *New England Journal of Medicine* 281, 488.

85. Aulenbacher, C. E. (1970). Hydrothorax from subclavian vein catheterization. *Journal of the American Medical Association* 214, 372.

86. Johnson, C. L., Lazarchick, J. and Lynn, H. B. (1970). Subclavian venipuncture: preventable complications. Report of two cases. *Mayo Clinic Proceedings* 45, 712.

87. Levinsky, W. J. (1969). Fatal air embolism during insertion of CVP monitoring apparatus. *Journal of the American Medical Association* 209, 1721.

88. Rosenfeld, L. E. (1985). Osteomyelitis of the first rib presenting as a cold abscess nine months after subclavian venous catheterization. *Pacing and Clinical Electrophysiology* 8, 897.

89. Rowley, S. and Downing, R. (1987). Breast 'abscess': an unusual complication of catheterisation of the subclavian vein. *British Journal of Radiology* 60, 773.

90. Friedman, A. P., Velcek, F. T., Haller, J. O. and Nagar, H. (1983). Clavicular periostitis: an unusual complication of percutaneous subclavian venous catheterization. *Radiology* 148, 692.

91. Klein, B., Mittelman, M., Katz, R. and Djaldetti, M. (1988). Osteomyelitis of both clavicles as a complication of subclavian venipuncture. *Chest* 86, 140.

92. Handsworth, J. L. (1981). An uncommon complication of central venous catheterization. *Anaesthesia and Intensive Care* **9**, 67.

93. Wang, L. P. and Einarsson, E. (1987). A complication of subclavian vein catheterisation. Extravascular knotting of a guidewire. *Acta Anaesthesiologica Scandinavica* **31**, 187.

94. Nicholas, F., Fenig, J. and Richter, R. M. (1970). Knotting of subclavian central venous catheter. *Journal of the American Medical Association* **214**, 373.

95. Longerbeam, J. K., Vannix, R., Wagner, W. and Joergenson, E. (1965). Central venous pressure monitoring. A useful guide to fluid therapy during shock and other forms of cardiovascular stress. *American Journal of Surgery* **110**, 220.

96. Massumi, R. A. and Ross, A. M. (1967). A traumatic non-surgical technic for removal of broken catheters from cardiac cavities. *New England Journal of Medicine* **277**, 195.

97. Johansen, J. R. and Jakobsen, H. (1982). Intravascular foreign body in subclavian vein catheterization by the Seldinger technique. *Acta Chirurgica Scandinavica* **148**, 297.

98. Kjeldsen, L. (1987). Transvenous misplacement and loop formation of spring guide wire. *Anaesthesia* **42**, 216.

99. Guin, J. D., Hutchins, L. and Johnson, J. L. (1990). Contact dermatitis from a subclavian catheter. *International Journal of Dermatology* **29**, 58.

100. Slezak, F. A. and Williams, G. B. (1984). Delayed pneumothorax: a complication of subclavian vein catheterization. *Journal of Parenteral and Enteral Nutrition* **10**, 542.

6

The Internal Jugular Vein

The internal jugular is a large vein which may be used (1) to introduce central venous catheters, (2) to obtain blood samples from infants and young children, or (3) to administer intravenous infusions through short cannulae.

Benotti *et al.*[1] advocated internal jugular vein cannulation for parenteral nutrition and used a subcutaneous tunnel so that the catheter's skin exit site was below the clavicle. Civetta and Gabel[2] introduced Swan–Ganz catheters via the internal jugular vein, using a spinal needle (22 gauge) to locate the vein. Hess and Tarnow[3] described a method for inserting both a central venous and a Swan–Ganz catheter into one internal jugular vein. In the United Kingdom, English and his colleagues[4] popularised the use of the internal jugular vein for central venous cannulation. Numerous alternative techniques have been described, sometimes with added refinements. Internal jugular vein cannulation has become more popular recently following reports of serious complications associated with subclavian vein cannulation.

The technique can be classified as high or low, which refers to the position of the needle's insertion in relation to the apex of the lung; a high approach has the advantage of avoiding the risk of pneumothorax. We have arbitrarily defined the high approach as being at or above the apex of the triangle formed by the two heads of the sternomastoid and the clavicle. A low approach is below the apex of the triangle. The cricoid cartilage is approximately level with the apex of the triangle. Techniques can also be classified as medial, lateral, or central depending upon their relation to the sternomastoid muscle.

ANATOMY

The sigmoid sinus passes through the mastoid portion of the temporal bone, emerging from the jugular foramen at the base of the skull as the internal jugular vein. Behind the sternal end of the clavicle it joins the subclavian vein to become the innominate vein. The internal jugular vein dilates at a valve 1 cm above the clavicle.

The internal jugular vein, the carotid artery, and the vagus nerve are contained together in the carotid sheath. The internal jugular vein at first lies posterior to the internal carotid artery, before becoming lateral and then anterolateral to the artery. The vein is capable of expanding mainly, then, on its lateral aspect to accommodate an increase in blood flow. The lower part of the vein lies behind the junction of the sternal and clavicular insertions of the sternomastoid muscle, loosely attached to the posterior surface of the muscle with fascia. Behind the vein are the prevertebral fascia, the prevertebral muscles, and the cervical transverse processes, and posteriorly, at the root of the neck, are the subclavian artery and its branches, the phrenic and vagus nerves, and the cupola of the pleura. On the left the thoracic duct and on the right the lymphatic duct drain into the junction of the internal jugular and subclavian veins.

The larger right jugular vein is believed to drain most of the blood from the cerebral hemispheres. Blood from the posterior fossa contents drains into the vein on the left.[11]

TECHNICAL CONSIDERATIONS

Time required

A number of authors have examined the time needed to cannulate the vein. One study compared a catheter over a needle method with a technique using a seeker needle followed by a Seldinger method.[5] In anaesthetised patients the mean times to cannulate the vein were 28·2 seconds and 141·6 seconds respectively. These differences are of no particular clinical significance. (Speed is only essential during resuscitation of patients who have suffered cardiac arrest.) Cannulating the right or left vein made no difference to the time of insertion. In another study 82% of cannulations were performed in less than 60 seconds; only 18% took from 60 seconds to several minutes.[6]

A different study investigated the time required to perform cut downs under local anaesthesia on the internal jugular and subclavian veins.[7] The mean time to insert internal jugular catheters was 28·7 minutes and 48·5 minutes for the subclavian catheters. The internal jugular catheters were not only quicker and easier to insert but also resulted in smaller and less conspicuous scars.

In an emergency in the absence of suitable apparatus a short catheter (5 cm) can be used to catheterise the internal jugular vein. This is adequate for infusions of drugs and will provide accurate measurements of central venous pressure.[8] Such catheters should not be left *in situ* for longer than necessary because of the risk of air embolus.

Our experience is that internal jugular catheterisation is usually a quick and easy procedure. Of course insertion can be unpredictably difficult in some patients and in some patients cannulation may not be possible at all.

Number of stabs to cannulate the vein

It is widely recognised that it is sensible to limit the number of stabs required to cannulate the vein. The upper limit is arbitrary and will depend on the size of the needle used, the urgency of the procedure, the availability of alternative veins and the equipment available. Many clinicians allow up to five attempts with a seeker needle but only three with the much larger introducer needle.

It is perhaps surprising that even after successful venepuncture with the seeker needle there may still be problems in locating the vein with the introducer needle.[9] (See page 131.) Some authors believe that

hitting the vein with a seeker needle may induce venospasm.

Other authors have suggested that abandoning venepuncture after only 3 failed attempts is premature if the carotid artery has not been inadvertently punctured. In a study of patients with coagulopathies, 3 or more attempts were made in over 40% of 1000 cannulations without apparent serious consequences.[10] In another series 1 or 2 punctures were required in 82% of cases and in the others it was stated that more than 5 attempts at cannulation were rarely required.[6]

Use of ultrasound

Ultrasound has been used to facilitate internal jugular vein cannulation[12-18] and to study different techniques of cannulation.[19]

Use of the Doppler facilitates cannulation and results in fewer passes per cannulation, a shorter time to cannulation and a lower incidence of carotid artery puncture.[14,18] Early use of ultrasound enabled localisation of the internal jugular vein; cannulation was subsequently performed blindly.[12-15] It is now possible to use a real-time technique to view the needle as it advances through the neck tissues and then through the vein wall.[17] The method would seem to be useful in facilitating venous cannulation if the anatomy is grossly abnormal.

Some points of practical value have emerged from the use of ultrasound.[13,19] The right internal jugular vein is usually bigger than that on the left. Palpation of the carotid artery and extreme head rotation can decrease vein diameter. The vein is wider below the cricoid cartilage than above it. Head-down tilt increases vein diameter. The mean skin to vein distance travelled by the needle was only 2·59 cm in a study comparing 15 different techniques.[19] The findings appear to recommend that palpation of the carotid artery should be performed routinely prior to cannulation and the arterial pulse used as a guide.

In clinical practice venous cannulation is usually a simple procedure and ancillary complex equipment is superfluous. Most clinicians on encountering difficulty with internal jugular vein cannulation would use an alternative vein. Ultrasound would seem to be helpful in cases of special difficulty and perhaps in training procedures.

Use of multi-lumen catheters

Some clinicians routinely use two or even three catheters in a single internal jugular vein.[20] This

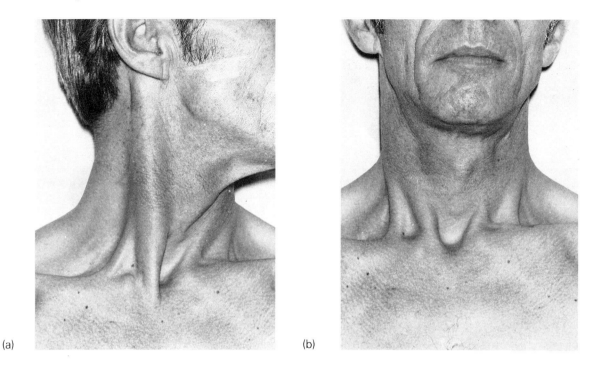

(a)   (b)

Figure 6.1.   Anatomical landmarks – the sternal and clavicular heads of the sternomastoid muscle: (1) with the head turned to the left; (b) from the front.

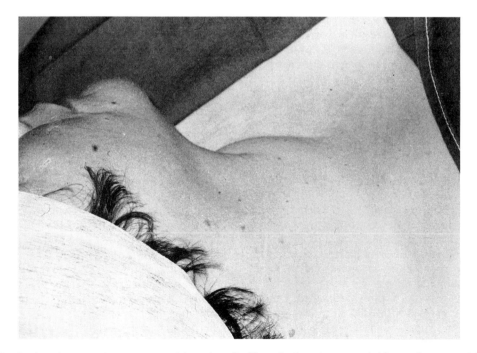

Figure 6.2.   In the obese patient, or one with a short 'bull' neck, the sternomastoid muscle may not be readily visible.

practice is likely to become less common with the introduction of double and triple lumen catheters. The disadvantage associated with the use of some multi-lumen catheters is that the introducer needle may be of large diameter. When using more than one catheter in a vein there is a possibility that the first catheter can be damaged by the second needle.

CHOICE OF TECHNIQUE

It is generally accepted that the incidence and severity of complications associated with cannulation of the internal jugular vein are lower than those for the subclavian vein. Consequently, internal jugular vein cannulation is now being employed with increasing frequency. If cannulation fails on one side, many authors then try the vein on the opposite site. This is an advantage not shared by the subclavian approach, where it is generally recommended that attempts should be restricted to one side to avoid the risk of bilateral pneumothorax.

The technique chosen is usually the one with which the operator is most familiar. However, it is not always possible or desirable to employ this approach. Most techniques rely on identifying the sternomastoid muscle and its sternal and clavicular insertions (Figure 6.1 a,b), but this muscle may not be readily visible in obese patients or in patients with short, 'bull' necks (Figure 6.2). In these circumstances a technique may be required which relies on **palpation** of an additional structure such as the thyroid cartilage,[21] the carotid artery,[22] the internal jugular vein and the carotid artery,[4] or the notch on the superior surface of the medial end of the clavicle.[23]

Techniques in which the needle is inserted well above the clavicle – a high approach – are less likely to cause major complications and are therefore preferable. Nevertheless, a pneumothorax can result from a high approach if a long needle is inserted at a narrow angle to the skin; the use of a short needle makes venous cannulation easier and decreases the frequency of carotid artery puncture.[24] With a low approach it is important to avoid hyperventilation during the cannulation so as to decrease the risk of a pneumothorax. Venous cannulation may be facilitated in the high approach by keeping the lung inflated for a short while or asking the patient to perform a Valsalva manoeuvre, thus distending the vein with minimal risk of pneumothorax.

We have chosen a representative selection of previously described techniques for internal jugular vein cannulation. Some of these were originally described only for use in adults, although this does not necessarily preclude their use in children.

Method preferred by authors

In our preferred technique the carotid artery is palpated to facilitate location of the internal jugular vein.[22] Despite the original authors' recommendation to use the left side, we find it much easier for a right-handed operator to cannulate the internal jugular vein on the patient's right side.

Method for describing the direction of the needle after positioning the patient for venepuncture

The approximate direction and points of insertion of the needle for the techniques described are shown in Figure 6.3. In each technique, the directions have five steps (see Figure 6.4):

1. Identify the point of insertion of the needle on the skin.
2. Place the needle tip on the skin at that point and direct the needle caudally (position A).
3. Swing the needle and syringe laterally or medially as instructed (A to B).
4. Elevate or depress the syringe to an appropriate degree above the coronal plane (the same plane as the surface of the operating table) or the skin (B to C).
5. Penetrate the skin with the needle and advance the needle into the vein. Then remove the syringe and thread the catheter centrally.

Points of management common to all techniques

To avoid unnecessary trauma, the vein can first be located with a fine needle using the chosen technique. The fine needle is then removed and the larger needle introduced. Alternatively the fine needle can be left in the vein and the larger needle introduced alongside, using the fine needle as a guide. Saline should be injected through the larger needle after puncturing the skin to clear the needle of any tissue. The catheter is fixed securely to the skin with a stitch to prevent movement. Alternatively, the catheter with its connection is looped down and fixed to the chest to allow free neck movement. A chest x-ray enables the position of the catheter to be determined.

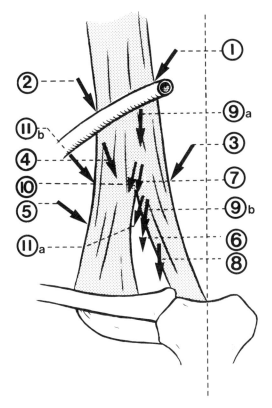

Figure 6.3. A selection of approaches to the catheterisation of the internal jugular vein. 1 = Boulanger et al. (1976)[21]; 2 = Brinkman and Costley (1973)[25]; 3 = Mostert et al. (1970)[22]; 4 = Civetta and Gabel (1972)[2]; 5 = Jernigan et al. (1970)[26]; 6 = Daily et al (1970)[33]; 7 = Vaughan and Weygandt (1973)[34]; 8 = Rao et al. (1977)[23]; 9a = English et al. (1969)[4]: elective method; 9b = English et al. (1969)[4]: alternative method, 10 = Prince et al. (1976)[35]; 11a = Hall and Geefhuysen (1977)[37]: elective method; 11b = Hall and Geefhuysen (1977)[37], alternative method.

Routes 1, 2, 3, 4 and 5 were originally described for adults; routes 6, 7, 8 and 9 for adults and children; and routes 10 and 11 for children.

HOW TO MAXIMISE THE CHANCES OF SUCCESS AND MINIMISE THE INCIDENCE OF COMPLICATIONS

Examine and position the patient before scrubbing up

1. Place patient in head-down position.
2. Slight extension of the head of table head may be helpful if the patient has short or 'bull' neck. Remove the pillow from behind the head. In children place a pillow or bolster behind the shoulders.

3. Mark position of the cricoid and thyroid cartilages with a marker pen. Draw a line across the neck at level of proposed catheterization.
4. Examine the carotid artery to assess ease of palpation (if this is used as part of technique).
5. See if the external jugular vein on same side will be suitable if failure occurs with internal jugular catheterization.

Equipment

Use a seeker needle to locate the vein. Use a short fine needle and a Seldinger technique. Avoid long catheter-over-needle devices. Avoid using large diameter needles to puncture the vein initially. Avoid rigid catheters particularly on the left side.

Operator and technique

1. For the Seldinger technique the clinician should use gown and gloves and full aseptic technique. Inexperienced clinicians should initially be carefully supervised.
2. Use a high approach in the neck to minimise risk of damage to the pleura.
3. Stay in 'safe area' (see Oda's technique). Avoid going too far medially (damage to artery, trachea or oesophagus). Avoid going too far posteriorly (damage to vertebral vessels and nerves).
4. If the patient is conscious perform catheterisation while a Valsalva manoeuvre is performed. If the patient is anaesthetised and ventilated perform venepuncture during inspiration.
5. Limit the number of stabs with both the seeker needle (maximum five) and the definitive needle (maximum three).
6. Have a plan for failure, i.e. try:

   (a) external jugular vein same side
   (b) internal jugular vein other side
   (c) external jugular vein other side.

HOW TO MINIMISE THE CHANCES OF SUCCESS AND MAXIMISE THE INCIDENCE OF COMPLICATIONS

Failure to examine and to position the patient before scrubbing up

This makes catheterisation more difficult and might prolong what could in any case be a difficult procedure.

Equipment

1. Failure to use a seeker needle.
2. Use of long catheter-over-long needle devices.
3. Use of rigid catheters particularly on the left side.

Operator and technique

1. Careless scrubbing up and lack of sterile precautions.

2. Failure to use a seeker needle.
3. Use of low approaches in the neck and straying outside the 'safe area', i.e. posteriorly and medially.
4a. Unsupervised inexperienced clinicians who persevere beyond the permitted number of attempts.
4b. Experienced clinicians who persevere beyond the permitted number of attempts.
5. Not having a plan for failure if initial attempt fails.

THE METHODS

A number of methods are described by various authors. IT IS CERTAINLY NOT NECESSARY FOR THE READER TO STUDY ALL THESE IN DETAIL. It is appropriate for an experienced clinician to have expertise in more than one method. The inexperienced clinician should first gain experience and confidence with a single suitable method. We recommend that a method in which the *carotid artery* is used as a primary landmark should be used initially. (See Mostert[22] and Oda's[6] techniques.)

HIGH TECHNIQUE: MEDIAL APPROACH
Boulanger et al. *(1976)*[21]

Patient category

Adults. The description of the technique by the original authors did not include its application in children, but this does not necessarily exclude its use in this age group.

Advantages and disadvantages

The high approach eliminates the risk of pneumo-thorax. The needle is pointed laterally, thus greatly decreasing the risk of puncturing the carotid artery. The vein is not transfixed with this method, which is claimed to be easy to teach and to learn. The internal jugular vein is at its widest (13–15 mm diameter) at this point. The method was also used to insert Swan–Ganz catheters.

Preferred side

The right.

Position of patient (Figure 6.4a)

Place the table in a 25° head-down position. Extend the patient's neck by placing a small towel under the shoulder and turn the head away from the side of the puncture. Place the patient's arms by his sides.

Position of operator (Figure 6.4a)

Stand at the head of the patient or on the opposite side to the puncture site.

Equipment used in original description

Catheter-through-needle.

Advice on current equipment

A guide wire technique is strongly recommended. Long rigid catheter over needle devices should be avoided especially on the left side.

Anatomical landmarks

The sternomastoid muscle, the thyroid cartilage, and the external jugular vein.

Preparation

Perform the puncture under sterile conditions using local anaesthesia if indicated.

Precautions and recommendations

If possible, maintain positive intrathoracic pressure during venous cannulation to distend the vein.

Point of insertion of needle (Figure 6.4b)

At the superior border of the thyroid cartilage (level with the 4th cervical vertebra) on the medial border of the sternomastoid muscle.

Initial location of vein with a small (21)-gauge needle

Locate the vein with a fine needle using the following directions. Then using the fine needle as a guide puncture the skin with the larger needle attached to a saline-filled syringe.

Direction of needle and procedure (Figure 6.4c,d,e)

Pinch the sternomastoid muscle to determine its thickness. Place the point of the needle at the entry site on the skin and point the needle and syringe caudally (A). Then swing the needle and syringe and point the needle laterally to make an angle of approximately 45° with the medial border of the sternomastoid (A to B). Elevate the syringe 10° above the skin (B to C). Direct the needle just underneath the sternomastoid, keeping close to its posterior aspect. The needle is directed superficially as if to come out 2 cm beyond the lateral border of the muscle. Maintain a slight negative pressure in the syringe as the needle is advanced. The vein is entered 2–4 cm from the puncture site. On entering the vein, direct the syringe and needle in the axis of the vein (that is, towards the midline) and advance the needle 1–2 cm into the vein. Introduce the wire centrally and remove the needle. Then thread the catheter centrally.

Success rate

A 94% success rate was achieved by 9 supervised residents with their first 100 attempted cannulations.

Complications

2% incidence of puncture of the carotid artery.

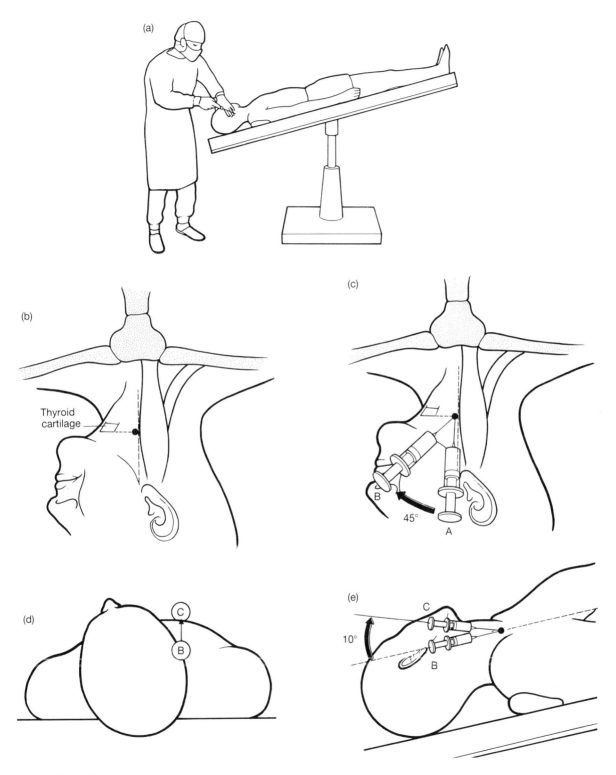

Figure 6.4. High technique: medial approach: Boulanger *et al.* (1976).[21]

HIGH TECHNIQUE: LATERAL APPROACH
Brinkman and Costley (1973)[25]

Patient category

Adults. The description of the technique by the original authors did not include its application in children, but this does not necessarily exclude its use in this age group.

Advantages and disadvantages

The high approach eliminates the risk of a pneumo-thorax. This technique cannot be used if the external jugular vein is not visible. If the approach via the internal jugular vein fails, the external jugular vein can be cannulated through the same skin puncture. The puncture in the vein wall is completely filled by a catheter outside a needle. This method was developed in response to failures with the method described by Jernigan and his colleagues.[26]

Preferred side

The right.

Position of patient (Figure 6.5a)

Place the table in a 25° head-down position. Extend the patient's neck by placing a small towel under the shoulders and turn the head away from the side of the puncture. Place the patient's arms by his sides.

Position of operator (Figure 6.5a)

Stand at the head of the patient.

Equipment used in original description

A 14 gauge 150 mm catheter-over-long needle.

Advice on current equipment

A guide wire technique is strongly recommended. Long rigid catheter over needle devices should be avoided especially on the left side.

Anatomical landmarks

The lateral border of the sternomastoid muscle, the external jugular vein, and the sternal notch.

Preparation

Perform the procedure under sterile conditions using local anaesthesia if indicated.

Precautions and recommendations

If possible, maintain positive intrathoracic pressure during venous cannulation to distend the vein.

Point of insertion of needle (Figure 6.5b)

Along the lateral border of the sternomastoid muscle cephalad to the junction of the external jugular vein and the muscle.

Initial location of vein with small (21)-gauge needle.

Locate the vein with a fine needle using the following directions. Then using the fine needle as a guide, puncture the skin with the larger needle attached to a saline-filled syringe.

Direction of needle and procedure

(Figure 6.5c,d,e)
Place the point of the needle at the entry site on the skin and point the needle and syringe caudally (A). Then swing the needle and syringe and point the needle towards the sternal notch (A to B). Elevate the syringe 10° above the coronal plane (B to C). Advance the needle, maintaining a slight negative pressure in the syringe, just beneath the belly of the sternomastoid muscle, aiming towards the sternal notch. The internal jugular vein is usually entered within 5–7 cm. Introduce the wire centrally and remove the needle. Then thread the catheter centrally.

Success rate

The technique was used in 180 punctures. The success rate was not specifically reported.

Complications

The carotid artery was punctured on 4 occasions (2·2%).

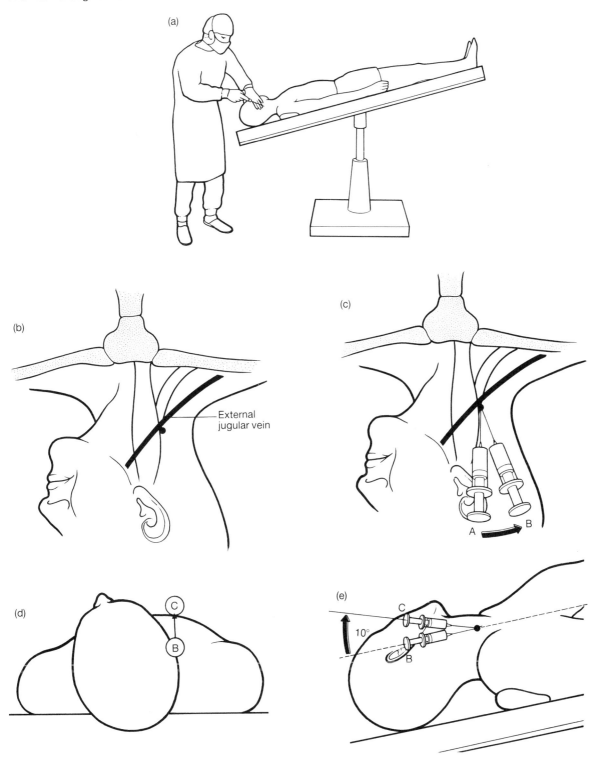

Figure 6.5. High technique: lateral approach: Brinkman and Costley (1973).[25]

HIGH TECHNIQUE: MEDIAL APPROACH
Mostert et al. (1970)[22]

Patient category

Adults. The description of the technique by the original authors did not include its application in children, but this does not necessarily exclude its use in this age group.

Advantages and disadvantages

This method relies on palpating the carotid artery, thus eliminating the need to identify the two heads of insertion of the sternomastoid muscle. The method was used successfully under local anaesthesia in conscious, critically ill patients. It was found to be acceptable to patients, who did not find it unduly painful. The stiff catheter was easily threaded beyond the bevel of the needle because the shaft of the needle was pointed in the same axis as the vein. This is the only approach which indicates preference for the vein on the left side, and in which the patient remains horizontal. We have found this method successful in adults under general anaesthesia and in children.

Preferred side

The left. We find it easier for a right-handed operator to use the vein on the right side.

Position of patient (Figure 6.6a)

Place the table in a 25° head-down position. Extend the patient's neck by placing a small towel under the shoulders and turn the head away from the side of the puncture. Place both arms by the sides.

Position of operator Figure 6.6a)

Stand at the head of the patient or on the opposite side to the puncture site.

Equipment used in original description

A 14 gauge O.D. needle with a 15 gauge O.D. 525 mm radiopaque catheter (catheter-through-needle).

Advice on current equipment

A guide wire technique is strongly recommended. Long rigid catheter over needle devices should be avoided especially on the left side.

Anatomical landmarks

The carotid artery and the midpoint of the sterno-mastoid muscle.

Preparation

Perform the puncture under sterile conditions using local anaesthesia if indicated.

Precautions and recommendations

It is technically easier for a right-handed operator to cannulate the patient's right internal jugular vein.

Point of insertion of needle (Figure 6.6b)

Along the medial border of the sternomastoid muscle at its midpoint just lateral to the carotid artery. This is above the level of the cricoid cartilage. In an adult this point should be at least 5 cm above the clavicle.

Initial location of vein with small (21)-gauge needle

Locate the vein with a fine needle using the following directions. Then using the fine needle as a guide, puncture the skin with the larger needle attached to a saline-filled syringe.

Direction of needle and procedure (Figure 6.6c,d,e)

Separate the sternomastoid muscle and the common carotid artery with the index and middle fingers of the left hand. The arterial pulsations should be felt by the tips of these fingers. Place the point of the needle at the entry site on the skin and point the needle and syringe caudally (A). Elevate the syringe 45° above the coronal plane (A to B). Swing the needle and syringe to point the needle towards the junction of the medial and middle thirds of the ipsilateral clavicle. Advance the needle, maintaining a slight negative pressure in the syringe until the vein is entered. *We prefer to keep the needle in the midline or pointing only slightly laterally as recommended by Hermosura and his colleagues.[27] On some occasions the vein may be transfixed and the lumen is entered only when the needle is slowly withdrawn.*Once the lumen is entered remove the syringe and thread the wire centrally. Then remove the needle from the vein and thread the catheter centrally.

Success rate

A success rate of 97·7% was reported in 133 patients aged 15 to 81 years (130 out of 133). On three occasions the catheter could not be advanced beyond the hub of the needle and the subclavian vein was used.

Complications

The carotid artery was punctured twice (1·5%).

There was a 34·5% incidence of tenderness at the catheter site when this was examined 24 hours after removal of the catheter. The incidence of tenderness was greater in patients in whom the catheter had been left *in situ* for at least 36 hours.

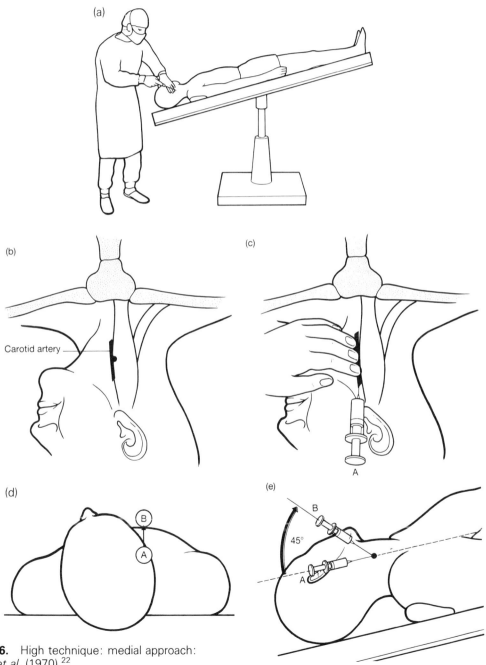

Figure 6.6. High technique: medial approach: Mostert *et al.* (1970).[22]

HIGH TECHNIQUE: MEDIAL APPROACH
Oda et al. (1981)[6]

Patient category

456 consecutive patients aged from less than 6 months to adults.

Advantages and disadvantages

The technique was used successfully in neonates, children and adults. It was used by junior trainees as well as senior anaesthetists. The carotid artery is palpated with the bare hand before skin preparation is undertaken to identify the course and depth of the artery and its lateral well. Palpation is applied by the finger tips perpendicular to the carotid artery. The method was used successfully in patients who were in the lateral position.

Preferred side

The right.

Position of patient

Place the patient in a slightly head-down position. The head is either not rotated or only slightly rotated to the contralateral side. Small children need hyperextension of the neck and a small pillow or towel is placed under the shoulders.

Position of operator

Stand at the head of the table.

Equipment used in original description

Hakko 'over the needle' catheters – 18 gauge × 130 mm catheters for adults, 21 gauge × 60 mm or 19 gauge × 50 mm catheters for small children. A 12 or 14 gauge × 80 mm catheter introducer was used for passing cardiac pacemakers or pulmonary artery catheters in adults. A flexible Teflon catheter guide was inserted into the 12, 14 and 18 gauge catheters after removal of the needle to facilitate catheter advancement.

Advice on current equipment

A guide wire technique is strongly recommended. Long rigid catheter over needle devices should be avoided especially on the left side.

Anatomical landmarks

The carotid artery and the laryngeal prominence of the thyroid cartilage (the cephalad portion).

Preparation

Perform the puncture under sterile conditions using local anaesthesia if indicated.

Precautions and recommendations

It is technically easier for a right-handed operator to cannulate the patient's right internal jugular vein. Avoid inserting the needle more deeply than the transverse processes of the cervical vertebrae to avoid damage to vertebral vessels and the cervical nerve plexus. Keep the needle in the safe puncture area (Figure 6.7a). Do not make more than five attempts at cannulation to minimise complications.

Point of insertion of needle

Just lateral to the carotid artery and level with the laryngeal prominence of the thryoid cartilage.

Initial location of vein with small (21)-gauge needle

A fine needle can be used to locate the vein using the following directions. The fine needle is then removed and the skin punctured with the large needle attached to a saline-filled syringe.

Direction of needle and procedure (Figure 6.7b)

Make a small incision in the skin at the needle insertion point. Palpate the right carotid artery with the tips of the fingers of the left hand pointing perpendicular to the coronal plane. Place the tip of the needle on the skin entry site and point the needle caudally. Then elevate the needle 30–45° to the skin. Advance the needle into the vein. If the initial puncture fails withdraw the needle and direct subsequent attempts gradually more laterally. Clicks may be noted on penetrating the cervical fascia, carotid sheath and the vein wall.

Success rate

Success rates in favourable clinical circumstances are shown in Table 6.1.
The success rate for patients in unfavourable clinical circumstances are shown in Table 6.2.

Complications

There were 5 (1·1%) carotid artery punctures. Haematomas occurred in two of these after prolonged cardiopulmonary bypass.

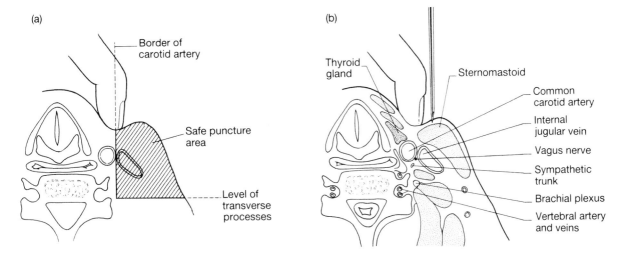

Figure 6.7. Cross-section of the neck. The direction of the fingers during palpation is perpendicular to the coronal plane. The direction fo the catheter is parallel with the patient's sagittal plane. The catheter should not be directed medially and should not be advanced deeper than transverse process of the cervical vertebra. The safe puncture area is also indicated schematically by hatching. From Oda et al. (1981)[6].

Table 6.1. Success rates for Oda's method in favourable clinical circumstances.

Age distribution	Number of cases	Success	Success rates
15 years–adult	408	396	97·1%
5 years–15 years	20	18	90·0%
1–5 years	14	13	92·9%
6 months–1 year	7	6	85·7%
Less than 6 months	7	4	57·1%
Total	456	437	95·8%

Table 6.2. Success rates for Oda's method in unfavourable clinical circumstances.

	Number of cases	Success	Success rates
Neuroanaesthesia patients (in horizontal position)	46	41	89·1%
Patients in pre-shock state	15	14	93·3%
Patients with extreme dehydration	12	11	91·6%
Patients in lateral or kidney position	8	8	100%
Cannulation with a 14 or 12 gauge catheter	13	11	84·6%

HIGH TECHNIQUE: CENTRAL APPROACH
Sharrock and Fierro (1983)[29]

Patient category

Adults aged from 22 to 95 years. Most were elderly and had either cardiac or respiratory problems.

Advantages and disadvantages

The authors claimed a low incidence of complications and a high success rate. They used a 'no touch' technique which is helpful for asepsis and avoids palpation of the carotid artery with its attendant complications.

Preferred side

The right.

Position of patient

Place the table in a slightly head-down position. If the vein is seen to collapse on expiration apply more head-down tilt. Turn the patient's head approximately 30° to the left. Examine the neck for venous pulsations. These are usually visible in the middle of the neck beneath the sternomastoid. The vein was located by inspection only.

Position of operation

Stand at head of the table.

Equipment used in original description

A 22 or 23 gauge seeker needle. A 14 or 8 French catheter.

Advice on current equipment

Suitable Seldinger wire equipment.

Anatomical landmarks

The pulsating internal jugular vein.

Preparation

Perform the punctures under sterile conditions using local anaesthesia if indicated. All patients in this series were anaesthetised and ventilated.

Precautions and recommendations

Always use a seeker needle. The fingers of the left hand were placed beneath the body of the mandible to retract the skin and stabilise the neck. Needle insertion should take place during the inspiratory phase of artificial ventilation when the vein is distended. This method should only be used if the vein is visible. If it is not visible use an alternative technique. Macdonald[30] noted that compression and release of the neck with three fingers in the anticipated line of the vein often demonstrated the vein as it refilled.

Point of insertion of needle

Directly over the venous pulsation (in the middle of the neck under the sternomastoid).

Direction of needle and procedure

Place the point of the 23 or 22 gauge seeker needle on the skin entry and point the needle caudally. Elevate the syringe to an angle of 45° to the neck. Advance the needle maintaining a slight negative pressure in the syringe until the vein is entered. Then repeat this procedure using the definitive needle and thread the catheter centrally.

Success rate

Successful venous cannulation was performed in 210 out of 212 patients (Table 6.3).

Complications

Cartoid artery puncture occurred in 3 patients.

Table 6.3. Number of needle insertions before successful internal jugular venous entry (a) or cannulation (b).

	No. patients	%
(a) 'Seeker' 22-or-23 gauge needle		
1st attempt	186	87·7
2nd attempt	14	6·6
3rd attempt	4	1·9
> 3 attempts	7	3·3
Failures	1	0·5
Total	212	
(b) 14 or 8 French catheters		
1st attempt	175	82·5
2nd attempt	13	6·1
3rd attempt	13	6·1
>3 attempts	7	3·3
Failures	1	0·5
Carotid punctures	3	1·4
Total	212	

HIGH TECHNIQUE: CENTRAL APPROACH
Civetta et al. *(1972)*[31]

Patient category

Adults. The description of the technique by the original authors did not include its application in children, but this does not necessarily exclude its use in this age group.

Advantages and disadvantages

The use of a spinal needle to locate the vein avoids excessive trauma with a large needle but it may be difficult to manipulate because of its length. This method has also been used to insert Swan–Ganz flow-directed pulmonary artery catheters through a 12 gauge needle introducer. A 90 mm spinal needle may not be long enough.

Preferred side

The right.

Position of patient (Figure 6.8a)

Place the table in a 25° head-down position. Extend the patient's neck by placing a small towel under the shoulders and turn the head away from the side of the puncture. Place the patient's arms by his sides.

Position of operator (Figure 6.8a)

Stand at the head of the patient or on the opposite side to the puncture site.

Equipment used in original description

A 22 gauge spinal needle threaded through a 14 gauge needle.

Advice on current equipment

A guide wire technique is strongly recommended. Long rigid catheter-over-needle devices should be avoided especially on the left side.

Anatomical landmarks

The sternomastoid muscle with its sternal and clavicular heads.

Preparation

Perform the puncture under sterile conditions using local anaesthesia if indicated.

Precautions and recommendations

This method is now likely to be less widely used with the common use of fine seeker needles and guide wire techniques.

Point of insertion of needle (Figure 6.8b)

5 cm above the clavicle and 1 cm medial to the lateral border of the sternomastoid muscle.

Initial location of the vein with the spinal needle

First locate the vein with the spinal needle threaded inside the 14 gauge needle using the following directions.

Direction of needle and procedure (Figure 6.8c,d,e)

Attach the spinal needle to a saline-filled syringe. Place the point of the spinal needle at the entry site on the skin and point the needle and syringe caudally (A). Swing the syringe and needle laterally until the needle is pointing parallel to the medial border of the sternomastoid muscle (A to B). Elevate the syringe 30° above the coronal plane (B to C). Then advance the spinal needle, maintaining a slight negative pressure in the syringe, until the vein is entered. Thread the 14 gauge needle over the spinal needle into the vein. Remove the spinal needle and thread the catheter centrally. Then remove the needle from the vein and fix the catheter securely.

Success rate

Not stated.

Complications

Not stated.

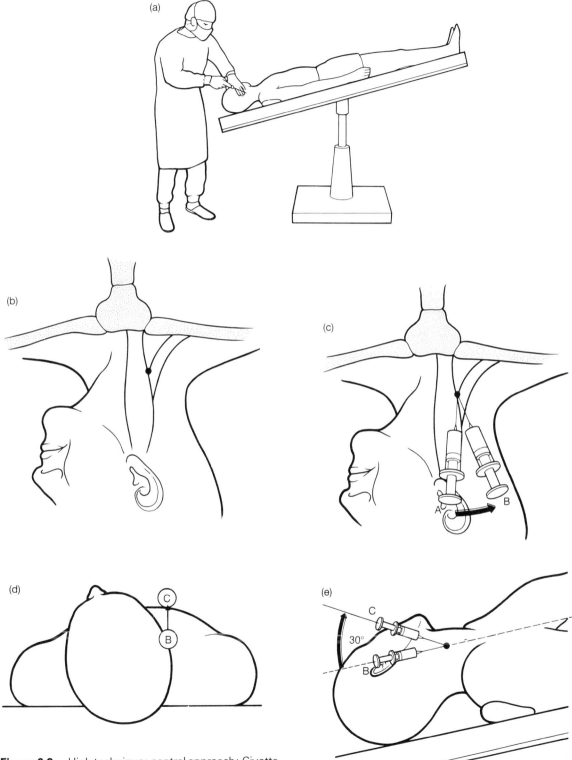

Figure 6.8. High technique: central approach: Civetta and Gabel (1972).[2]

LOW TECHNIQUE: LATERAL APPROACH
Jernigan et al. *(1970)*[26]

Patient category
Adults.

Advantages and disadvantages
Catheters inserted by this route were left *in situ* for 2–3 weeks without complications. The internal jugular route was particularly indicated in a patient with extensive burns because it was the only unburned site available. Other authors often failed to enter the internal jugular vein using this technique and developed alternative modifications.[25] A report has been published of a case of arterial pseudoaneurysm in which a similar technique was used.[32] It was claimed that a Valsalva manoeuvre in the Trendelenburg position distends the vein to a diameter of approximately 2.5 cm. Other authors have found it difficult to thread stiff catheters centrally since the vein is approached almost at a right angle.

Preferred side
Not stated.

Position of patient (Figure 6.9a)
Place the table in a 25° head-down position. Extend the patient's neck by placing a small towel under his shoulders and turn the head away from the side of the puncture. Place both arms by the sides.

Position of operator (Figure 6.9a)
Stand at the head of the patient or on the same side as the puncture site.

Equipment used in original description
Catheter-through-needle.

Advice on current equipment
A guide wire technique is strongly recommended. Long rigid catheter over needle devices should be avoided especially on the left side.

Anatomical landmarks
The sternal and clavicular heads of the sterno-mastoid muscle and the clavicle.

Preparation
Perform the puncture under sterile conditions using local anaesthesia if indicated.

Precautions and recommendations
Avoid hyperinflation of the lung to minimise the risk of a pneumothorax.

Point of insertion of needle (Figure 6.9b)
Two finger breadths above the clavicle on the lateral border of the clavicular head of the sterno-mastoid muscle.

Initial location of vein with small (21)-gauge needle
A fine needle can be used to locate the vein using the following directions. Then, using the fine needle as a guide, puncture the skin with the larger needle attached to a saline-filled syringe.

Direction of needle and procedure (Figure 6.9c,d,e)
Place the point of the needle at the entry site on the skin and point the needle and syringe caudally (A). Swing the syringe and needle laterally to point the needle towards the suprasternal notch (A to B). Elevate the syringe 15° above the coronal plane (B to C). Then advance the needle towards the suprasternal notch, maintaining a slight negative pressure in the syringe. Once the needle enters the vein remove the syringe and thread the wire centrally. Then remove the needle and thread the catheter centrally.

Success rate
Not stated.

Complications
Three major complications occurred during 3 years' use of the technique in 1000 patients (0·3%). All were considered preventable. One patient suffered an air embolus. A second patient developed thrombophlebitis of the internal jugular vein and septicaemia. The infected vein was surgically excised. A catheter should be removed if there is evidence of skin sepsis. In a third patient a central vein was perforated with consequent mediastinal infusion of fluid and a pleural effusion. All patients made a full recovery. The incidence of minor complications was not stated.

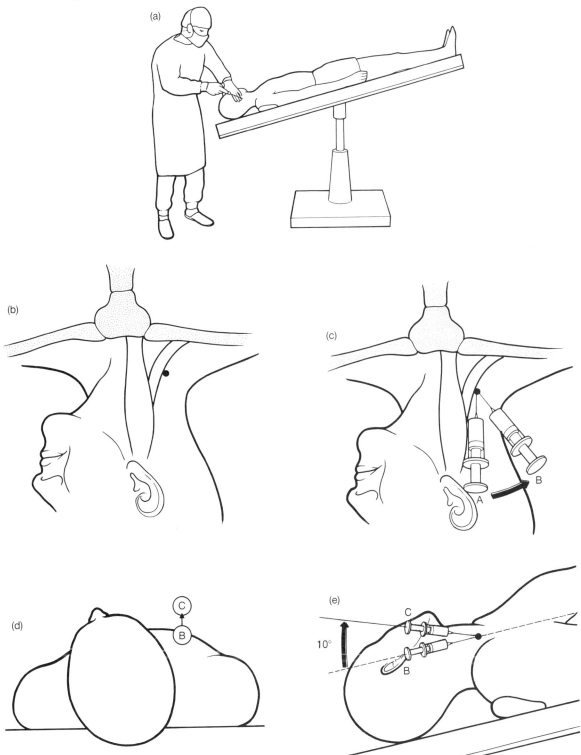

Figure 6.9. Low technique: lateral approach: Jernigan *et al.* (1970)[26].

LOW TECHNIQUE: CENTRAL APPROACH
Daily et al. *(1970)*[33]

Patient category
Adults and children.

Advantages and disadvantages
These authors prefer the internal jugular to the subclavian route for venous catheterisation. The internal jugular vein is more superficial and accessible than the subclavian vein in obese patients. In five patients undergoing cardiac transplantation the internal jugular vein had been previously ligated. The catheters were successfully introduced below the point of ligation. Patients are routinely positioned supine.

Preferred side
The right.

Position of patient (Figure 6.10a)
The patient is placed in a head-down position only if the neck veins collapse during inspiration with the patient horizontal. Extend the patient's neck by placing a small towel under the shoulders and turn the head away from the side of the puncture. Place both arms by the sides.

Position of operator (Figure 6.10a)
Stand at the head of the patient or on the opposite side to the puncture site.

Equipment used in original description
Catheter-through-needle.

Advice on current equipment
A guide wire technique is strongly recommended. Long rigid catheter over needle devices should be avoided especially on the left side.

Anatomical landmarks
The sternal and clavicular heads of the sternomastoid muscle and the clavicle.

Preparation
Perform the puncture under sterile conditions using local anaesthesia if required.

Precautions and recommendations
Avoid hyperinflation of the lung to minimise the risk of pneumothorax.

Point of insertion of needle (Figure 6.10b)
At the centre of the triangle bounded below by the inner edge of the sternal insertion and the outer edge of the clavicular insertion and above by the junction of the two heads of the sternomastoid muscle.

Initial location of vein with small (21)-gauge needle
A fine needle can be used to locate the vein using the following directions. Then, using the fine needle as a guide, puncture the skin with the larger needle attached to a saline-filled syringe.

Direction of needle and procedure
Place the point of the needle at the entry site on the skin and point the needle caudally (A). Elevate the syringe 30° above the coronal plane (A to B). Advance the needle maintaining a slight negative pressure in the syringe. Once the needle enters the vein, remove the syringe and thread the wire centrally. Then remove the needle and thread the catheter centrally. If the vein is not entered initially, redirect the needle 5–10° laterally. Do not direct the needle medially or the artery will be punctured.

Success rate
This technique was used in approximately 100 patients. In 9 patients, puncture of the right internal jugular vein was unsuccessful. In 8 of these, puncture of the left internal jugular vein was then successful.

Complications
In one case cannulation of the left internal jugular vein was performed during operation with a 50 mm catheter. A postoperative chest x-ray showed a left-side pleural effusion and mediastinal widening. This was presumed to be due to fluid infiltrating into the mediastinum. Short cannulae are thus contraindicated. No cases of pneumothorax or air embolism were observed. Cannulae were left *in situ* for from 2 days to 3 weeks without local or systemic infection. Arterial puncture occurred in some cases.

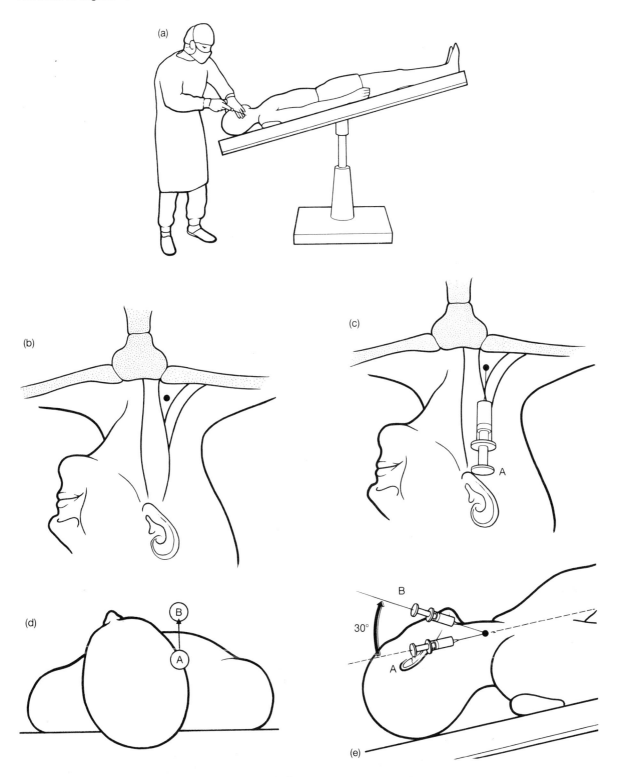

Figure 6.10. Low technique: central approach: Daily
et al (1970)[33].

HIGH TECHNIQUE: CENTRAL APPROACH
Vaughan and Weygandt (1973)[34]

Patient category
Adults and children.

Advantages and disadvantages
The head is positioned in the midline. A very high failure rate (86·5%) with this technique in children under age 2 years led the authors to use a cut-down and abandon this percutaneous technique. It is recommended that the ECG be monitored during cannulation to detect dysrhythmias caused by the catheter tip. In some patients an intravascular ECG was used to check the position of the catheter tip.

Preferred side
The right.

Position of patient (Figure 6.11a)
Place the table in a 15–20° head-down position. Extend the patient's neck by placing a small towel under the shoulders. These authors position the head in the *midline* with the arms by the sides.

Position of operator (Figure 6.11a)
Stand at the head of the patient or on the opposite side to the puncture site.

Equipment used in original description
Catheter-through-needle.

Advice on current equipment
A guide wire technique is strongly recommended. Long rigid catheter over needle devices should be avoided especially on the left side.

Anatomical landmarks
The sternal and clavicular heads of the sterno-mastoid muscle and the clavicle.

Preparation
Perform the puncture under sterile conditions using local anaesthesia if indicated.

Precautions and recommendations
Avoid hyperinflation of the lung to minimise the risk of pneumothorax.

Point of insertion of needle (Figure 6.11b)
At the apex of the triangle bounded below by the inner edge of the sternal insertion and the outer edge of the clavicular insertion and above by the junction of the two heads of the sternomastoid muscle.

Initial location of vein with small (21)-gauge needle
A fine needle can be used to locate the vein using the following directions. Then, using the fine needle as a guide, puncture the skin with the larger needle attached to a saline-filled syringe.

Direction of needle and procedure
Place the point of the needle at the entry site on the skin and point the needle caudally (A). Elevate the syringe about 30° above the skin (A to B). Inject 0.5 ml of saline after the needle has punctured the skin. Advance the needle maintaining a slight negative pressure in the syringe. A click is noted both when the cervical fascia and when the vein wall are punctured. When the vein is entered, remove the syringe and thread the wire centrally. Then remove the needle and thread the catheter centrally. If the first attempt fails, redirect the needle more laterally.

Success rate
The technique was used by junior and senior anaesthetists on 242 cardiac patients aged from 0–65 years with an overall success rate of 93·8% (15 failures). Thirteen failures occurred in 15 attempts (86·5% failure rate) in children aged from 1–2 years, and the authors now avoid percutaneous cannulation in this age group. In 14 adults, right-sided cannulation was unsuccessful but an attempt on the left side succeeded.

Complications
There were 4 (1·6%) major complications, 3 of which required surgical correction. In 2 adults there was persistent bleeding from the left internal jugular vein requiring exploration postoperatively. A 13-month-old child bled from the right pleura as a result of a pulmonary puncture. In a 4-year old child with a ventricular septal defect the catheter tip precipitated a supraventricular tachycardia. In 26 patients (11%) the carotid artery was punctured.

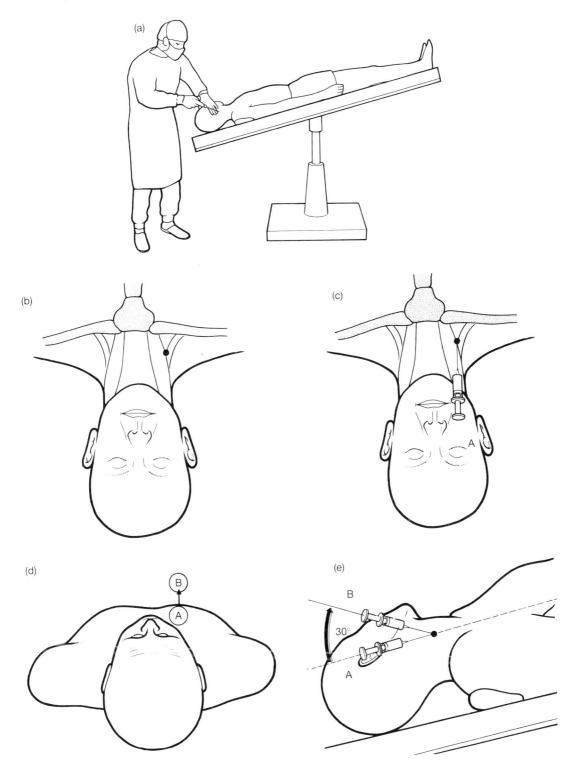

Figure 6.11. High technique: central approach: Vaughan and Weygandt (1973)[34].

LOW TECHNIQUE: CENTRAL APPROACH
Rao et al. *(1977)*[23]

Patient category
Adults and children.

Advantages and disadvantages
This technique avoids the need to identify the sternomastoid muscle, which may be difficult to see or to palpate in obese patients and children. An easily palpable notch on the superior surface of the medial end of the clavicle must be identified. This method gives the highest success rate of all published methods but the low approach introduces a small risk of pneumothorax and trauma. In a comparative trial of this low technique with two high techniques[4,35] in children, the authors recommended using a high approach as it was associated with a lower incidence of significant clinical morbidity.[36] Coté and his colleagues,[36] using this low technique, reported a lower success rate and a higher incidence of major complications than were found by Rao and his colleagues.[23] One death in a child was reported with the use of the low approach.

Preferred side
The right.

Position of patient (Figure 6.12a)
Place the table in a 25° head-down position. Extend the patient's neck by placing a small towel under the shoulders and turn the head away from the side of the puncture. Place both arms by the sides.

Position of operator (Figure 6.12a)
Stand at the head of the patient or on the opposite side to the puncture site.

Equipment used in original description
19 gauge O.D. needle and 22 gauge O.D. catheter for infants younger than 3 months old. 17 gauge O.D. needle and 19 gauge O.D. catheter in children between 4 months and 6 years old. 14 gauge O.D. needle and 17 gauge O.D. catheter for patients older than 6 years.

Advice on current equipment
A guide wire technique is strongly recommended. Long rigid catheter-over-needle devices should be avoided especially on the left side.

Anatomical landmarks (Figure 6.12f)
A notch, 0.25–1 cm from the medial end of the clavicle, is bounded medially by the upward curve of the clavicle and below by its superior surface.

Preparation
Perform the puncture under sterile conditions using local anaesthesia if indicated. All catheterisations in this series were performed under endotracheal anaesthesia.

Precautions and recommendations
Ventilate the lungs manually and avoid hyperinflation to minimise the risk of pneumothorax.

Point of insertion of needle (Figure 6.12b)
Just above the notch on the upper surface of the clavicle.

Initial location of vein with small-gauge needle
A fine needle can be used to locate the vein using the following directions. Then, using the fine needle as a guide, puncture the skin with the larger needle attached to a saline-filled syringe.

Direction of needle and procedure (Figure 6.12c,d,e)
Identify the notch on the clavicle with the left thumb. Place the point of the needle at the entry site on the skin and point the needle caudally (A) with the needle bevel facing medially. Elevate the syringe 30–40° above the coronal plane (A to B). Then advance the needle caudally and posteriorly. A clicking sensation may be noted as the needle penetrates the cervical fascia and also as it penetrates the vein at a depth of 2–4 cm. Remove the syringe and thread the wire centrally. Then remove the needle and thread the catheter centrally.

If the vein is not located, redirect the needle in a slightly lateral direction to the saggital plane. Take a chest x-ray after insertion to exclude a pneumothorax.

Success rate
The procedures were performed both by anaesthesia trainees and by consultants.

There was a 93% success rate on the first attempt

in 192 paediatric patients (ages 21 days to 12 years), and a 97% success rate on the second attempt.

A 94% success rate was achieved on the first attempt in 124 adults, and a 99% success rate on the second attempt.

Complications

The overall complication rate was 2% (6 out of 315). One patient (0·3%) developed a pneumothorax. In two patients (0·6%) the thoracic duct was punctured. In three patients (1%) the carotid artery was punctured.

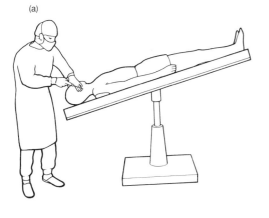

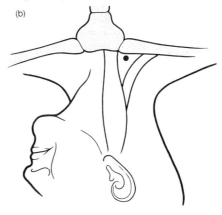

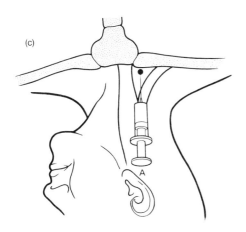

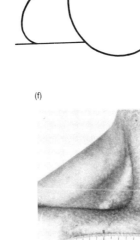

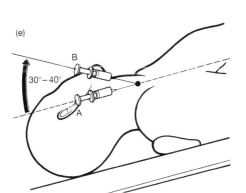

Figure 6.12.   Low technique: central approach: Rao *et al.* (1977)[23].

HIGH TECHNIQUE: CENTRAL APPROACH
English et al. *(1969)[4]: elective method*

Patient category

Adults. This technique is not often used in infants as it is difficult to feel the vein.

Advantages and disadvantages

The elective technique requires muscle relaxation and is the preferred method with general anaesthesia. Both the carotid artery and the internal jugular vein should be palpated. If the vein was not palpable the authors used the alternative technique (see below). In some patients 2 catheters were inserted into the vein, one by the elective technique and one by the alternative technique.

Preferred side

The right.

Position of patient (Figure 6.13a)

Place the table in a 25° head-down position. The neck is extended by placing a small towel under the shoulders and the head is turned away from the side of the puncture. Both arms are placed by the sides.

Position of operator (Figure 6.13a)

Stand at the head of the patient.

Equipment used in original description

200 mm catheter-through-14 gauge needle. Catheters without stylets are recommended for observing the immediate reflux of blood into the catheter.

Advice on current equipment

A guide wire technique is strongly recommended. Long rigid catheter-over-needle devices should be avoided especially on the left side.

Anatomical landmarks

The internal jugular vein, the carotid artery, and the sternomastoid muscle.

Preparation

Perform the puncture under sterile conditions using local anaesthesia if indicated.

Precautions and recommendations

Make sure there is full muscle relaxation. Maintain positive intrathoracic pressure during venous cannulation to distend the vein.

Point of insertion of needle (Figure 6.13b)

Cephalad and medial to where the vein is most clearly felt.

Initial location of the vein with small (21)-gauge needle

Locate the vein with a fine needle using the following directions. Then, using the fine needle as a guide, puncture the skin with the larger needle attached to a saline-filled syringe.

Direction of needle and procedure (Figure 6.13c,d,e)

First palpate the carotid artery and the internal jugular vein with the fingers of the left hand. Place the point of the needle at the entry site on the skin and point the needle caudally (A). Swing the syringe and point the needle slightly laterally (A to B). Elevate the syringe 30–40° above the skin surface (B to C). The needle may pierce the sternomastoid muscle if the internal jugular vein is palpated lateral to its medial edge. Advance the needle, maintaining a slight negative pressure in the syringe. A sensation of 'give' is usually noted both as the deep cervical fascia is pierced and as the vein is entered. Once the needle enters the vein, remove the syringe and thread the wire centrally. Then remove the needle and thread the catheter centrally.

Success rate

The results of the elective and alternative techniques are presented together.

The techniques were used for 500 cannulations of the internal jugular vein in unselected cases of all ages by all members of the anaesthetic department. There were 26 failures (5·2%): 8 (9·4%) failures in 85 patients aged 0–15 years and 18 (4·3%) failures in 415 patients over 15 years. The failure rate was reduced with increasing experience. In 12 cases the vein was entered but the catheter could not be threaded down it.

Complications

Three arterial punctures occurred (0·6%). There was one pneumothorax (0·2%). Internal jugular vein thrombosis did not occur. In one patient the vein was cannulated on four occasions and appeared undamaged by the procedure. The average duration of venous cannulation was 48 hours.

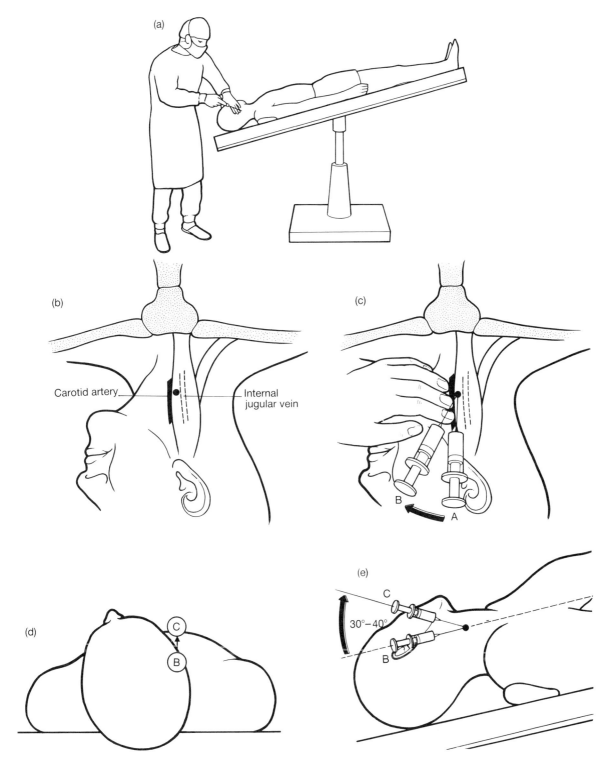

Figure 6.13. High technique: central approach:
English *et al.* (1969)[4], elective method.

LOW TECHNIQUE: CENTRAL APPROACH
English et al. *(1969)*[4]*:alternative method*

Patient category
Adults and children.

Advantages and disadvantages
This method does not require muscular relaxants or palpation of the vein and is used under local anaesthesia in awake patients and in emergencies such as cardiac arrest. It is used when the elective technique has failed or the internal jugular vein is not palpable. It is normally used in children as the vein is difficult to palpate.

Preferred side
The right.

Position of patient
Place the table in a 25° head-down position. The neck is extended by placing a small towel under the shoulders and the head is turned away from the side of the puncture. Both arms are placed by the sides.

Position of operator (Figure 6.14a)
Stand at the head of the patient.

Equipment used in original description
20 mm catheter (without stylet)-through-needle; 14 gauge needle for adults and most children; 17 gauge needle for small children, infants and neonates.

Advice on current equipment
A guide wire technique is strongly recommended. Long rigid catheter-over-needle devices should be avoided especially on the left side.

Anatomical landmarks
The clavicle and the sternal and clavicular heads of insertion of the sternomastoid muscle.

Preparation
Perform the puncture under sterile conditions using local anaesthesia if indicated.

Precautions and recommendations
Avoid hyperventilation of the lung to decrease the risk of pneumothorax.

Point of insertion of needle (Figure 6.14b)
Near the apex of the triangle formed by the sternal and clavicular heads of the sternomastoid muscle and the clavicle.

Initial location of vein with small (21)-gauge needle
Locate the vein with a fine needle using the following directions. Then using the fine needle as a guide, puncture the skin with the larger needle attached to a saline-filled syringe.

Direction of needle and procedure (Figure 6.14c,d,e)
Place the point of the needle at the entry site on the skin and point the needle caudally (A). Swing the syringe and point the needle laterally (A to B). Elevate the syringe 30–40° above the skin surface (B to C). Advance the needle towards the inner border of the anterior end of the first rib behind the clavicle. Once the vein is entered, introduce the wire. Then remove the needle and thread the catheter centrally.

Success rate
See under elective method.

Complications
See under elective method.

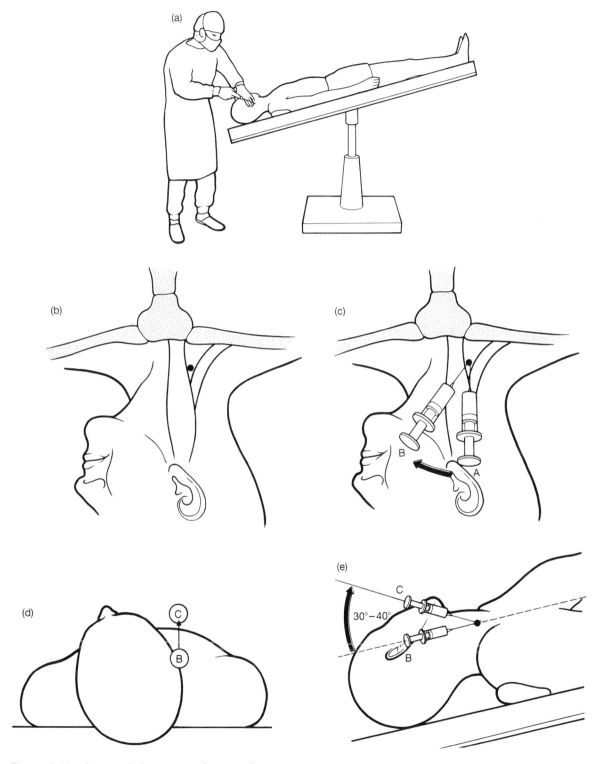

Figure 6.14. Low technique: central approach:
English *et al.* (1969)[4], alternative method.

HIGH TECHNIQUE: CENTRAL APPROACH
Prince et al. *(1976)*[35]

Patient category

Infants and children.

Advantages and disadvantages

This technique was performed under general anaesthesia. Puncture of the internal jugular vein is more difficult in infants than in older children as the landmarks are less apparent and there is often difficulty in threading the catheter into the vein. Internal jugular vein cannulation is considered to be preferable to subclavian vein cannulation in infants. The technique is similar to that used by Daily and his colleagues,[33] who strongly recommended using a fine needle to locate the vein.

Preferred side

The right.

Position of patient (Figure 6.15a)

Place the table in a 15° or 20° head-down position. Extend the patient's neck by placing a small towel under the shoulders and turn the head away from the side of the puncture. Place both arms by the sides.

Position of operator (Figure 6.15a)

Stand at the head of the patient or on the opposite side to the puncture site.

Equipment used in original description

Catheter-through-needle.

Advice on current equipment

A guide wire is strongly recommended. Long rigid catheter-over-needle devices should be avoided especially on the left side.

Anatomical landmarks.

The sternal and clavicular heads of insertion of the sternomastoid muscle and the clavicle.

Preparation

Perform the puncture under sterile conditions.

Precautions and recommendations

Avoid hyperinflation of the lung to minimise the risk of pneumothorax. Care should be taken to avoid the prevertebral area as trauma here can cause Horner's syndrome.

Point of insertion of needle (Figure 6.15b)

At the apex of the triangle formed by the two heads of the sternomastoid muscle and the clavicle.

Initial location of vein with small (21)-gauge needle

Locate the vein with a fine needle using the following directions. Then, using the fine needle as a guide, puncture the skin with the larger needle attached to a saline-filled syringe.

Direction of needle and procedure (Figure 6.15c,d,e)

Place the point of the needle at the entry site on the skin and point the needle caudally (A). Swing the syringe and needle and point the needle laterally towards the ipsilateral nipple (A to B). Elevate the syringe 45° above the skin surface (B to C). Then advance the needle, maintaining a slight negative pressure in the syringe. A loss of resistance is frequently noted on entering the vein, usually within 1–2 cm of the skin surface. Remove the syringe and thread the wire centrally. Then remove the needle and thread the catheter centrally.

Take a chest x-ray to check the position of the catheter tip.

Success rate

The technique was performed by supervised residents familiar with the technique of internal jugular vein cannulation in adults. If cannulation of the right internal jugular vein failed, an attempt was made on the left side. If this failed, an attempt was made to cannulate the external jugular vein. This technique was used on 52 patients aged from 6 weeks to 14 years. Cannulation of right or left vein was successful in 40 patients (77%); 31 on the right and 9 on the left. The success rate in 19 infants aged 6 weeks to 2 years was 68% and in 33 patients aged 2 to 14 years was 82%.

A higher but statistically insignificant success rate was achieved in infants of over 10 kg and in those patients with a central venous pressure higher than 10 cm H_2O.

In 9 of the 12 failures the external jugular vein was then cannulated. One of the left internal jugular vein catheters passed down the left subclavian vein. All the others passed to the superior vena cava or right atrium.

Complications.

The carotid artery was punctured in 12 patients (23%) and resulted in a cervical haematoma in 3 instances (5.7%). Horner's syndrome developed in 2 patients (4%) but both recovered completely.

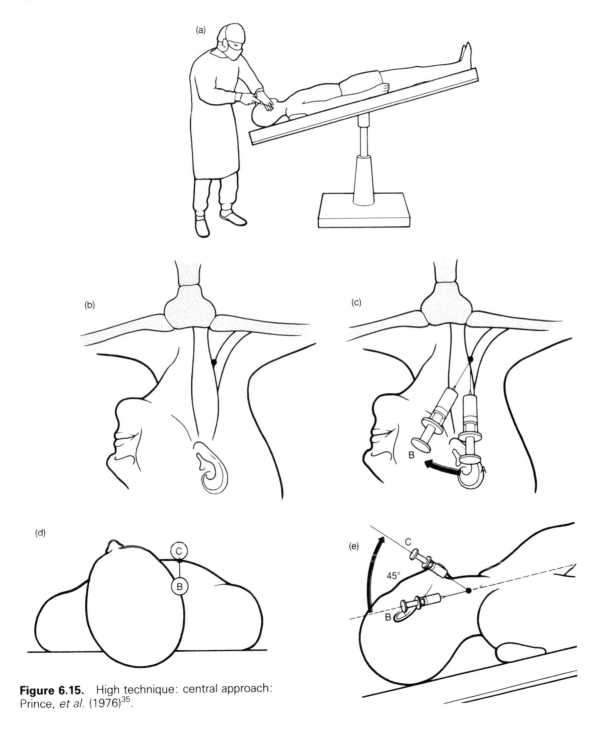

Figure 6.15. High technique: central approach: Prince, *et al.* (1976)[35].

LOW TECHNIQUE: CENTRAL APPROACH
Hall and Geefhuysen (1977)[37]:elective method

Patient category
Children and neonates.

Advantages and disadvantages
This technique has been used for resuscitation on at least 20 occasions, although it was observed that some ill patients were not always able to tolerate the head-down position. It is advisable to learn the technique under favourable conditions before using it in emergencies. (It should be noted that some authors have recommended that subclavian vein cannulation should not be used in emergencies.[38]) The method is easily learned. To avoid infection in these ill, malnourished patients, an arbitrary time limit of 6 days was set, after which the catheter was removed and a fresh catheter inserted.

Preferred side
The right.

Position of patient (Figure 6.16a)
Place the table in a 25° head-down position. Extend the patient's neck by placing a small towel under the shoulders and turn the head away from the side of the puncture. If the procedure is done on the ward, place the head downwards over the edge of the bed. Place both arms by the sides.

Position of operator (Figure 6.16a)
Stand at the head of the patient or on the opposite side to the puncture site.

Equipment used in original description
Catheter (with stylet)-through-needle.

Advice on current equipment
A guide wire technique is strongly recommended. Long rigid catheter-over-needle devices should be avoided especially on the left side.

Anatomical landmarks
The triangle formed by the sternal and clavicular heads of insertion of the sternomastoid muscle and the clavicle.

Preparation
Perform the puncture under sterile conditions using local anaesthesia, except in emergencies.

Precautions and recommendations
The catheter tip should lie in the superior vena cava above the atrium to avoid the risk of atrial perforation and cardiac tamponade.

Point of insertion of needle (Figure 6.16b)
Near the apex of the triangle formed by the two heads of insertion of the sternomastoid muscle.

Initial location of vein with small-gauge needle
Locate the vein with a fine needle using the following directions. Then, using the fine needle as a guide, puncture the skin with the larger needle attached to a saline-filled syringe.

Direction of needle and procedure (Figure 6.16c,d,e)
Place the point of the needle at the entry site on the skin and point the needle caudally (A). Swing the syringe and needle and point the needle slightly laterally (A to B). Elevate the syringe 30° above the skin surface (B to C). Advance the needle maintaining a slight negative pressure in the syringe. The vein is entered behind the medial edge of the clavicular head of the sternomastoid muscle just above the clavicle. Once the vein is entered, remove the syringe and thread the wire centrally. Then remove the needle and thread the catheter centrally. The catheter is connected to the administration set and blood should flow into the set if it is lowered below the head.

Success rate
The combined results of the elective and alternative methods are given together. The technique was used on the ward on 100 frequently critically ill children aged from 2 weeks to 9 years. Venous cannulation was successful in over 90% of attempts. If the elective approach failed, the alternative method was tried.

Complications
No serious complications occurred. Arterial puncture occurred in 3 cases (3%). Bacterial cultures were positive in over 10% of catheter tips removed; in only one was there a correlation between the culture obtained from the catheter tip and a positive blood culture. Conversely, blood cultures were sometimes positive when the tip of the catheter was sterile.

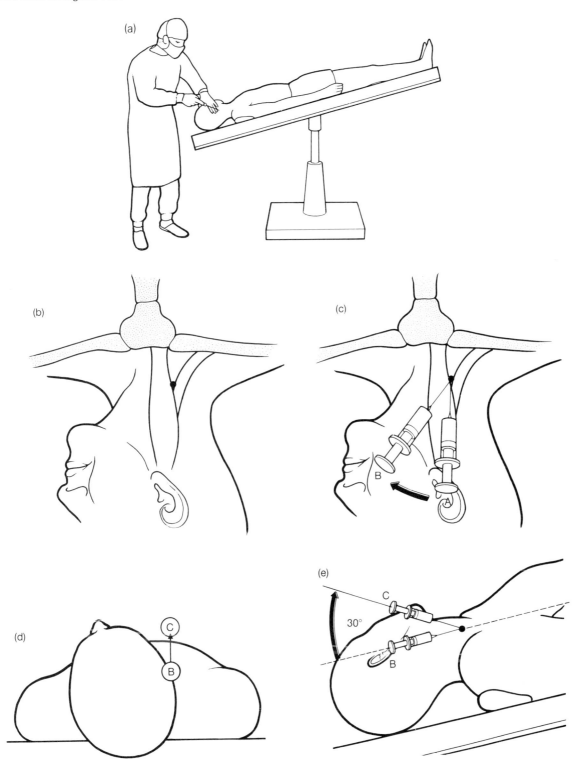

Figure 6.16. Low technique: central approach: Hall and Geefhuysen (1977)[37], elective method.

HIGH APPROACH: LATERAL APPROACH
Hall and Geefhuysen (1977)[37]: alternative method

Patient category
Children and neonates.

Advantages and disadvantages
This technique was used when the elective method failed. The number of elective and alternative attempts is not given.

Preferred side
The right.

Position of patient (Figure 6.17a)
Place the table in a 25° head-down position. Extend the patient's neck by placing a small towel under the shoulders and turn the head away from the side of the puncture. If the procedure is done in the ward, place the head downwards over the edge of the bed. Place both arms by the sides.

Position of operator (Figure 6.17a)
Stand at the head of the patient or on the same side as the puncture site.

Equipment used in original description
Catheter (with stylet)-through-needle.

Advice on current equipment
A guide wire technique is strongly recommended. Long rigid catheter-over-needle devices should be avoided especially on the left side.

Anatomical landmarks
The triangle formed by the sternal and clavicular heads of insertion of the sternomastoid muscle and the clavicle.

Preparation
Perform the puncture under sterile conditions using local anaesthesia, except in emergencies.

Precautions and recommendations
The catheter tip should lie in the superior vena cava above the atrium to avoid the risk of atrial perforation and cardiac tamponade.

Point of insertion of needle (Figure 6.17b)
At the midpoint of the sternomastoid muscle on its lateral edge.

Initial location of vein with small-gauge needle
Locate the vein with a fine needle using the following directions. Then, using the fine needle as a guide, puncture the skin with the larger needle attached to a saline-filled syringe.

Direction of needle and procedure (Figure 6.17c,d,e)
Place the point of the needle at the entry site on the skin and point the needle caudally (A). Swing the syringe and needle and point the needle towards the suprasternal notch (A to B). Elevate the syringe slightly (B to C). Advance the needle maintaining a slight negative pressure in the syringe. Once the vein is entered, proceed as with the elective method.

Success rate
See under elective method.

Complications
See under elective method.

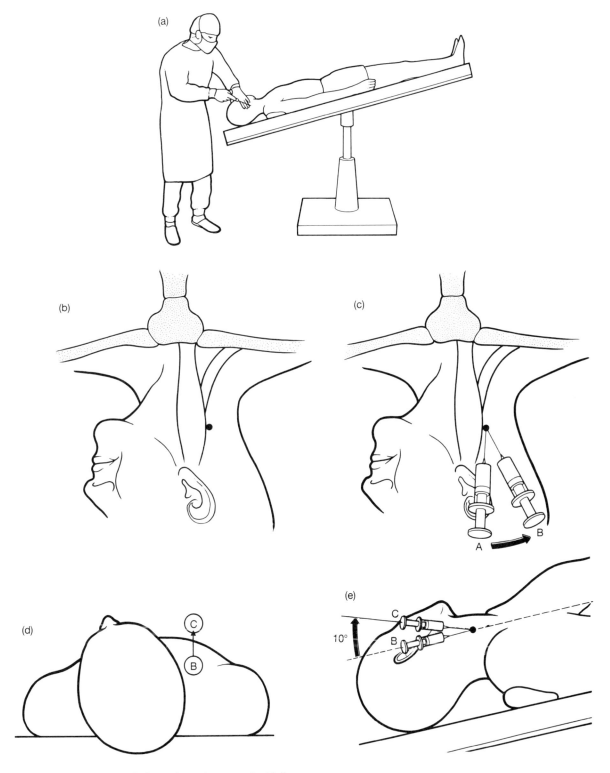

Figure 6.17. High technique: lateral approach: Hall and Geefhuysen (1977),[37] alternative method.

SUMMARY OF TECHNIQUES

The techniques are summarised for comparison in Tables 6.4, 6.5, and 6.6. Although some techniques are described for use in the anaesthetised patient, there is no obvious reason why they cannot be used in conscious patients using local anaesthesia. Other techniques have been described for cannulation of the internal jugular vein.[27,36,39,40-46,119]

Factors influencing the incidence of successful cannulation

A number of factors have been described as increasing the chance of successful venous cannulation and catheter replacement. These include the increasing experience of the operator,[4] cannulation in adults as compared with children,[4,34,40] particularly in children more than 2 years old,[34] and in patients over 10 kg,[35] if the central venous pressure is greater than 10 cm H_2O,[35] using a short 4 cm 18 gauge needle and the Seldinger wire technique,[24] in anaesthetised patients,[41] using the right side,[24,35,40] and using an ultrasound Doppler blood flow detector.[39]

Some factors have been reported to make venous cannulation and central catheter placement less easy. These include severe obesity,[42,43] a short thick neck,[43,44] the presence of a tracheostomy,[42] cannulation of the left side,[24,35,40,45] hypovolaemia[45] and lack of clinical experience. The route has, however, been successfully used in severe hypovolaemia.[46]

Central placement of the catheter tip

Many techniques have been described for cannulating the internal jugular vein. In only a few of these has the position of the catheter tip been fully documented (Table 6.7). The success rate for central placement varies from 100% to 66%. For right-sided cannulation, success rates vary from 100% to 94·3%. The right internal jugular route appears to give the highest incidence of central placement of all routes.

Function of central catheters

It is not uncommon with arm vein catheters inserted centrally to find that either blood cannot be aspirated or the catheters stop giving accurate measurements of the central venous pressure. These catheters have a single distal orifice and it is probable that this is occluded against the vessel wall. Once the position of the catheter is adjusted, blood can often be aspirated. In one report[47] 10% of external jugular vein catheters inserted centrally did not give satisfactory pressure readings until the position was adjusted. We have not found this to be a problem with catheters introduced through the right internal jugular vein, possibly because the catheter comes straight down into the superior vena cava and the distal end does not press against the vein wall. The problem is less likely to occur with catheters possessing side holes as well as a distal orifice.[48]

Complications

The complications and their incidences in the techniques described are shown in Tables 6.4, 6.5 and 6.6. The commonest complication is puncture of the carotid artery; this has an average incidence of approximately 2% but ranges with different techniques from 0%–30% of catheters inserted. Pneumothorax occurred in only 2 of the techniques and in both of these the site of insertion of the needle was low. The incidence in the two techniques was 0·2%[4] and 0.3% respectivey. Other complications reported with these techniques included malposition of the catheter, air embolus, catheter-related infecton, thrombophlebitis of the internal jugular vein, infusion of fluid into the mediastinum or pleural cavity, trauma to the lung, supraventricular tachycardia, puncture of the thoracic duct, Horner's syndrome, and postoperative venous bleeding.

There have been other case reports of complications associated with internal jugular cannulation.[32,49-72] These are shown in Table 6.8. It is important to be aware that these complications can occur, to be able to recognise them, and to be able to institute prompt and effective treatment if required. Some can be avoided by a knowledge and understanding of their aetiology and by using a technique in which the needle has a high point of insertion. As with any technique of central venous cannulation, the distal end of the catheter should not be more than 2 cm below a line joining the lower end of the clavicles, to avoid the possibility of cardiac tamponade.

The list of complications described is formidable. It is noteworthy, however, that we very rarely see major or significant complications in our clinical practice.

We believe that this is because guide wire techniques are now widely used and attention is paid to the recommendations of Table 8.

Conclusion

The internal jugular vein can be successfully cannulated both as an elective procedure and in an emergencey. Catheters can be left *in situ* either for the short term or for the long term. The incidence of central placement of the catheter is greater when the vein on the right, rather than the left, is used.

The overall complication rate for internal jugular vein techniques is much lower than with the subclavian route and the incidence of major complications is very low. Nearly all major complications can be avoided by using a technique in which the needle is inserted high above the clavicle. Proficiency in the selected technique is easily acquired. The internal jugular vein is now used confidently, routinely and safely by anaesthetists all over the world.

Table 6.4. Internal jugular vein – results and complications of techniques used in adults.

Author and year	Point of insertion of needle		Distance between skin and vein (cm)	No. patients or cannulation attempts	No. Successes (%)	Complications	No. complications (as % of catheters inserted)	Personnel	Comments	State of consciousness
	Height	Position								
Boulanger et al. (1976)[21]	High	Medial	2–4	100 cannulation attempts	94 (94)	Carotid artery puncture	2 (2·1)	Supervised inexperienced residents	Method claimed easy to learn	Not stated. Probably both awake or under anaesthesia
Brinkman and Costley (1973)[25]	High	Lateral	5–7	180 cannulation attempts	Not given	Carotid artery puncture	4 (2·2)	Authors	Technique can be used when access to arm and subclavian veins is limited	Awake or under anaesthesia
Mostert et al. (1970)[22]	High	Medial	Not given	133 patients	130 (97·7)	Carotid artery puncture Local tenderness following puncture	2 (1·5) 46 (35·4)	Authors	Technique relies on palpation of carotid artery. This is the technique we use	Awake; we have frequently used this technique under anaesthesia
Civetta et al. (1972)[31]	High	Central	Not given	Not given	Not given	Not given	Not given	Authors and residents	Spinal needle used as alternative to using needle to locate the vein. Technique has also been used for introducing Swan–Ganz catheters.	Awake

| Jernigan et al. (1970)[26] | Low | Lateral | Not given | 1000 patients | Not given | 3 non-fatal major complications in 3 years: (a) Air embolus (b) Thrombophlebitis of the internal jugular vein with septicaemia (c) Mediastinal widening and fluid in left pleural space | 3 (0·3) 1 (0·1) 1 (0·1) 1 (0·1) | Authors | These authors consider the internal jugular vein the first choice for central cannulation | Probably awake |
| Sharrock and Fierro (1983)[29] | High | Central | Not given | 212 patients | 210 (99) | 3 carotid artery punctures | 3 (1·4) | Authors | Used a technique in which the vein was located by inspection only | Under anaesthetic |

Table 6.5. Internal jugular vein – results and complications of techniques used in adults and children.

Author and year	Point of insertion of needle		Distance between skin and vein (cm)	No. patients or cannulation attempts	No. Successes (%)	Complications	No. complications (as % of catheters inserted)	Personnel	Comments	State of consciousness
	Height	Position								
Daily et al. (1970)[33]	Low	Central	Not given	100 patients, ages not given	91 (91) after 1st attempt	Carotid artery puncture	Not given	Authors	Recommended that use of short catheters be avoided	Awake or under anaesthesia
					99 (99) after 2nd attempt	Mediastinal fluid infusion due to use of short catheter	1 (1)			
Vaughan and Weygandt (1973)[34]	High	Central	Not given	242 patients, ages 0–65 + years	227 (93·8)	Carotid artery puncture	26 (11)	Authors	Head positioned in *midline*	Awake or under anaesthesia
				15 patients, ages 1–2 years	2 (13·3)	Bleeding from internal jugular vein postoperatively (adult)	2 (0·9)		These authors had high failure rate in children under 2 years and subsequently introduced catheters using surgical cut-down	
						Supraventricular tachycardia (child)	1 (0·45)			
						Trauma to right lung (child)	1 (0·45)			

Study		Approach		Numbers	Success (%)	Complications n (%)	Operators	Comments	Anaesthesia
Rao et al. (1977)[23]	Very low	Central	2–4	316 patients: 124 adults. 192 children (0–11 years)	311 (98) 123 (99) 188 (97) same after 2nd attempt	Arterial puncture 3 (1·0) Pneumothorax 1 (0·3) Thoracic duct puncture 2 (0·6)	Authors and residents	Bony landmark used. This technique has highest success rate of all methods reviewed. Avoid hyperventilation during insertion	Under anaesthesia
English et al. (1969)[4]	Elective technique High / Alternative technique Low	Central / Central	Not given / Not given	500 patients: 415 adults, 85 children	474 (94·8) 397 (95·6) 77 (90·6)	Arterial puncture with haematoma 3 (0·6) Pneumothorax 1 (0·2)	All members of anaesthetic department	Elective technique requires profound muscle relaxation for palpation of vein. Artery should also be palpated. Alternative technique recommended in small children	Under anaesthesia for elective technique. Awake or under anaesthesia for alternative technique
Oda et al. (1981)[28]	High	Medial	Not given	15 years–adult: 408 5–15 years: 20 1–5 years: 14 6 months–1 year: 7 0–6 months: 7 Totals: 456	396 (97) 18 (90) 13 (92·9) 6 (85.7) 4 (57.1) 437 (95·8)	5 carotid artery punctures 5 (1·1)	Authors	A safe puncture area was described lateral to the carotid artery	Not stated

Table 6.6. Internal jugular vein – results and complications of techniques used in children.

Author and year	Point of insertion of needle		Distance between skin and vein (cm)	No. patients or cannulation attempts	Successes (%)	Complications	No. complications (as % of catheters inserted)	Personnel	Comments	State of consciousness
	Height	Position								
Prince et al. (1976)[35]	High	Central	1–2	52 patients:	40 (77)	Carotid artery puncture	12 (30)	Residents supervised by staff anaesthesiologists	These authors argued strongly against the use of subclavian catheterisation in children	Under anaesthesia
				19 aged between 6 weeks and 2 years	13 (68)	Haematoma Horner's syndrome	3 (7·5) 2 (5)			
				33 aged between 2 years and 14 years	27 (82)					
Hall and Geefhuysen (1977)[37]	*Elective technique* Low Central *Alternative technique* High Lateral		Not given	100 patients ages 2 weeks to 9 years	90 (90)	Carotid artery puncture	3 (3·3)	Authors	Positive bacterial culture in more than 10% of catheter tips removed. These authors avoid the use of rigid cannulae. No serious complications occurred in this series	Awake

Table 6.7. Success rate for central placement of the catheter tip.

Author and year	No. attempted cannulations	No. successful cannulations (%)	No. on right (R) and left (L)	No. central placements: right atrium, superior vena cava, or innominate vein (% of successful venous cannulations)	Position of non-central catheters (No.)	
English et al. (1969)[4]	500	474 (94·8)	Not given	472 (99·6)	Subclavian vein	(2)
Belani et al. (1980)[24]	125	114 (91·2)	111 R	111 (100)	Left superior intercostal vein	(1)
			3 L	2 (66)		
Prince et al. (1976)[35]	52	40 (76·9)	31 R	31 (100)	Subclavian vein	(1)
			9 L	8 (88·9)		
McConnell and Fox (1972)[42]	Not given	70 (–)	Not given	70 (100)		
Baker and Wallace (1976)[43]	100	88 (88)	88 R	83 (94·3)	Not given	(5)
Korshin et al. (1978)[40]	168	156 (92·9)	145 R	141 (97·2)	Subclavian vein	(2)
					Loop in innominate vein	(2)
			11 L	9 (81·8)	Subclavian vein	(1)
					Internal thoracic vein	(1)
Coté et al. (1979)[36]	122	97 (79·5)	Not given	97 (100)		(0)
Malatinsky et al. (1976)[73]	Not given	87 (–)	Not given	82 (94·3)	Loop formation—	
					left	(3)
					right	(2)
Kuramoto and Sakabe (1975)[74]	Not given	50 (–)	25 R	24 (96)	Axillary vein	(1)
			25 L	20 (80)*	Catheter coiled	(5)
Fischer et al. (1977)[75]	Not given	262 (–)	247 R	231 (93·5)	Subclavian vein	(6)
					Internal jugular vein	(10)
			15 L	9 (60)	Subclavian vein	(4)
					Internal jugular vein	(2)

* Central position defined as right atrium, superior vena cava, inferior vena cava, innominate vein, subclavian vein.

Table 6.8. Complications following internal jugular vein cannulation.

Complication	Comments
	ARTERIAL COMPLICATIONS
Carotid artery puncture	This is the commonest complication associated with internal jugular cannulation and occurs in 0.6%[4]–30%[35] of catheters inserted. In most series the incidence varies between 1% and 5%. The severity of ensuing complications is related to the size of the needle entering the artery. If a small gauge seeker needle is used initially the chances of sequelae are minimised. With larger needles severe damage may result. Use if possible a short fine needle and a Seldinger wire technique. If the pleura is also damaged there is the possibility of massive haemorrage and the formation of a haemothorax. If the pleura is not damaged the blood loss will be less and restricted to the tissues in the neck
	There also exists the hazard of unappreciated arterial cannulation which occurred in approximately 0.5% of cases in two reported series [76, 77]
Carotid artery laceration[78]	The carotid artery was entered in two patients with a 16-gauge cannula. In one patient direct repair of the laceration was required. In the other the large haematoma slowly reabsorbed spontaneously. It was recommended that if the artery is damaged with a large needle the patient should not be heparinised and any cardiopulmonary bypass procedure be postponed for a few days. The needle should be left *in situ*, the area explored and the defect repaired before the definitive surgical procedure is commenced
Carotid artery cannulation with 8F catheter sheath[76]	Out of 1021 attempted internal jugular cannulation there were 43 (4·2%) arterial punctures. In five patients this was unrecognised and an 8F catheter sheath was threaded into the carotid artery. Three patients underwent the proposed surgery after delays of 2 hours, 5 days and 13 days. One died 48 hours later of his ischaemic heart disease (perhaps due to the delay), and the other died of hemorrhage (a haemothorax) 12 hours later
	It was recommended that a pressure wave form should initially be obtained before passing the sheath. If an 8F sheath is accidentally placed in the carotid artery the neck should be explored and any arterial damage repaired
	However, in three other patients accidental carotid artery puncture with a 7·5F introducer sheath was treated by 5 minutes compression over the artery after immediate removal of the sheath. The patients were heparinised within 2 hours and no adverse sequelae were observed[79]
Avoidance of carotid artery puncture sequelae[77]	Following the above study the authors used the external jugular vein as the first choice route and the internal jugular vein as the second choice. In addition when using the internal jugular vein the intravascular wave form was monitored from the 20-gauge catheter before inserting the 8 introducer sheath. The incidence of carotid artery puncture was 4·5%. There were 4/710 clinically inapparent carotid artery punctures in which carotid artery damage with the 8F introducer was avoided by detection of arterial placement of the 20-gauge catheter by wave form monitoring
Carotid artery aneurysm[80]	Cannulation of the right internal jugular vein of a patient with an abdominal aortic aneurysm was performed during resuscitation. The cannulation was apparently uneventful but the patient developed a dissecting aneurysm of the common carotid artery. This was thought to have been due to the catheterisation procedure
Fistula between the common carotid artery and the internal jugular vein[81]	This was treated surgically and there were no further complications

Table 6.8. Continued.

Complication	Comments
	ARTERIAL COMPLICATIONS (continued)
Cervical *arteriovenous fistulae* following internal jugular vein catheterisation[82]	Five cases were treated by percutaneous transarterial occlusion with a detachable balloon. Such fistulae are most common between the vertebral artery and vein but may also form between the inferior thyroid artery and internal jugular vein. Such fistulae can also be closed by surgical ligation
Fistula between right *vertebral artery* and vertebral venous plexus[83]	Produced by unsuccessfully attempting to thread a 14-gauge needle over a spinal needle as described by Civetta *et al*[31]. The patient complained of tinnitus postoperatively and a continuous to-and-fro mumor was audible in the neck. A surgical repair was required
Severed *thyro-cervical artery*[84]	Carotid artery puncture occurred at attempted internal jugular catheterisation and resulted in haematoma formation. After open heart surgery anticoagulants were started and the haematoma increased in size and became tense. At surgical exploration the thyro-cervical artery was found to be severed
Laceration of *vertebral artery* near its origin with the subclavian artery[85]	An unsuccessful attempt was made to cannulate the right internal jugular vein with a 14-gauge introducer needle. At the end of the operation there was cervical bruising and a large haematoma was drained. Two hours later the patient collapsed and internal cardiac massage was performed. The patient also required large volume infusions of blood, colloid and crystalloid. Exploration of the neck revealed that lacerated vertebral artery which was tied off. The patient recovered
Disconnected *right subclavian artery*[86]	Three Wallace cannula inserted into one internal jugular vein caused a large right sided haemothorax. The patient required large quantities of blood, FFP and platelets. Surgical exploration revealed that the subclavian artery was disconnected at its junction with the common carotid. This was repaired and the patient spent 8 days on intensive care. The use of Seldinger techniques was advocated
Damage to *ascending cervical artery*[58]	The ascending cervical artery was damaged prior to cardiac surgery when an unsuccessful attempt was made to cannulate the right internal jugular vein. Fatal post-operative haemorrhage occurred. Early surgical exploration is mandatory if this complication is suspected
Aortic catheterisation[67]	Occurred in child with transposition of great arteries with use of low approach to vein on right side
Aortic dissection[68]	Followed a number of attempts at venous catheterisation when using 7 cm needle and catheter
Pseudoaneurysm of the brachiocephalic arteries[32]	Three cases of cervical arterial pseudoaneurysms occurred due to arterial laceration following low lateral approach for cannulation of vein. Pseudoaneurysms were treated surgically. It appears that this approach should be avoided
Cardiac arrest[69]	Compression of carotid artery following accidental arterial puncture resulted in cardiac arrest. ECG monitoring is recommended during cannulation for early diagnosis
Ventricular fibrillation[70]	Ventricular fibrillation during carotid artery palpation prior to internal jugular vein cannulation. Care during arterial palpation was advocated

Table 6.8. Continued.

Complication	Comments
	VENOUS COMPLICATIONS
Post-operative cervical haematoma requiring surgical evacuation[63]	This occurred after an unsuccessful attempt at internal jugular vein cannulation in a patient who underwent coronary artery surgery. The haematoma was removed 6 weeks post-operatively
Respiratory obstruction due to cervical haematoma[64]	A large cervical haematoma followed venous cannulation in a patient with coagulation defects. It was recommended that arm veins should be used in such patients for central venous cannulation
Cervical haematoma[87]	This occurred in 10 out of 1000 patients with coagulopathies after internal jugular vein cannulation. It was not stated if the carotid artery had been punctured in any of these 10 patients. In one patient the haematoma compressed the airway and required surgical drainage. The carotid artery had not been punctured in this patient
Superior vena cava thrombosis[65]	This developed 5 days after venous cannulation in a 72-year-old woman. Thrombectomy was undertaken using cardiopulmonary bypass
Superior vena cava syndrome[66]	The catheter passed through a narrowed segment of the superior vena cava and symptoms of obstruction developed. These resolved on removal of the catheter
Cardiac tamponade[71]	This can be caused by central venous catheters, introduced by any route, if the catheter tip lies below the line of pericardial reflection and perforates the vascular wall. However, this is least likely to arise with the right internal jugular vein route, probably because the catheter tip lies clear of vessel wall
Fatal tamponade after left internal jugular catheter[88]	Five days after a left-sided internal jugular vein catheter was inserted a 74-year-old woman developed a cardiac tamponade and died. A tract was demonstrated linking the superior vena cava with the pericardial cavity which contained 450 ml of blood. *Avoid rigid catheters* particularly on the *left* side and keep the tip of the catheter above the line of the pericardial reflection
Axillary vein thrombosis[89]	This occurred in 2 of 63 patients with long-term (mean 93 days) Hickman catheters
Internal jugular vein thrombosis following insertion of PA catheters[90]	These authors found a 66% incidence of internal jugular vein thrombosis demonstrated either by venography or at autopsy
Failure to demonstrate internal jugular vein thrombosis following insertion of PA catheters[91-93]	Late studies however have failed to demonstrate evidence of venous thrombosis when using ultrasound or venography after short-term (1–3 days) catheterisation
Bilateral thrombosis of internal jugular veins[94]	This is very rare and occurred in a 75-year-old man who had both veins catheterised twice in a 14-day period. The patient developed a hemiparesis and died. At autopsy both veins were occluded by thrombosis but there was no obvious cerebral pathology
Atrial thrombus[125,126]	A prospective study of postmortems in patients with a central venous catheter showed a 5% incidence of right atrial thrombus.[125] Diagnosis in vivo is by echocardiography and treatment is by anticoagulation, thrombolysis or surgery.[126] There was a 29% mortality in patients with atrial thrombus diagnosed in vivo.
Septic atrial thrombus[127]	This developed postoperatively in a 77-year-old man and was demonstrated by echocardiography. A pulmonary artery catheter was inserted postoperatively to facilitate haemodynamic management. Treatment with heparin and antibiotics was successful.

Table 6.8. Continued.

Complication	Comments
	VENOUS COMPLICATIONS (continued)
Jugular vein thrombosis and hydrocephalus	See Neurological section

PLEURAL COMPLICATIONS

One of the factors that encouraged the move from subclavian to internal jugular vein catheterisation was the latter's apparent freedom from pleural complications especially pneumothorax. These complications are rare and nearly always avoidable with internal jugular cannulation. A short needle and a high approach in the neck should be used. They are, however, relatively frequent and unavoidable when the subclavian vein is cannulated

Tension pneumothorax[54]	After preperative insertion of a cannula into the right internal jugular vein a tension pneumothorax was diagnosed during operation. Nitrous oxide administration should be discontinued if this occurs and the pneumothorax should be released
Bilateral hydrothorax[55]	The internal jugular vein catheter slipped out of the vein and intravenous fluid accumulated in the pleural spaces
Bilateral hydrothorax[56]	It is sometimes possible for fluid under pressure in one pleural cavity to flow into the opposite plural cavity
Mediastinal fluid extravasation in 2 infants following the use of the infusion pump (1 fatality)[57]	Extravasation of fluid into the mediastinum was reported in two infants associated with the use of an infusion pump. Only gravity-fed devices for delivering fluid should be used in infants and neonates
Fatal haemothorax following damage to the ascending cervical artery[58]	The ascending cervical artery was damaged prior to cardiac surgery when an unsuccessful attempt was made to cannulate the right internal jugular vein. Fatal postoperative haemorrhage occurred. Early surgical exploration is mandatory if this complication is suspected
Contralateral effusion of Intralipid[120]	Late perforation of the innominate vein probably occurred following the use of a rigid 5 inch catheter in the right internal jugular vein
Contralateral hydrothorax[95]	Six cases were described of the development of delayed right-sided hydrothorax after *left* jugular cannulation. All patients recovered uneventfully after removal of the catheters and placement of chest drains. A stiff catheter can produce gradual vein wall erosion and perforation. Avoid rigid polyethylene or Teflon catheters and use soft polyurethane catheters and Seldinger techniques
	Naturally if the perforation occurs below the line of the pericardial reflection tamponade can result
	This complication is unlikely to occur with right internal jugular catheter as the catheter goes straight down the lumen of the vein and the tip does not abut against the vein wall
Catheter tip not recognised as being in pleural cavity[28]	The catheter entered the pleural cavity in a patient with a traumatic heamopneumo thorax. Blood could be aspirated from the cavity. Check rate of drainage from the chest against the rate of infusion of fluid via the catheter
Contralateral hydrothorax[96]	Five out of eight patients who had a left-sided Teflon (Wallace Flexihub) internal jugular vein catheter inserted showed evidence of venous wall perforation two days after insertion of the catheter. None of nine patients with right-sided catheters showed evidence of perforation. Four of five patients who developed confirmed perforations had either no symptoms or mild shoulder tip pain. *Avoid* using *rigid* Teflon *catheters* on the *left* side

Table 6.8. Continued.

Complication	Comments
	NEUROLOGICAL COMPLICATIONS
Bilateral vocal cord paralysis[59]	This occurred after bilateral attempts at internal jugular vein cannulation. Cervical haematomas caused temporary dysfunction of the recurrent laryngeal nerves and a tracheostomy was required
Extensive neurological damage[60]	Lesions of the left 9–12 cranial nerves, anterior primary rami of the left 2–4 cervical nerves and a left Horner's syndrome occurred after jugular cannulation. These were caused by pressure from haematoma or by chemical damage from extravasated fluid and the drugs it contained. These lesions resulted in chronic pulmonary aspiration and contributed to the patient's death
Horner's syndrome[61]	This was caused by damage to the cervical sympathetic trunk either by needle or from a haematoma. The sympathetic trunk lies behind the carotid artery but outside the carotid sheath
Ipsilateral mydriasis following accidental carotid artery puncture[97]	A dilated pupil unreactive to light was noted 1 hour after accidental carotid artery puncture. Pupil size spontaneously returned to normal over the next 10 days. Transient irritation of the sympathetic trunk occurred secondary to needle trauma or haematoma. Such mydriasis could proceed to a typical Horner's syndrome
Permanent right phrenic nerve injury[98]	This occurred following repeated unsuccessful attempts to insert a temporary transvenous pacemaker into the right internal jugular vein. The patient developed rapid onset shortness of breath and hypoxaemia. The symptoms rapidly improved but the paralysis of the right hemidiaphragm persisted
Transient phrenic nerve paralysis[99]	Right shoulder tip pain was experienced during insertion of a seeker needle. Two ml of 1% lignocaine were injected as the needle was removed. The catheter entered the vein but could not be advanced into the vein. Shortness of breath was noticed 15 minutes after the lignocaine injection. An x-ray showed an elevated right hemidiaphragm. This had returned to normal 10 hours later
Intermittent hiccups for 8 days[24]	Following accidental carotid artery puncture a right paratracheal haematoma developed which caused phrenic nerve irritation. The hiccups ceased when the haematoma resolved
Transient brachial plexus lesions[100]	Paraesthesiae or muscle weakness occurs after cardiac surgery in 5–13% of cases. This may be due to sternal retraction, fractured ribs, or to trauma to the phrenic nerve during internal jugular vein cannulation
Paralysis of C5[101]	A flaccid paralysis of the arm developed 24 hours after uneventful left-sided internal jugular cannulation. 20 days later EMG analysis showed complete denervation of C5. The possible causes of nerve damage are: – Needle trauma – Diffusion of local anaesthetic – Haematoma compressing a nerve – Action of drugs or fluids escaping from the vein.
Isolated hypoglossal nerve palsy[102]	A right hypoglossal nerve palsy was noted after right internal jugular vein cannulation. This recovered spontaneously over 8 weeks. The patient noted difficulties in moving his tongue and in mastication. A high medial approach was used and the cause of the palsy was thought to be due to direct trauma or haematoma around an aberrant hypoglossal nerve
Lesion of vagus nerve[103]	This occurred in five patients after internal jugular vein cannulation. The main symptoms were hoarseness, problems with deglutition and aspiration into the respiratory tract

Table 6.8. Continued.

Complication	Comments
NEUROLOGICAL COMPLICATIONS (continued)	

Complication	Comments
Cerebrovascular accident during jugular vein cannulation[104]	Six cases were reviewed where carotid artery puncture occurred followed by manual compression of the puncture site. Contralateral hemiparesis ensued. The cause was thought to have been dissection of the intima of the carotid artery, dislodgment of atheromatous plaques or manual pressure. Haematoma compressing the carotid artery was not thought to be a common contributing cause of the problem. One patient developed the hemiparesis immediately and died 8 hours later. The mean age of the patients involved was 68 years
	Stroke has also been reported as a complication of carotid sinus massage and it was recommended that such massage should be avoided in elderly patients[105]
Cerebral embolus resulting in hemiparesis[106]	The right carotid artery was accidentally cannulated with a large French Cordis introducer. Removal was delayed for 96 hours and a left hemiparesis developed 18 hours after surgery for removal. The authors stressed the need for recognition of arterial puncture and immediate removal of cannulae inadvertently placed in the carotid artery
Bilateral thrombosis of internal jugular veins[94]	This is very rare and occurred in a 75-year-old man who had both veins catheterised twice in a 14-day period. The patient developed a hemiparesis and died. At autopsy both veins were occluded by thrombosis but there was no obvious cerebral pathology
Air embolus after accidental removal of catheter with cannula left in vein[62]	Cardiac arrest occurred secondary to air embolus. The patient suffered cerebral damage and failed to regain consciousness. Introducing cannulae should be removed from the vein after the catheter has been inserted and the catheter should be securely stitched in place
Earache following internal jugular vein cannulation[107] (auricular branch of X, tympanic branch of IX)	The adventitial sheath of the vein is supplied by unmyelinated nerve fibres that are stimulated if the vein is distended. The proximal jugular vein is supplied by the vagus and the distal part of the vein is supplied by the glossopharyngeal nerve. Venous distention and stimulation of the auricular branch of the vagus and or the tympanic branch of the glossopharyngeal nerve resulted in referred pain in the ear. The arm vein catheter had gone up into the internal jugular vein and its tip lay level with the mastoid. Pain relief was obtained by withdrawing the catheter a few cm
The 'ear-gurgling' sign[108]	In five cases catheters inserted into the infraclavicular subclavian vein went up the internal jugular vein. On administration of fluid an unpleasant gurgling or swishing sound was heard by the patient. The sound was magnified by increasing fluid flow and stopped when the infusion was clamped
	A buzzing sensation in the ear on the rapid insertion of 10 ml of saline into such a catheter has been described.[109] This was thought to have been due to turbulence in the internal jugular vein being transmitted to the auditory ossicles. If the neck is compressed when an arm vein catheter goes into the internal jugular vein then there is a rise of central venous pressure of approximately 10 cm of water
Unsuspected cerebral perfusion of noradrenaline and lignocaine[110]	This occurred following insertion of a subclavian catheter to help in the resuscitation of a 48-year-old female. The catheter went up into the internal jugular vein. The patient complained of headache prior to a systemic pressor effect with the noradrenaline and later became stuporose following infusion of lignocaine

Table 6.8. Continued.

Complication	Comments

NEUROLOGICAL COMPLICATIONS (continued)

Unsuspected cerebal perfusion of hyperosmolar alimentation fluid[111]	A subclavian feeding catheter went up into the jugular vein. Six days after starting the infusion the patient developed pain in the ear and neck. Five days later she developed an upper motor neuron lesion of the V and VII cranial nerves and a right parietal infarct was demonstrated associated with a cortical venous thrombosis. It was recommended that the catheter tip should be demonstrated to be in the superior vena cava before infusion of hyperosmolar fluid is started
Pseudo tumour cerebri[112]	A left subclavian catheter used for feeding accidentally went into the left internal jugular vein. The patient developed headache, diplopia, bilateral papilloedema and a partial right VI nerve paresis. A thrombosis of the internal jugular vein and the transverse sinus was demonstrated. The patient recovered after treatment with steroids and anticoagulants
Communicating hydrocephalus related to prolonged total parenteral nutrition (TPN) and jugular vein thrombosis[113]	Four cases were described of communicating hydrocephalus in very young children. It was believed that this occurred after both internal jugular veins had been used for TPN and the veins had subsequently thrombosed
Accidental insertion of a Swan–Ganz catheter into the intrathecal space[114]	A guide wire was threaded centrally after an attempt to locate the internal jugular vein. The Swan–Ganz catheter was advanced 20 cm centrally. When the balloon was inflated it was noticed that the patient's right leg twitched. An x-ray showed that the catheter was in the spinal canal and it was immediately removed. No permanent neurological sequelae were noted. Guide wires should never be advanced unless there is free flow of blood

Miscellaneous

Infection[37,89,124,115]	The incidence of positive tip culture has been reported as 5·6%[124], 6%[115], and greater than 10%[37] in catheters removed from children. This incidence did not imply catheter related septicaemia or endocarditis. In a series of long-term catheters (mean 98 days) in adults five out of 71 catheters had to be removed as a result of sepsis[89]
Puncture of cuff of tracheal tube[49]	A complication which results if the needle is directed too far medially. No other complication resulted from puncture of the trachea in this patient
Tracheal perforation and puncture of cuff of tracheal tube[116]	This occurred in two patients when a posterior approach was used to catheterise the jugular vein. It was recommended that the posterior route should be avoided if possible. Both patients recovered uneventfully. Subcutaneous emphysema, pneumomediastinum or air trapping between the pleura and the chest wall can follow this complication
Oesophageal perforation[117]	A 17-year-old girl had an oesophageal stricture and a pre-stenotic dilation. The dilated oesophagus was perforated three times during attempted right sided venous cannulation. A large amount of thick clear fluid was aspirated. Eight hours later she developed chest pain, and an elevated temperature. She was treated with antibiotics and recovered

REFERENCES

1. Benotti, P. N., Bothe, A., Miller, J. D. B. and Blackburn, G. L. (1977). Safe cannulation of the internal jugular vein for long term hyperalimentation. *Surgery, Gynecology and Obstetrics*, **144**, 574.

2. Civetta, J. M. and Gabel J. C. (1972). Flow directed pulmonary artery catheterization in surgical patients: indications and modifications of technic. *Annals of Surgery* **176**, 753.

3. Hess, W. and Tarnow, J. (1978). Ein Verfahren zur gleichzeiter Pazierung von zwei zentralen Katheteren über ein V. jugularis interna. *Anaesthesist* **27**, 579.

4. English, I. C. W., Frew, R. M., Pigott, J. F. and Zaki, M. (1969). Percutaneous catheterization of the internal jugular vein. *Anaesthesia* **24**, 521.

5. Escarpa, A. and Gomez-Arnau, J. (1983). Internal jugular vein catheterization: time required with several techniques under different clinical situations. *Anesthesia and Analgesia* **62**, 97.

6. Oda, M., Fukushima, Y., Hirota, T., Tanaka, A., Aono, M. and Sato, T. (1981). The para-carotid approach for internal jugular catheterization. *Anaesthesia* **36**, 896.

7. Stotter, A. T., Sim, A. J. W. and Dudley, H. A. F. (1984). The insertion of intravenous feeding catheters: comparing internal jugular and subclavian approaches. *British Journal of Parenteral Therapy* 193.

8. Reynolds, A. D., Cross, R. and Latto, I. P. (1984). Comparison of internal jugular and central venous pressure measurements. *British Journal of Anaesthesia* **56**, 267.

9. Sharrock, N. E. and Fierro, L. E. (1983). Jugular venous pulsations as the sole landmark for percutaneous internal jugular cannulation. *British Journal of Anaesthesia* **55**, 1213.

10. Goldfarb, G. and Lebrec, D. (1982). Percutaneous cannulation of the internal jugular vein in patients with coagulopathies: an experience based on 1000 attempts. *Anesthesiology* **56**, 321.

11. Andrews, P. J. D., Dearden, N. M. and Miller, J. D. (1991). Jugular bulb cannulation: description of a cannulation technique and validation of a new continuous monitor *British Journal of Anaesthesia* **67**: 55.

12. Bazaral, M. and Harlan, S. (1981). Ultrasonographic anatomy of the internal jugular vein relevant to percutaneous cannulation. *Critical Care Medicine* **9**, 307.

13. Tryba, M., Kleine, P. and Zenz, M. (1982). Sonographic studies for optimizing the cannulation of the internal jugular vein. *Anaesthetist* **31**, 626.

14. Legler, D. and Nugent, M. (1984). Doppler localization of the internal jugular vein facilitates central venous cannulation. *Anesthesiology* **60**, 481.

15. Ullman, J. I. and Stoelting, R. K. (1978). Internal jugular vein location with the ultra-sound Doppler blood flow detector. *Anesthesia and Analgesia* **57**, 118.

16. Lee, K. C. and Chinyanga, M. (1985). Use of a modified doppler flow detector for percutaneous cannulation of the internal jugular vein. *Canadian Anaesthetists' Society Journal* **32**, 548.

17. Bond, D. M., Champion, L. K. and Nolan, R. (1989). Real-time ultrasound imaging aids jugular venipuncture. *Anesthesia and Analgesia* **68**, 698.

18. Troianos, C. A., Jobes, D. R. and Ellison, N. (1990). Ultrasound guided cannulation of the internal jugular vein. *Anaesthesiology* **72**, A450.

19. Metz, S., Horrow, J. C. and Balcar, I. (1984). A controlled comparison of techniques for locating the internal jugular vein using ultrasonography. *Anesthesia and Analgesia* **63**, 673.

20. Latto, I. P. and Hilton, P. J. (1986). Multiple cannulation of a single vein. *Anaesthesia* **41**, 559.

21. Boulanger, M., Delva, E., Mailléet, J. G. and Paiment, B. (1976). Une nouvelle voie d'abord de la veine jugulaire interne. *Canadian Anaesthetists' Society Journal* **23**, 609.

22. Mostert, J. W., Kenny, G. M. and Murphy, G. P. (1970). Safe placement of central venous catheter into internal jugular veins. *Archives of Surgery* **101**, 431.

23. Rao, T. L. K., Wong, A. Y. and Salem, M. R. (1977). A new approach to percutaneous catheterization of the internal jugular vein. *Anesthesiology* **46**, 362.

24. Belani, K. G., Buckley, J. J., Gordon, J. R. and Castaneda, W. (1980). Percutaneous cervical central venous line placement: a comparison of the internal and external jugular vein routes. *Anesthesia and Analgesia* **59**, 40.

25. Brinkman, A. J. and Costley, D. O. (1973). Internal jugular venipuncture. *Journal of the American Medical Association* **223**, 182.

26. Jernigan, W. R., Gardner, W. C., Mahr, M. M. and Milburn, J. L. (1970). Use of the internal jugular vein for placement of central venous catheter. *Surgery, Gynecology and Obstetrics* **130**, 520.

27. Hermosura, B., Vanags, L. and Dickey, M. W. (1966). Measurement of pressure during intravenous therapy. *Journal of the American Medical Association* **195**, 321.

28. Pina, J. Morujao, N. and Castro-Tavares, J. (1992) Internal jugular catheterisation. Blood reflux is not a reliable sign in patients with thoracic trauma. *Anaesthesia* **47**: 30.

29. Sharrock, N. E. and Fierro, L. E. (1983). Jugular venous pulsations as the sole landmark for percutaneous internal jugular cannulation. *British Journal of Anaesthesia* **55**, 1213.

30. Macdonald, D. J. F. (1984). Locating the internal jugular vein. *British Journal of Anaesthesia* **56**, 1447.

31. Civetta, J. M., Gabel, J. C. and Gemer, M. (1972). Internal-jugular-vein puncture with a margin of safety. *Anesthesiology* **36**, 622.

32. Shield, C. F., Richardson, J. D., Buckley, C. F. and Hagood, C. O. (1975). Pseudoaneurysm of the brachiocephalic arteries: a complication of percutaneous internal jugular vein catheterization. *Surgery* **78**, 190.

33. Daily, P. O., Griepp, R. B. and Shumway, N. E. (1970). Percutaneous internal jugular vein cannulation. *Archives of Surgery* **101**, 534.

34. Vaughan, R. W. and Weygandt, G. R. (1973). Reliable

percutaneous central venous pressure measurement. *Anesthesia and Analgesia, Current Researches* **52**, 709.

35. Prince, S. R., Sullivan, R. L. and Hackel, A. (1976). Percutaneous catheterization of the internal jugular vein in infants and children. *Anesthesiology* **44**, 170.

36. Cote, C. J., Jobes, D. R., Schwartz, A. J. and Ellison, N. (1979). Two approaches to cannulation of a child's internal jugular vein. *Anesthesiology* **50**, 371.

37. Hall, D. M. B. and Geefhuysen. J. (1977). Percutaneous catheterization of the internal jugular vein in infants and children. *Journal of Pediatric Surgery* **12**, 719.

38. Groff, D. B. and Ahmed, N. (1974). Subclavian vein catheterization in the infant. *Journal of Pediatric Surgery* **9**, 171.

39. Ullman, J. I. and Stoelting, R. K. (1978). Internal jugular vein location with the ultrasound Doppler blood flow detector. *Anesthesia and Analgesia, Current Researches* **57**, 118.

40. Korshin, J., Klauber, P. V., Christensen, V. and Skovsted, P. (1978). Percutaneous catheterization of the internal jugular vein. *Acta Anaesthesiologica Scandinavica, Supplement* **67**, 27.

41. Johnson, F. E. (1978). Internal jugular vein catheterization. *New York State Journal of Medicine*, **78**, 2168.

42. McConnell, R. Y. and Fox, R. T. (1972). Experience with percutaneous internal jugular-innominate vein catheterization. *California Medicine* **117**, 1.

43. Baker, J. D. and Wallace, C. T. (1976). Internal jugular central venous pressure monitoring. A panacea? *Anesthesiology Review* March, 15.

44. Defalque, R. J. (1974). Percutaneous catheterization of the internal jugular vein. *Anesthesia and Analgesia. Current Researches* **53**, 116.

45. Stevens, J. C. and Hamit, H. F. (1978). A simple method for percutaneous cannulation of the internal jugular vein. *American Journal of Surgery* **135**, 722.

46. Masud, K. Z. and Forster, K. J. (1973). Percutaneous internal jugular vein catheterization. *Michigan Medicine* **72**, 699.

47. Blitt, C. D., Wright, W. A., Petty, W. C. and Webster, T. A. (1974). Central venous catheterization via the external jugular vein. A technique employing the J-wire. *Journal of the American Medical Association* **229**, 817.

48. Stoelting, R. K. and Haselby, K. A. (1974). Evaluation of a catheter with two side holes for external jugular vein catheterization. *Anesthesia and Analgesia. Current Researches* **53**, 628.

49. Blitt, C. D. and Wright, W. A. (1974). An unusual complication of percutaneous internal jugular vein cannulation, puncture of an endotracheal tube cuff. *Anesthesiology* **40**, 306.

50. Lingenfelter, A. L., Guskiewicz, R. A. and Munson, E. S. (1978). Displacement of right atrial and endotracheal catheters with neck flexion. *Anesthesia and Analgesia. Current Researches* **57**, 371.

51. Khalil, K. G., Parker, F. B., Mukherjee, N. and Webb, W. R. (1972). Thoracic duct injury. A complication of jugular vein catheterization. *Journal of the American Medical Association* **221**, 908.

52. Majek, M., Malatinský, J. and Kadlic, T. (1977). Inadvertent thoracic duct catheterization during trans-jugular central venous cannulation. A case report. *Acta Anaesthesiologica Scandinavica* **21**, 320.

53. Arnold, S., Feathers, R. S. and Gibbs, E. (1973). Bilateral pneumothoraces and subcutaneous emphysema: a complication of internal jugular venepuncture. *British Medical Journal* **1**, 211.

54. Cook, T. L. and Dueker, C. W. (1976). Tension pneumothorax following internal jugular cannulation and general anesthesia. *Anesthesiology* **45**, 554.

55. Koch, M. J. (1972). Bilateral 'I. V. hydrothorax'. *New England Journal of Medicine* **286**, 218.

56. Carvell, J. E. and Pearce, D. J. (1976). Bilateral hydrothorax following internal jugular catheterization. *British Journal of Surgery* **63**, 381.

57. Ayalon, A., Anner, H., Berlatzky, Y. and Schiller, M. (1978). A life-threatening complication of the infusion pump. *Lancet* **1**, 853.

58. Wisheart, J. D., Hassan, M. A. and Jackson, J. W. (1972). A complication of percutaneous cannulation of the internal jugular vein. *Thorax* **27**, 496.

59. Butsch, J. L., Butsch, W. L. and Da Rosa, J. F. T. (1976). Bilateral vocal cord paralysis. A complication of percutaneous cannulation of the internal jugular veins. *Archives of Surgery* **111**, 828.

60. Briscoe, C. E., Bushman, J. A. and McDonald, W. I. (1974). Extensive neurological damage after cannulation of internal jugular vein. *British Medical Journal* **1**, 314.

61. Parikh, R. K. (1972). Horner's syndrome. A complication of percutaneous catheterisation of internal jugular vein. *Anaesthesia* **27**, 327.

62. Ross, S. M., Freedman, P. S. and Farman, J. V. (1979). Air embolism after accidental removal of intravenous catheter. *British Medical Journal* **1**, 987.

63. Brown, C. S. and Wallace, C. T. (1976). Chronic hematoma – a complication of percutaneous catheterization of the internal jugular vein. *Anesthesiology* **45**, 368.

64. Knoblanche, G. E. (1979). Respiratory obstruction due to haematoma following internal jugular vein cannulation. *Anaesthesia and Intensive Care* **7**, 286.

65. Schuster, W., Vennebusch, H., Doetsch, N. and Taube, H. D. (1978). Vena cava superior thrombosis following placement of internal jugular vein catheter. *Anaesthesist* **27**, 546.

66. Nottage, W. M. (1976). Iatrogenic superior vena cava syndrome. A complication of internal jugular venous catheters. *Chest* **70**, 566.

67. Schwartz, A. J. (1977). Percutaneous aortic catheterisation – a hazard of supraclavicular internal jugular vein catheterization. *Anesthesiology* **46**, 77.

68. McDaniel, M. M. and Grossman, M. (1978). Aortic dissection complicating percutaneous jugular-vein catheterisation. *Anesthesiology* **49**, 213.

69. Ohlgisser, M., Kaufman, T. S., Taitelman, U., Burzstein, S. and Birkhan, J. H. (1979). Cardiac arrest following a complication of internal jugular vein cannulation. *Anaesthesia* **34**, 1035.

70. Sprigge, J. S. and Oakley, G. D. G. (1979). Carotid artery

palpation during internal jugular vein cannulation and subsequent ventricular fibrillation. *British Journal of Anaesthesia* **51**, 807.

71. Greenall, M. J., Blewitt, R. W. and McMahon, M. J. (1975). Cardiac tamponade and central venous catheters. *British Medical Journal* **2**, 595.

72. Defalque, R. J. and Campbell, C. (1979). Cardiac tamponade from central venous catheters. *Anesthesiology* **50**, 249.

73. Malatinský, J., Kadlic, T., Májek, M. and Sámel, M. (1976). Misplacement and loop formation of central venous catheters. *Acta Anaesthesiologica Scandinavica* **20**, 237.

74. Kuramoto, T. and Sakabe, T. (1975). Comparison of success in jugular versus basilic vein technics for central venous pressure catheter position. *Anesthesia and Analgesia. Current Researches* **54**, 696.

75. Fischer, J., Lundstrom, J. and Ottander, H. G. (1977). Central venous cannulation: a radiological determination of catheter positions and immediate intrathoracic complications. *Acta Anaesthesiologica Scandinavica* **21**, 245.

76. Schwartz, A. J., Jobes, D. R., Greenhow, E., Stephenson, L. W. and Ellison, N. (1979). Carotid artery puncture with internal jugular cannulation using the Seldinger technique: incidence, recognition, treatment and prevention. *Anesthesiology* **51** S160.

77. Ellison, N., Schwartz, A. J., Jobes, D. R., Greenhow, D. E. and Stephenson, L. W. (1982). Avoidance of carotid artery puncture sequelae during internal jugular cannulation. *Anesthesia and Analgesia* **61**, 181.

78. McEnany, M. T. and Austen, W. G. (1977). Life threatening haemhorrage from inadvertent cervical arteriotomy. *Annals of Thoracic Surgery* **24**, 233.

79. Shah, K. B., Tadikonda, L. K., Rao, M. D., Laughlin, S. and El-Etr, A. (1984). A review of Pulmonary Artery Catheterization in 6245 Patients. *Anaesthesiology* **61**, 271.

80. Peters, J., Steinhoff, H. and Sandmann, W. (1984). Carotid aneurysm after jugular vein catheterization. *Anaesthetist* **33**, 330.

81. Burri, C. and Ahnefeld, F. W. (1978). *The Caval Catheter*, p. 45. Berlin: Springer-Verlag.

82. Verrieres, D., Bernard, C. and Dacheux, J. (1986). Cervical arteriovenous fistulas following internal jugular catheterisation. *Anesthesia Reanimation* **5**, 162.

83. Ellison, N., Jobes, D. R. and Schwartz, A. J. (1981). Cannulation of the internal jugular vein: a cautionary note. *Anesthesiology* **55**, 336.

84. Tyden, H. (1982). Cannulation of the internal jugular vein – 500 cases. *Acta Anaesthesiologica Scandinavica* **26**, 485.

85. Morgan, R. N. W. and Morell, D. F. (1981). Internal jugular catheterisation: a review of a potentially lethal hazard. *Anaesthesia* **36**, 512.

86. Powell, H. (1988). Safety first with triple lumen catheters. *Murmurs* **5**, 4.

87. Goldfarb, G. and Lebrec, D. (1982). Percutaneous cannulation of the internal jugular vein in patients with coagulopathies: an experience based on 1000 attempts. *Anesthesiology* **56**, 321.

88. Sheep, R. E. and Guiney, W. B. (1982). Fatal cardiac tamponade. Occurrence with other complications after left internal jugular vein catheterisation. *Journal of the American Medical Association* **248**, 1632.

89. Sagor, G. Mitchelmere, P., Layfield, J., Prentice, P. and Kirk, R. M. (1983). Prolonged access to the venous system using the Hickman right atrial catheter. *Annals of the Royal College of Surgeons of England* **65**, 47.

90. Chastre, J., Cornud, F., Bouchama, A., Viau, F., Benacerraf, R. and Gibert, C. (1982). Thrombosis as a complication of pulmonary-artery catheterization via the internal jugular vein. *New England Journal of Medicine* **306**, 278.

91. Elinger, J. H., Bedford, R. F. and Buschi, A. J. (1981). Do pulmonary artery catheters cause internal jugular vein thrombosis. *Anesthesiology* **57**, A118.

92. Perkins, N. A. K., Bedford, R. F., Buschi, A. J. and Cail, W. S. (1983). Internal jugular vein function after Swan–Ganz catheterization studied by venography and ultrasound. *Anesthesiology* **59**, A145.

93. Perkins, N. A. K., Cail, W. S., Bedford, R. F., Elinger, J. H. and Buschi, A. J. (1984). Internal jugular vein function after Swan–Ganz catheterization. *Anesthesiology* **61**, 456.

94. de Bruijn, N. R. and Stadt, H. H. (1981). Bilateral thrombosis of internal jugular veins after multiple percutaneous cannulations. *Anaesthesia and Analgesia* **60**, 448.

95. Barra, D. P., Dru, M. and Freffe, B. (1986). Late venous perforations due to percutaneous central venous cannulation. *Canadian Anaesthetists' Society Journal* **33**, 225.

96. Punt, C. D., Swen, J., Bovill, J. G. and Obermann, W. R. (1990). Delayed perforations of intrathoracic veins: a comparison between right- and left-sided internal jugular cannulation. *European Journal of Anaesthesiology* **7**, 25.

97. Forestener, J. E. (1980). Ipsilateral mydriasis following carotid-artery puncture during attempted cannulation of the internal jugular vein. *Anesthesiology* **52**, 438.

98. Vest, J. V., Pereira, M. B. and Senior, R. M. (1980). Phrenic nerve injury associated with venipuncture of the internal jugular vein. *Chest* **78**, 777.

99. Stock, M. C. and Downs, J. B. (1982). Transient phrenic nerve blockade during internal jugular vein cannulation using the anterolateral approach. *Anesthesiology* **57**, 230.

100. Lange, L. S. and Rees, A. (1986). Preventing early neurological complications of coronary artery bypass surgery. *British Medical Journal* **292**, 27.

101. Frasquet, F. J. and Belda, F. J. (1981). Permanent paralysis of C5 after cannulation of the internal jugular vein. *Anesthesiology* **54**, 528.

102. Whittet, H. B. and Boscoe, M. J. (1984). Isolated palsy of the hypoglossal nerve after central venous catheterisation. *British Medical Journal* **41**, 288.

103. Feldmann, H. and Seetzen-Kanaan, G. (1984). Lesion of vagus nerve: a complication following cannulation of internal jugular vein? *Anaesthetist* **33**, 322.

104. Anagnou, J. (1928). Cerebrovascular accident during percutaneous cannulation of internal jugular vein. *Lancet* **2**, 377.

105. Bastulli, J. A. and Orlowski, J. P. (1985). Stroke as a complication of carotid sinus massage. *Critical Care Medicine* **13/10**, 867.

106. Brown, C. Q. (1982). Inadvertent prolonged cannulation of the carotid artery. *Anesthesia and Analgesia* **61**, 150.

107. Cozanitits, D. A. (1981). Earache following caval catheterization. *Anaesthetist* **30**, 150.

108. Gilner, L. I. (1977). The 'ear-gurgling' sign (Letter to Editor), *New England Journal of Medicine* **296**, 1301.

109. Polglase, A. (1976). Malpositioned central venous cannulae and the internal jugular vein. *Medical Journal of Australia* **2**, 714.

110. Klein, H. O., Di Segni, E. and Kaplinski, E. (1978). Unsuspected cerebral perfusion: a complication of the use of a central venous pressure catheter. *Chest* **74**, 109.

111. Souter, R. G. and Mitchell, A. (1982). Spreading cortical venous thrombosis due to infusion of hyperosmolar solution into the internal jugular vein. *British Medical Journal* **285**, 935.

112. Saxena, V. K. Heilpern, J. and Murphy, S. F. (1976). Pseudotumour cerebri. A complication of parenteral hyperalimentation. *Journal of the American Medical Association* **235**, 2124.

113. Stewart, D. R., Johnson, D. G. and Myers, G. G. (1975). Hydrocephalus as a complication of jugular catheterization during total parenteral nutrition. *Journal of Pediatric Surgery* **10**, 771.

114. Nagai, K. and Kemmotsu, O. (1985). An inadvertent insertion of a Swan–Ganz catheter into the intrathecal space. *Anesthesiology* **62**, 48.

115. Damen, J. (1987). Positive bacterial cultures and related risk factor associated with percutaneous internal jugular vein catheterization in pediatric cardiac patients. *Anesthesiology* **66**, 558.

116. Konichezky, S., Saguib, S. and Soroker, D. (1983).

117. Tracheal puncture. A complication of percutaneous jugular vein cannulation. *Anaesthesia* **38**, 572.

117. Levin, H., Bursztein, S. and Heifetz, M. (1986). Prestenotic dilatation of the oesophagus: a hazard of internal jugular vein cannulation. *Anesthesia and Analgesia* **65**, 901.

118. Royster, R. L., Johnston, W. E., Gravlee, G. P., Brauer, S. and Richards, D. (1985). Arrhythmias during venous cannulation prior to pulmonary artery catheter insertion. *Anesthesia and Analgesia* **64**, 1214.

119. Petty, C. (1975). An alternate method for internal jugular venipuncture for monitoring central venous pressure. *Anesthesia and Analgesia. Current Researches* **54**, 157.

120. Gilston, A. (1982). Internal jugular vein catheterisation. A right sided pleural effusion. *Anaesthesia* **37**, 221.

121. Gomez-Amau, J., Escarpa, A. and Burgos, R. (1987). Placement of the catheter tip in open heart surgery. *Anaesthesia* **37**, 221.

122. Bromley, L. (1989). Fracture of internal jugular catheters: five case reports. *British Journal of Hospital Medicine* **42**, 491.

123. Munro, H. (1990). An unusual complication of a central venous line. *Anaesthesia* **45**, 334.

124. Berlatzky, Y., Freund, H. and Schiller, M. (1976). Percutaneous internal jugular vein cannulation in children. *Zeitschrift fuer Kinderchir* **18**, 237.

125. Ducatman, B. S., McMichan, J. C. and Edwards, W. D. (1985). Catheter induced lesions of the right side of the heart. *Journal of the American Medical Association* **253**: 791.

126. Crowell, R. H., Adams, G. S., Koilpillai, C. J. McNutt, E. J. and Montague, T. J. (1988). In vivo right heart thrombus: precursor of life-threatening pulmonary embolism. *Chest* **94**: 1236.

127. Joshi, P., Bullingham, A. and Soni, N. (1991). Septic atrial thrombus: a complication of central venous catheterisation. *Anaesthesia* **46**: 1030.

7

The External Jugular Vein

Cannulation of the external jugular vein for central venous pressure monitoring and fluid infusion was first described by Rams and his colleagues in 1966.[1] They used a surgical cut-down technique. A percutaneous variation of this technique was later described to avoid the disadvantages of a surgical cut-down.[2] Subsequent authors described percutaneous techniques for external jugular vein cannulation both in adults[3-6] and in children.[7-9] The route however remained relatively unpopular for at least another eight years because of the difficulty in successfully threading catheters past the sharply angulated junction of the external jugular and subclavian veins.

In 1974 Blitt and his colleagues described the value of a J-wire in improving the incidence of successful central placement of catheters when using the external jugular route.[10] They achieved a previously unattainable incidence of central placement of 96%. Their four failures were attributed to the presence of a venous plexus formed by the external jugular vein above the clavicle.

In the last few years the J-wire kit has become a freely available and affordable item for the British anaesthetist. A number of authors[11-13] have suggested that the external jugular vein route should be more widely adopted because of its low incidence of serious complications. Indeed, there does appear to be a trend towards an increasing use of the external jugular vein in anaesthetic practice.

This change in clinical practice is due to the appreciation of the low risk of complications during insertion; to the increasing availability of J-wires and thus an improved success rate in satisfactory central placement; it has also been shown that valid venous pressure measurements can be made from catheters whose tips are placed just above the junction of the external jugular and subclavian veins.[14]

PRESSURE MONITORING

Although measurements of central venous pressure can be made with short cannulae in the external jugular vein in anaesthetised patients,[15,16] they may be unreliable since they may be affected by changes in the position of the head as the patient moves around. Improved results are obtained using a catheter with two side holes near its distal end.[17] Reliable measurements cannot be obtained with short cannulae after the chest has been opened.[15]

A later study has shown that accurate pressure measurements can be obtained with the catheter tip just above the obstruction at the external jugular–subclavian junction.[14] Measurements were unaffected by head position or the side of catheterisation. A round-tipped catheter with two side holes was used. This means that by using such a catheter satisfactory pressure measurements can be obtained in 100% of cases if external jugular venous catheterisation is possible.

CLINICAL USES OF THE EXTERNAL JUGULAR VEIN

Since the external jugular vein lies superficially in the neck, the traumatic complications associated with blind venepuncture of deep veins are avoided. This vein, therefore, may be specifically indicated as an alternative to arm veins, particularly if expertise in internal jugular and subclavian vein cannulation is lacking. A short venous catheter can usually be readily inserted into the external jugular vein for intraoperative infusion of drugs or volume replacement. Such a catheter provides a convenient intraoperative access site. The tip of such a short catheter is near the external jugular subclavian junction and thus approximates to a 'half-way' catheter.[18] Such a catheter should be removed immediately at the end of the anaesthetic because of the risk of air embolus in the sitting position if a disconnection occurs. This technique may be particularly useful in cardiac arrest patients for 'central' infusion of drugs if a central venous catheter is not immediately available. It should also be recognised that attempts to insert central venous catheters by house officers during a cardiac arrest have a low success rate and a high complication rate.[19]

The vein can also be used for the insertion of one or more single lumen central venous catheters, a double or triple lumen catheter, a haemodialysis catheter, a pacemaker or a Swan–Ganz catheter.

The external jugular vein can be used as a route for long-term (9–50 days) parenteral nutrition in adults.[20] The vein has also been used for inserting Hickman catheters by a surgical cut down technique in children requiring bone marrow transplant.[21] The catheters were left *in situ* from 1 to 3½ months. The procedure was done under fluoroscopic control and the catheter tip advanced to the mid-atrial position.

The external jugular vein was the preferred route for percutaneous insertion of flexible, soft silastic central venous catheters in 15 newborn infants.[22] The fine bore flexible catheters passed without difficulty into the right atrium and were left *in situ* for a mean of 24·8 days. They were used for administration of total parenteral nutrition. No thrombophlebitis, infection or caval thrombosis was detected.

Some patients do not have a visible or palpable vein on either side. In other patients the vein on one side is visible but not on the other side. It has been claimed that about 90% of people have a single prominent external jugular vein running down from the angle of the jaw across the sternomastoid muscle to the subclavian vein.[13] There is no difference in the success of central placement between the vein on the right or left sides and therefore the most prominent vein should be selected.

In practice the right side of this neck is commonly draped for the more frequently used internal jugular route. The patient should be carefully examined before this is carried out to assess the size of external jugular vein. If cannulation of the internal jugular vein is difficult and the attempt abandoned, then the external jugular vein can be used.

CLINICAL EXPERIENCE

When external jugular veins are used by junior staff in emergency situations the results are worse than for experienced staff under elective circumstances.

A success rate of only 53% (18/34) was achieved by house officers on an intensive care unit.[23] It was stressed that operator inexperience was a most important factor and that considerable manipulation of the J-wire was often required.

In another study inexperienced house officers attempted central venous cannulation.[19] Their success rate with the external jugular vein was 61% (51/84). Surprisingly failure was attributed most commonly to inability to thread the catheter into the vein. Their success rate was lower than that for internal jugular and subclavian routes.

PRACTICAL POINTS

Various authors have made recommendations to facilitate puncture of the external jugular vein and to advance a guide wire or catheter centrally. These recommendations appear arbitrary and their validity has not been confirmed by clinical evaluation.

Patient preparation and examination

Place the patient in the Trendelenburg position and examine the neck to determine the degree of venous prominence. If necessary a stethoscope or a finger may be used to further distend the vein by obstructing venous return. In some patients the vein is prominent with the patient in the horizontal position and therefore the Trendelenburg position is not required.

A conscious patient can be asked to perform a Valsalva manoeuvre both before venepuncture and while the J-wire is being threaded centrally. In an anaesthetised patient the lungs can be momentarily held in inflation to distend the vein, both during venous catheterisation and while the J-wire is threaded centrally. Although the vein is only loosely fixed in the subcutaneous tissues it is not always easy to distend.[13]

Some cardiac patients are unable to tolerate either a Trendelenburg or even a flat position. The external jugular veins may however be dilated in these patients even in the sitting position. In the absence of a suitable arm vein the external jugular vein can be catheterised in the sitting position but great care must be taken to avoid the risk of air embolus. Turning the head fully on to one side can stretch the skin over the vein on the side to be cannulated and make the vein less visible. Bringing the head back towards the mid-line will in some patients make the vein more easily visible.

Getting into the vein

Use a catheter-over-needle for venepuncture. A steel needle is more likely to cause vein wall puncture and haematoma.[12] Advance the catheter only a few cm into the vein to prevent the catheter tip entering a small tributary.[12] Enter the vein from the side rather than on top to minimise transfixion and haematoma formation.[13]

Threading wire or catheter centrally

Repeated insertion of guide wires is required in a third of all cases.[12] If the wire cannot be threaded centrally retract it fully before making another attempt.[12] If the wire sticks it can be withdrawn and rotated through 180° before a further attempt is made.[13] Alternatively the J-wire can be advanced or withdrawn while it is being gently rotated.[24] Avoid prolonged or forceful manipulation of wires and make a skin incision to facilitate easy insertion of the catheter or vein dilator over the guide wire.

Turning the head to the side being catheterised and medial traction on the skin of the neck will make the angle between the external jugular and subclavian veins less acute.[13,24,25] In addition external manipulation by finger tip pressure may be helpful; saline can be injected to distend the veins locally. If the arm is raised and pulled to the same side the subclavian, external jugular vein angle is made less acute.

Do not advance the catheter with any force past points of obstruction as it may become angulated and stuck and difficult to remove.[26] Such catheters may require surgical intervention to facilitate removal.

Choice of equipment

A number of studies using different catheters and wires are summarised in Table 7.1. Early studies compared the use of catheter through cannula and catheter through needle devices.[25,27] In both studies round-ended rather than open-ended catheters gave a higher incidence of successful central placement. The use of catheter-through-cannula rather than through-needle devices will prevent shearing of catheters and the potential for catheter embolisation.

The use of J-wires improves the success rate of central placement. Berthelsen et al. in 1986[12] concluded that it was nearly always possible to insert a central venous catheter past the external jugular subclavian junction if the vein could be cannulated. More and more authors are recommending the external jugular vein as the route of first choice.

Comparisons have been made between J-wires of different radii. It has been suggested by Humphry and Blitt[28] that a radius of 1·5 mm may increase the incidence of successful central placement in children: the standard size radius used is 3 mm. A curved J-wire has been shown to result in a high incidence of successful central placement than a straight Seldinger wire.[29]

As always the clinician may be limited in his choice of equipment. If a J-wire kit is available this should be used in preference to simple catheter-through-cannula devices. If a J-wire is not available the use of a round-ended catheter with side holes is preferable to the use of an open-ended catheter.[27,28]

Anatomy

The external jugular vein is formed by the junction of the posterior division of the posterior facial vein and the posterior auricular vein. It receives blood from the deep parts of the face and the surface of the cranium, and runs down the neck from the angle of the mandible, crosses the sternomastoid muscle obliquely, and terminates behind the middle of the clavicle on joining with the subclavian vein. The vein is variable in size and possesses valves 4 cm above the clavicle and just before its junction with the subclavian vein. Natural variations and disease states are responsible for the wide range in the degree of prominence of the external jugular vein.

EXTERNAL JUGULAR VEIN APPROACH
Authors' method (if J-wire is unavailable)

Patient category

Adults and children.

Advantages and disadvantages

The only contraindication to using the external jugular vein is local sepsis. When catheters or cannulae are used without J-wires there is a substantially lower incidence of central placement than when J-wires are used. The only reason for using catheters alone therefore is if J-wires are unavailable. However round-ended catheters placed approximately 1 cm above the clavicle will give accurate central venous pressure readings.[14] Such catheters have their tips close to the lateral region of the first rib, and therefore function in a similar way to the 'half-way' catheters described by Gustavsson *et al.* in 1985.[18] The frequency of use of J-wires in the developed world is likely to increase. However, in Third World countries catheters alone will still be frequently required.

Preferred side

Either side may be used.

Position of patient (Figure 7.1a)

Place the table in a 25° head-down position. Turn the patient's head away from the side of puncture and place both arms by his sides.

Position of operator (Figure 7.1a)

Stand at the head of the patient.

Equipment used

Catheter-through-cannula.

Anatomical landmarks (Figure 7.1b)

The external jugular vein and sternomastoid muscle. (The external jugular vein is not always palpable or visible; if this is the case, cathererisation should not be attempted.)

Preparation

Perform the puncture under sterile conditions using local anaesthesia if indicated.

Precautions and recommendations

Distend the vein if necessary by holding the lungs in inflation for a short time if the patient is anaesthetised, or by asking the patient to perform a Valsalva manoeuvre if awake. Place a finger on the lower portion of the vein to impede venous drainage so as to distend the vein.

Point of insertion of needle (Figure 7.1b.)

In the line of the vein where it is most easily seen. Cannulate well above the clavicle to avoid the risk of pneumothorax.

Direction of needle and procedure (Figure 7.1c,d,e)

Attach the needle to a saline-filled syringe. Place the point of the needle on the skin entry site and point the needle caudally (A). Swing the needle and syringe to point the needle in the axis of the vein (A to B). Elevate the syringe just above the skin (B to C). Advance the needle and syringe maintaining a slight negative pressure in the syringe. When the vein is entered, remove the needle from the cannula and thread the catheter centrally. Fix the catheter securely. If resistance is encountered when threading the catheter centrally, inject fluid into the catheter as it is advancd, rotate the catheter, and press on the skin just above the clavicle. If central placement proves impossible, leave the catheter at the position reached as this will frequently be satisfactory during anaesthesia for making measurements of central venous pressure and for taking blood samples.

Success rate

72% central placement in 50 patients.[27]

Complications

None.

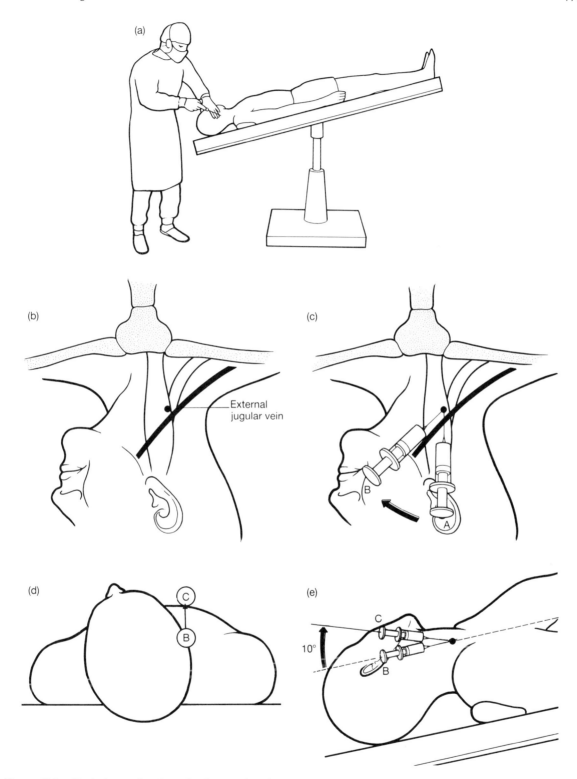

Figure 7.1. Technique of catheterisation: authors' method.

EXTERNAL JUGULAR VEIN APPROACH: J-WIRE TECHNIQUE
Blitt et al. (1974)[10]

Patient category

Adults and children.

Advantages and disadvantages

This technique greatly increases the rate of central placement.

Preferred side

Either side may be used. The choice may be influenced by the prominence of the external jugular vein.

Position of patient (see Figure 7.1a)

Place the table in a 30° head-down position. Turn the patient's head away from the side of puncture and place both arms by his sides.

Position of operator (see Figure 7.1a)

Stand at head of patient.

Equipment used in original description (Figure 7.2)

14 or 16 gauge. 14 cm Teflon catheter-over-needle. A 35 cm, 0.089 cm-diameter, flexible wire catheter guide with a distal radius of curvature of 3 mm (the J-wire). This equipment is supplied complete with instructions in a single pack.

Advice on current equipment

Use a small needle, a J-wire and a soft flexible non-thrombogenic catheter.

Anatomical landmarks

The external jugular vein and the sternomastoid muscle.

Preparation

Perform the puncture under sterile conditions using local anaesthesia if indicated.

Precautions and recommendations

Distend the vein if necessary by holding the lungs in inflation for a short time if the patient is anaesthetised, or by asking the patient to perform a Valsalva manoeuvre if awake. Place a finger on the lower portion of the vein to impede venous drainage and so distend the vein.

Point of insertion of needle (see Figure 7.1b)

In the line of the vein where it is easily seen. The point of insertion should be well above the clavicle to avoid the risk of pneumothorax.

Direction of needle and procedure (see Figure 7.1c, d, e)

Attach the needle to a saline-filled syringe. Place the point of the needle on the skin entry site and point the needle caudally (A). Swing the needle and syringe to point the needle in the axis of the vein (A to B). Elevate the syringe just above the skin (B to C). Advance the needle and syringe maintaining a slight negative pressure in the syringe. When the vein is entered, advance the needle assembly approximately 2·5 cm into the vein. Straighten the J-tip of the wire by sliding the plastic insertion sleeve to its end. Remove the needle from the catheter and place the tip of the plastic sleeve into the hub of the catheter. This allows the J-wire to be pushed through the catheter and then into the vein. When the wire emerges from the end of the catheter its tip reverts to the original 'J' shape. Advance the wire into the intrathoracic vein, rotating it if obstruction is encountered. Once the wire is in an intrathoracic vein, advance the catheter over the wire. Remove the wire and connect the catheter to the infusion system. Fix the catheter securely and check its position with a chest radiograph.

Results

Central placement was achieved in 96 of 100 attempts. In 5 of the 96 cases, measurement of central venous pressure was initially unsatisfactory and alteration of the position of the catheter was needed.

Complications

No complications were reported.

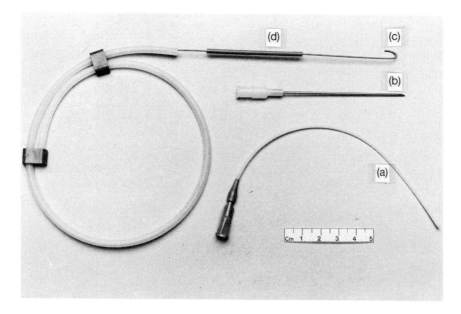

Figure 7.2.   The J-wire technique: Blitt *et al.* (1974).[10] (a) Soft flexible catheter; (b) needle; (c) J-wire; (d) plastic insertion sleeve.

COMPLICATIONS

As with any technique a haematoma can cause localised swelling. The incidence of major complications with this technique is very low and most serious complications can be avoided by using soft non-thrombogenic catheters. A summary of the complications reported in the literature is shown in Table 7.2.

CONCLUSION

The external jugular vein provides safe and convenient access to the central cirulation. The most important disadvantage is the difficulty in a significant per cent of patients in threading the catheter centrally after venous cannulation. The introduction of the J-wire has substantially increased the incidence of successful central placement. It can be confidently predicted that this route will be used more frequently in the future.

Table 7.1.

Author and year	Equipment used or cannulation attempts	No. of patients	Successful central placements and number (%)	Comments
		DIFFERENT CANNULAE		
Riddell et al. (1982)[27]	Catheter-through-cannula (closed tip)	114 patients with 100 venous cannulations	36/50 (72) (closed tip)	Choice of catheter may influence the success rate
	Catheter-through-needle (open-ended)		30/50 (62) (open-ended)	
Schaps et al. (1988)[25]	Closed-tip catheter 60	125	51/60 (85) (closed tip)	Central catheter placement was helped by:
	Open-ended catheter 65		44/65 (67.7) (open-ended)	(1) Fingertip pressure at external jugular subclavian junction
				(2) Injection of saline through the catheter to expand the vein
				(3) Pulling the arm to the side to improve the angle between external jugular and subclavian veins
				(4) Turning the head to the side of catheterized vein
		PAEDIATRIC SELDINGER WIRE		
Giesy (1972)[6]	Soft pliable silicone elastomer catheter	112	101/112 (90)	
Humphrey and Blitt (1982)[28]	J-wire with 3 mm radius of curvature	20 children with 17 venous cannulations (mean age 56 months, mean wt 18·9 kg)	10/17 (59)	They suggested that the use of a J-wire with a 1.5 mm radius of curvature wire may improve the success rate in children

Reference	Seldinger wires		Age	Attempt	Success	Comments
Nicolson et al. (1985)	Seldinger wires		<1 month	1	1 (100)	No difference between right and left external jugular vein. They preferred the IJV to the EJV route in children (the IJV route gave an 86% incidence of successful cannulations and a 99.9% incidence of central placement of the catheter tip)
	117 patients for EJV study. (An investigation in children comparing the IJV and EJV routes)		1 month–1 year	17	6 (35)	
			1–5 years	22	13 (59)	
			>5 years	77	56 (76)	
			Total	117	76 (65)	
			14% of successful cannulations had catheter tips incorrectly positioned			

ADULT SELDINGER WIRE

Reference	Seldinger wires	Number	Success	Comments
Blitt et al. (1974)[10]	J-wire with 3 mm radius of curvature	100	96/100(96)	The first reported use of the J-wire in the external jugular vein. The technique is easy to teach to residents and free of complications. The 4 failures occurred in patients with a venous plexus above the clavicle
Abadair et al. (1979)[24]	J-wire 0·035 inch diameter	108	99/108 (91·6) 96 first attempt 3 on opposite side Failures 3 failed both EJV 5 no visible EJV 1 advanced to basilic vein	The external jugular vein is suitable for Swan–Ganz catheters
Belani et al. (1980)[31]	J-wire 0·089 cm O.D.	42	32/42 (76) 30 intrathoracic catheter tips 2 malpositioned tips	Lower success rate than Blitt et al., possibly due to less vigorous attempts to get the J-wire past venous obstructions. This study also compared external and internal jugular routes. The external route was safe but had a lower incidence of central catheter placements
Blyth (1985)[32]	J-wire 0·899 mm diameter	100	90/100 (90) Cannulation of vein unsuccessful in 3 cases Unable to pass wire centrally in 7 cases	Most important advantage is the absence of major complications. If cannulation of EJV is unsuccessful IJV cannulation can be performed without the need to redrape

Table 7.1. Continued.

Author and year	Equipment used or cannulation attempts	No. of patients	Successful central placements and number (%)					Comments
			Number	J-wire used 1st	Success	J-wire used 2nd	Success	
Nordstrom and Fletcher (1983)[33]	Patients randomised to get J-wire of either: (a) 6 mm diameter or (b) 3 mm diameter. If allocated J-wire could not passed then other wire was tried	138	77 61	6 mm 3 mm	54/77 (70%) 55/61 (88%)	3 mm 6 mm	13/23 (56%) 0/6 (0%)	Success
			Difference between two wires was statistically significant $P < 0.05$					
Schwartz et al (1982)[11]	(a) Straight wire — straight central venous catheter (b) J-wire — straight central venous catheter (c) Straight wire — PA catheter with curved tip	163	(a) 19/31 (61) (b) 25/29 (86%) (c) 91/103 (88) 135/163 (83%)					The J-wire is not necessary for PA catheterization. J-wire more successful than straight wire $P < 0.05$. PA catheter with curved tip sufficient. This technique was recommended as the initial approach in all patients with an appropriate EJ vein
Blitt et al. (1982)[29]	(a) Straight wire (0·035 inch diameter) was first passed if possible (b) If this failed a J-wire (3 mm radius) was used (successful in all remaining cases)	36	16/36 (44) 20/20 (100)					*Study to compare straight with J-wires. The J-wire was thought to 'bounce off' or 'roll through' angles and bends in the vein*
Berthelson et al. (1986)[12]	First — Straight wire (then if unsuccessful) Second — J-modified wire; end of straight wire angulated (then if unsuccessful) Third — proper J — wire	115 bilateral attempts in 35 patients	Wire past SC–EJV junction in 148/150 attempts (98·6%). Successful central placements in 146/150 attempts (97%)					*They concluded that it is nearly always possible to insert a central venous catheter in an adult if the EJV can be cannulated. No difference found between right and left sides*

Table 7.2. Complications of external jugular vein cannulation.

Reference	Complication	Comments
Ghani and Berry (1983)[34]	*Right hydrothorax* secondary to *left* external jugular vein cannulation in 4 patients	The superior vein cava was eroded by the tip of the catheter 24–48 hours after insertion and fluid infusion resulted in hypotension. They recommended using 8 inch rather than 6 inch catheters. It is particularly important to avoid using stiff catheters on the left side
Eichold and Berryman (1985)[35]	*Right hydrothorax* secondary to *left* external jugular vein cannulation in 1 patient	The catheter probably eroded the vein and entered the right pleura. Acute dyspnoea and chest pain developed 4 days after catheter insertion. The clinician should check for lack of venous return and inspect the chest x-ray for evidence of pleural effusion
Molinari *et al.* (1984)[36]	*Right plural effusion* in 3 patients. Hyperalimentation fluid *in right lung* in one patient which was coughed up. *Left*-sided venous cannulation	Use of stiff 6 inch polytetrafluoroethylene (PTFE) catheters should be avoided on the left side. Perforation of vein wall can occur with insecure catheter fixation and head, neck or cardiopulmonary movement resulting in movement of the tip of the catheter
Fischer and Scherz (1973)[37]	Haemopericardium and *death* occurred on the fourth postoperative day in a 12-month-old boy. A right-sided external jugular cannulation had been performed using a 2 inch rigid catheter	This might have resulted from catheter tip movement or due to trauma at the time of insertion. An autopsy study showed that extreme neck movement could result in 2–3 cm movement of the catheter tip and that venous or atrial perforation occurred 60% of the time
Lingenfelter *et al* (1978)[38]	Catheter tip movement occurred during neck flexion and extension	With jugular catheters the catheter tip may advance into the ventricle during neck flexion
Moore *et al.* (1985)[39]	Clinically silent *venous thrombosis* in paediatric cardiac surgery patients. Teflon non-heparin-bonded catheters were used	This was diagnosed by dye wash out at catheter removal. Thrombosis occurred in 27% of patients (4 out of 15). No significant differences were found between patients with and without silent thrombosis. Thrombosis was more likely to occur if the catheter tip was outside the thoracic cavity. Such catheters should be removed as soon as possible
Jobes *et al.* (1983)[40]	Occasional small *subcutaneous haematoma* at failed insertion sites	A comparison was made between internal and external jugular routes. The lower success rate and lack of arterial complications with the EJV route must be balanced against the higher success rate and incidence of arterial complications of the IJV route
Berry and Ghani (1982)[41]	*Venous occlusion* of the left external jugular vein occurred after central venous cannulation. The vein of a jejunal graft was anastomosed to the external jugular vein. The graft became engorged, was not viable and had to be replaced	This case demonstrated the need to understand the surgical procedure thoroughly before inserting cannulae

Table 7.2. Continued.

Reference	Complication	Comments
Stewart *et al.* (1975)[7]	Hydrocephalus. This was reported in a child aged 9 months in whom catheters had been inserted first into the right external jugular vein and later into the left external jugular vein for parenteral nutrition	Hydrocephalus was thought to have resulted from jugular venous thrombosis and impaired cerebral venous return

Monitoring and removal complications

Reference	Complication	Comments
McKenzie and Latto (1981)[26]	Difficult removal of soft pliable central venous catheters occurred in two patients. In one the catheter needed to be surgically removed	Accurate radiographic assessment of the catheter deformity may be helpful. No force should be used if resistance to insertion of the catheter occurs. Non-central placement of round-ended catheter tips is usually satisfactory for pressure monitoring
Finley (1988)[42]	Problem with removal of a 0·018 inch diameter J-wire used to insert a double lumen catheter	Clinicians should exercise caution when using thin flexible guide wires. If difficulties with removal occurs the wire and catheter should be removed together
Lawson and Kushins (1985)[43]	Difficulty in removal of a PA catheter inserted via the right external jugular vein. The catheter and introducer wire were then withdrawn at the same time	Multi-purpose pacing pulmonary artery catheters should be used with caution if there is an acute angle between the external jugular and subclavian veins (Probably best avoided in the external jugular vein)
Bromley and Moorthy (1983)[44]	Intraoperative problems: – Pulmonary artery pressure trace damping – Resistance to injection of cold fluid for cardiac outputs – Difficulty in advancing or withdrawing the catheter	Acute catheter angulation at the subclavian external jugular junction can lead to kinking of the catheter and monitoring problems

REFERENCES

1. Rams, J. J., Daicoff, G. R. and Moulder, P. V. (1966). A simple method for central venous pressure measurements. *Archives of Surgery* 92, 886.
2. Craig, R. G., Jones, R. A., Sproul, G. J. and Kinyon, G. E. (1968). Alternative methods of central venous system catheterization. *American Surgeon* 34, 131.
3. Jernigan, W. R., Gardner, W. C., Mahr, M. M. and Milburn, J. L. (1970). Use of the internal jugular vein for placement of central venous catheters. *Surgery, Gynecology and Obstetrics* 130, 520.
4. Malatinsky, J., Kadlic, M., Majek, M. and Samel, M. (1976). Misplacement and loop formation of central venous catheters. *Acta Anaesthesiologica Scandinavica* 20, 237.
5. Deitel, M. and McIntyre, J. A. (1971). Radiographic confirmation of site of central venous pressure catheters. *Canadian Journal of Surgery* 14, 42.
6. Giesy, J. (1972). External jugular vein access to central venous system. *Journal of the American Medical Association* 219, 1216.
7. Stewart, D. R., Johnson, D. G. and Myers, G. G. (1975). Hydrocephalus as a complication of jugular catheterization during total parenteral nutrition. *Journal of Pediatric Surgery* 10, 771.
8. Prince, S. R., Sullivan, R. L. and Hackel, A. (1976). Percutaneous catheterization of the internal jugular vein in infants and children. *Anesthesiology* 44, 170.
9. Cockington, R. A. (1979). Silicone elastomer for nasojejunal intubation and central venous cannulation in neonates. *Anaesthesia and Intensive Care* 7, 248.
10. Blitt, C. D., Wright, W. A., Petty, W. C. and Webster, T. A. (1974). Central venous catheterisation via the external jugular vein. A technique employing the J-wire. *Journal of the American Medical Association* 229, 817.

11. Schwartz, A. J., Jobes, D. R., Levy, W. J., Palermo, L. and Ellison, N. (1982). Intrathoracic vascular catheterisation via the external jugular vein. *Anesthesiology* 56, 400.

12. Berthelsen, P., Hansen, B., Howardy-Hansen, P. and Moller, J. (1986). Central venous access via the external jugular vein in cardiovascular surgery. *Acta Anaesthesiologica Scandinavica* 30, 470.

13. Dailey, R. H. (1988). External jugular vein cannulation and its use for CVP monitoring. *Journal of Emergency Medicine* 6, 133.

14. Shah, M. V., Swai, E. A. and Latto, I. P. (1986). Comparison between pressures measured from the proximal external jugular vein and a central vein. *British Journal of Anaesthesia* 58, 1384.

15. Briscoe, C. E. (1973). A comparison of jugular and central venous pressure measurements during anaesthesia. *British Journal of Anaesthesia* 45, 173.

16. Stoelting, R. K. (1973). Evaluation of external jugular venous pressure as a reflection of right atrial pressure. *Anesthesiology* 38, 29.

17. Stoelting, R. K. and Haselby, K. A. (1974). Evaluation of a catheter with two side holes for external jugular vein catheterization. *Anesthesia and Analgesia: Current Researches* 53, 628.

18. Gustavsson, B., Linder, L. E., Hultman, E. and Curelaru, I. (1985). 'Half-way' venous catheters. I. Theoretical premises and aims. *Acta Anaesthesiologica Scandinavica Suppl* 80, 30.

19. Bo-Linn, G. W., Anderson, D. J., Anderson, K. C., McGoon, M. D. and the Osler Medical House Staff (1982). Percutaneous central venous catheterization performed by medical house officers: a prospective study. *Catheterization and Cardiovascular Diagnosis* 8, 23.

20. Wilmore, D. W. and Dudrick, S. J. (1969). Safe long-term venous catheterization. *Archives of Surgery* 98, 256.

21. El-Gohary, M. A. (1985). The external jugular vein – a simple access to the central venous system. *British Journal of Parenteral Therapy* 154.

22. Dolcourt, J. L. and Bose, C. L. (1982). Percutaneous insertion of silastic venous catheters in newborn infants. *Pediatrics* 70, 484.

23. Sessler, C. N. and Glauser, F. L. (1987). Central venous cannulation done by house officers in the intensive care unit: a prospective study. *Southern Medical Journal* 80, 1239.

24. Abadair, A. R., Kwong, A. U. and Chaudry, R. (1979). Evaluation of external jugular vein for Swan–Ganz catheter insertion. *Anesthesiology* 51, S159.

25. Schaps, D., Ajman, A., Mehler, D. and Dransmann, N. F. (1988). External jugular vein catheterisation: a comparison of two different catheter types. *Care of the Critically Ill* 4, 21.

26. McKenzie, B. J. and Latto, I. P. (1981). Difficult removal of external jugular vein catheters. *Anaesthesia and Intensive Care* 9, 158.

27. Riddell, G. S., Latto, I. P. and Ng, W. S. (1982). External jugular vein access to the central venous system — a trial of two types of catheter. *British Journal of Anaesthesia* 54, 535.

28. Humphrey, M. J. and Blitt, C. D. (1982). Central venous access in children via the external jugular vein. *Anesthesiology* 57, 50.

29. Blitt, C. D., Carlson, G. L., Wright, W. A. and Otto, C. (1982). J-wire versus straight wire for central venous system cannulation via the external jugular vein. *Anesthesia and Analgesia* 61, 536.

30. Nicolson, S. C., Sweeney, M. F., Moore, R. A. and Jobes, D. R. (1985). Comparison of internal and external jugular cannulation of the central circulation in the pediatric patient. *Critical Care Medicine* 13, 747.

31. Belani, K. G., Buckley, J. J., Gordon, J. R. and Castaneda, W. (1980). Percutaneous cervical central venous line placement: a comparison of the internal and external jugular vein routes. *Anesthesia and Analgesia* 59, 40.

32. Blyth, P. L. (1985). Evaluation of the technique of central venous catheterisation via the external jugular vein using the J-wire. *Anaesthesia and Intensive Care* 13, 131.

33. Nordstrom, L. and Fletcher, R. (1983). Comparison of two different J-wires for central venous cannulation via the external jugular vein. *Anesthesia and Analgesia* 62, 365.

34. Ghani, G. A. and Berry, A. J. (1983). Right hydrothorax after left bilateral jugular vein catheterisation. *Anesthesiology* 58, 93.

35. Eichold, B. H. and Berryman, C. R. (1985). Contralateral hydrothorax: an unusual complication of central venous catheter placement. *Anesthesiology* 62, 673.

36. Molinari, P. S., Belani, K. G. and Buckley, J. J. (1984). Delayed hydrothorax following percutaneous central venous cannulation. *Acta Anaesthesiologica Scandinavica* 15, 107.

37. Fischer, G. W. and Scherz, R. G. (1973). Neck vein catheters and pericardial tamponade. *Pediatrics* 52, 868.

38. Lingenfelter, A. L., Guskiewicz, R. A. and Munson, E. S. (1978). Displacement of right atrial and endotracheal catheters with neck flexion. *Anesthesia and Analgesia* 57, 371.

39. Moore, R. A., McNicholas, K. W., Naidech, H., Flicker, S. and Gallagher, J. D. (1985). Clinically silent venous thrombosis following internal and external jugular central venous cannulation in pediatric cardiac patients. *Anesthesiology* 62, 640.

40. Jobes, D. R., Schwartz, A. J., Greenhow, D. E., Stephenson, L. V. and Ellison, N. (1983). Safer jugular vein cannulation: recognition of arterial puncture and preferential use of the external jugular route. *Anesthesiology* 59, 353.

41. Berry, A. J. and Ghani, G. A. (1982). An unusual complication following cannulation of an external jugular vein. *Anesthesiology* 56, 411.

42. Finley, G. A. (1988). A complication of external jugular vein catheterization in children. *Canadian Journal of Anaesthesia* 35, 536.

43. Lawson, D. and Kushins, L. G. (1985). A complication of multi purpose pacing pulmonary artery catheterization via the external jugular vein approach. *Anesthesiology* 62, 377.

44. Bromley, J. L. and Moorthy, S. S. (1983). Acute angulation of a pulmonary artery catheter. *Anesthesiology* 59, 367.

8

The Femoral Vein

The technique of introducing a catheter into the inferior vena cava through a percutaneous puncture of the femoral vein, introduced by Duffy[1] in 1949, was once popular. It was used when patients required long-term intravenous therapy or when markedly hypertonic sugar solutions were being administered to patients in acute renal failure. Peripheral veins quickly became thrombosed by these solutions, but it was found that treatment could be maintained for long periods by catheters introduced into the inferior vena cava through the femoral vein.[2–4] Some authors reported that percutaneous catheterisation of the femoral vein was relatively free from immediate complications or serious late complications.[1,4,6,7] Others recorded an incidence of serious venous thrombosis, thromboembolism, and thrombophlebitis.[8,9] The technique received severe criticism from Bansmer and his colleagues,[10] although they did believe that inferior caval catheterisation represented an advance in clinical treatment. Among 24 of their patients in whom an inferior vena caval catheter had been inserted through the femoral vein, 11 suffered serious complications, with three subsequent deaths.

However, because of adverse reports and the practical difficulty of keeping the site of skin puncture free from infection, the technique of placing central venous catheters through the femoral vein was largely superseded by the introduction of subclavian venous catheterisation by Wilson in 1962.[11] One of the alleged advantages of subclavian catheters was the reduced risk of venous thrombosis and pulmonary embolism. Experience has not borne this out. Femoral vein catheterisation is still occasionally performed in adults when other routes cannot be used. Nevertheless, the femoral vein remains an important alternative to the subclavian and internal jugular routes, especially in cases of emergency and cardiac surgery.[12]

The femoral vein route is still favoured in paediatric practice because of the relatively straightforward nature of femoral venepuncture in such small patients. The anatomy is constant and the femoral arterial pulse provides a very reliable landmark. Should accidental arterial trauma occur, it becomes obvious at an early stage and management is facilitated by its relatively superficial position. During resuscitation involving cardiac massage and intubation in these small patients, the femoral vein is conveniently out of the way so is an eminently suitable route for inserting a venous line if needed. The femoral vein has been used with success and low morbidity by paediatric house staff,[13] and is the site of choice for inserting cardiac catheters in infants and older children.[14]

A study involving cannulation during cardiopulmonary resuscitation in adults, though, showed that the femoral vein was rather less successfully catheterised compared to cannulation through the subclavian vein.[15]

In a recently published prospective study involving a large number of paediatric cases receiving intensive care, the femoral vein route proved to compare very favourably with catheters placed through the jugular veins, subclavian and arm veins.[16] All catheters were introduced with a guide wire technique; tunnelling was not employed. No difference was found in any of the complication rates including that of infection. Importantly, none of the femoral vein catheterisations was complicated by Gram-negative enteric infections. It appears that provided adequate attention is paid to perineal hygiene then stool contamination does not appear to be an important factor in the development of femoral vein catheter-related infection.

It is probable that more recent developments in catheter materials and techniques could decrease the incidence of infection complicating the use of the femoral vein route. Hohn and Lambert[17] introduced Teflon catheters through the femoral vein in 8 children, and left them *in situ* for 2 to 6 weeks without complications. Indeed in one recent careful study silastic catheters were inserted in the femoral vein and led out through a subcutaneous tunnel remote from the groin.[18] The lines were all inserted by surgical cut down so the results are not necessarily applicable to lines inserted percutaneously. A high standard of management of the lines (all long term) was maintained with the result that only a small number of complications arose: one case each of infection in the subcutaneous tunnel and the catheter and two cases of thrombosis of the inferior vena cava. The use of silastic catheters could result in even further improvement. It might also be useful in longer-term infusions to consider subcutaneous tunnelling so as to move the catheter entry site to a point further from the perineum.

ANATOMY

Venous drainage of the leg takes place through a superficial and a deep system of veins. The superficial veins are situated immediately beneath the skin whilst the deep veins accompany the main arteries. The great (long) saphenous vein together with its tributaries provide the main superficial venous drainage: the vein originates in the foot and runs upwards and to the medial side of the thigh,

passes through the saphenous opening, and ends in the femoral vein. The femoral vein – the main deep vein – accompanies the femoral artery in the thigh and ends at the level of the inguinal ligament, where it becomes the external iliac vein.

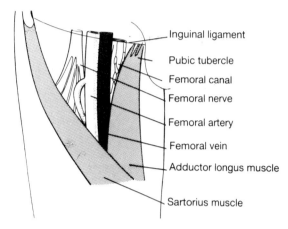

Figure 8.1.   Anatomy of the femoral vein.

In the femoral triangle (Figure 8.1) the femoral vein is medial to the artery. Here it occupies the middle compartment of the femoral sheath, lying between the femoral artery and the femoral canal. It receives the great saphenous vein on its anterior aspect just below the inguinal ligament. Several smaller superficial veins also enter the femoral vein as it lies in the femoral triangle. The femoral nerve lies lateral to the femoral artery. The femoral vein is separated from the skin by superficial and deep fasciae: these layers contain lymph nodes, various superficial nerves, superficial branches of the femoral artery, and the upper part of the saphenous vein before it joins the femoral vein.

FEMORAL VEIN APPROACH
Duffy (1949)[1]

Patient category
Adults and infants.

Advantages and disadvantages
The femoral route is associated with a high incidence of serious complications (Table 8.1); therefore it should be used only when venous catheterisation is not possible through other veins.

Preferred side
Either side may be used.

Position of patient Figure (8.2a)
Place the patient in a supine position. Put a pillow under the patient's buttocks to thrust the groin upwards. Abduct and externally rotate the thigh slightly.

Position of operator Figure (8.2a)
Stand on the same side as the puncture site, facing the patient's head. For a right-handed operator, cannulation of the left vein may be more comfortably performed from the patient's right.

Equipment used in original description
Polyethylene catheter through 14 gauge O.D. needle (in adults).

Advice on current equipment
Adults. 14 gauge O.D. needle or introducer, length 40 mm (minimum). Catheter length 600 mm (minimum).
Neonates. 20 or 18 gauge O.D. needle or introducer, length 20 mm (minimum). Catheter length 200 mm (minimum).

Anatomical landmarks Figure (8.2b)
Identify the femoral artery below the inguinal ligament by palpation. The vein is medial to the artery.

Preparation
Perform the puncture under sterile conditions using local anaesthetic if indicated.

Precautions and recommendations
Perform the venepuncture with care to avoid puncturing the femoral artery, thereby causing haemorrhage or arterial spasm.

Point of insertion of needle Figure (8.2b)
Adults. About 1 cm medial to the artery just below the inguinal ligament.
Neonates and infants. Immediately medial to the artery just below the inguinal ligament.

Direction of needle and procedure Figure (8.2c,d)
Adults. Place the point of the needle at the entry site on the skin (A) and point the needle cephalad; swing the needle and syringe slightly laterally (A to B). Elevate the needle and syringe above the skin (20–30° to the skin surface) and advance the needle. Maintain a negative pressure in the syringe as the needle is advanced. The vein is usually entered at a depth of between 2 and 4 cm. Insert the catheter to the required distance.
Infants. As above, but elevate the needle and syringe to less of an angle to the skin (10–15° to the skin surface), as the vein is more superficial.

Success rate
100% (28 cases).

Complications
None.

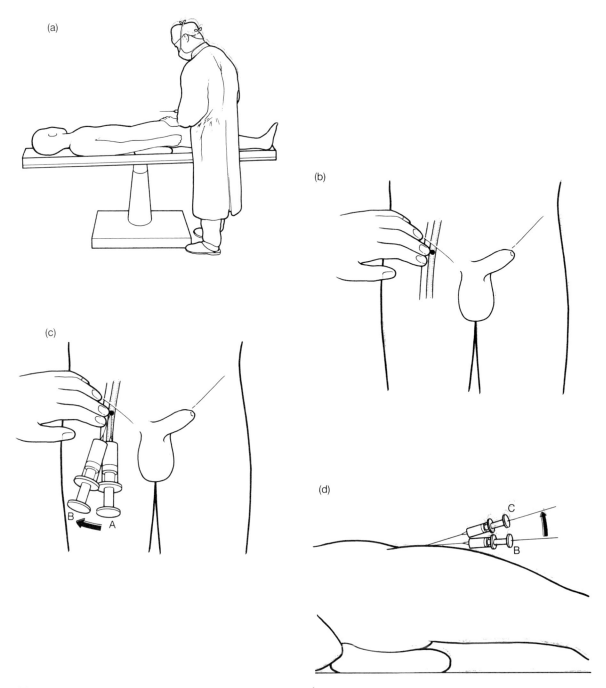

Figure 8.2. Technique of catheterisation: Duffy (1949).[1]

FEMORAL VEIN APPROACH: GUIDE WIRE TECHNIQUE
Hohn and Lambert (1966)[17]

Patient category

Children over 3 years of age.

Advantages and disadvantages

This technique employs a modified guide wire (Seldinger) technique. No infants weighing less than 10 kg were included in the original series.

Preferred side

Either side may be used.

Position of patient (Figure 8.3a)

Place the patient in the supine position. Put a pillow under the patient's buttocks to make the groin prominent. Abduct and externally rotate the thigh slightly.

Position of operator (Figure 8.3b)

Stand on the same side as the puncture site, facing the patient's head.

Equipment used in original description

19 gauge O.D. needle, length 40 mm. Nylon filament (continuous nylon, monofilament, 40 lb test fishline). 19 or 17 gauge O.D. Teflon catheter. Length 500 mm.

Advice on current equipment

20 or 18 gauge O.D. needle or introducing cannula in infants. 200–300 mm catheter or longer in larger children. Guide wire or nylon filament.

Anatomical landmarks (Figure 8.3c)

Identify the femoral artery below the inguinal ligament by palpation. The vein lies immediately medial to the artery.

Precautions and recommendations

Perform the puncture under sterile conditions using local anaesthetic if indicated.

Point of insertion of needle (Figure 8.3c)

Immediately medial to the femoral artery, below the inguinal ligament (about 2 cm in a 7-year-old child).

Direction of the needle and procedure (Figure 8.3d)

Place the point of the needle at the entry site on the skin (A) and point the needle cephalad; then swing the needle and syringe slightly laterally (A to B). Elevate the needle and syringe above the skin (10–15° to the skin surface) and advance the needle. Maintain a negative pressure in the syringe as the needle is advanced until the vein is entered. Pass the nylon filament (or guide wire) into the vein through the needle. Enlarge the skin puncture 1–2 mm on each side of the needle with a scalpel blade to help the catheter to pass easily through the skin. Remove the needle. Thread the catheter over the nylon filament (or guide wire) and advance both into the vein to the required distance. Withdraw the filament (or guide wire). Confirm the position of the catheter with a chest x-ray.

Success rate

The technique was successful in 8 patients (3–15 years). The rate of successful cannulation was not stated. Catheters were left in for an average of 28 days (range 15–43 days).

Complications

None.

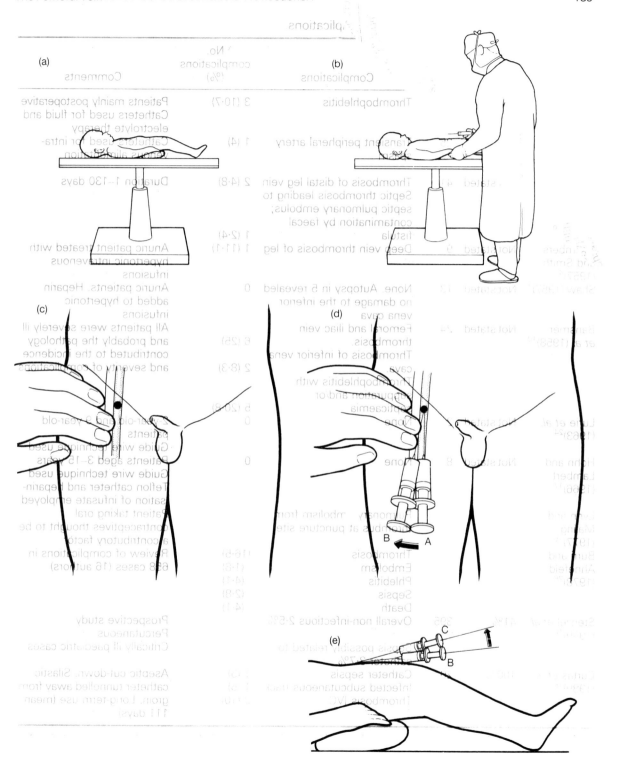

Figure 8.3. Guide wire technique: Hohn and Lambert (1966).[16]

Table 8.1. Femoral vein – results and complications.

Author and year	Success rate	No. cases	Complications	No. complications (%)	Comments
Duffy (1949)[1]	100%	28	Thrombophlebitis	3 (10·7)	Patients mainly postoperative. Catheters used for fluid and electrolyte therapy
Ladd and Schreiner (1951)[6]	Not stated	25	Transient peripheral artery spasm	1 (4)	Catheters used for intra-venous alimentation
Bonner (1951)[8]	Not stated	41	Thrombosis of distal leg vein. Septic thrombosis leading to septic pulmonary embolus; contamination by faecal fistula	2 (4·8); 1 (2·4)	Duration 1–130 days
Chambers and Smith (1957)[4]	Not stated	9	Deep vein thrombosis of leg	1 (11·1)	Anuric patient treated with hypertonic intravenous infusions
Shaw (1957)[7]	Not stated	13	None. Autopsy in 5 revealed no damage to the inferior vena cava	0	Anuric patients. Heparin added to hypertonic infusions
Bansmer et al (1958)[10]	Not stated	24	Femoral and iliac vein thrombosis. Thrombosis of inferior vena cava. Thrombophlebitis with suppuration and/or septicaemia	6 (25); 2 (8·3); 5 (20·8)	All patients were severely ill and probably the pathology contributed to the incidence and severity of complications
Lurie et al. (1963)[24]	Not stated	2	None	0	2-year-old and 9-year-old patients. Guide wire technique used
Hohn and Lambert (1966)[17]	Not stated	8	None	0	Patients aged 3–15 years. Guide wire technique used. Teflon catheter and heparin-isation of infusate employed
Lynn and Maling (1977)[25]	–	–	Pulmonary embolism from thrombus at puncture site		Patient taking oral contraceptives thought to be a contributory factor
Burri and Ahnefeld (1978)[26]	–	–	Thrombosis; Embolism; Phlebitis; Sepsis; Death	(16·5); (1·8); (4·1); (2·8); (4·1)	Review of complications in 658 cases (16 authors)
Stenzel et al. (1989)[16]	41%	395	Overall non-infectious 2·5%. Sepsis possibly related to catheter 3·7%		Prospective study. Percutaneous. Critically ill paediatric cases
Curtas et al. (1989)[18]	100%	20	Catheter sepsis; Infected subcutaneous track; Thrombosis IVC	1 (5); 1 (5); 2 (10)	Aseptic cut-down. Silastic catheter tunnelled away from groin. Long-term use (mean 111 days)

CASE REPORTS OF COMPLICATIONS FOLLOWING FEMORAL VEIN CATHETERISATION

Ischaemic leg in infant.[19]
Accidental femoral arterial puncture and periarterial haematoma.[12]
Retroperitoneal haematoma following perforation of the iliac vein.[21]
Transient A–V fistula.[21]
Delayed (7 months) A–V fistula.[22]
Peritonitis from dislodged catheter.[23]

REFERENCES

1. Duffy, B. J. (1949). The clinical use of polyethylene tubing for intravenous therapy. *Annals of Surgery* 130, 929.
2. Bull, G. M. (1952). Discussion on the treatment of anuria. *Proceedings of the Royal Society of Medicine* 45, 848.
3. Chalmers, J. A. and Fawns, H. T. (1955). Prolonged anuria treated by infusion into the vena cava. *Lancet* 1, 79.
4. Chambers, J. W. and Smith G. (1957). The use of caval catheterisation in cases of severe oliguria and anuria. *British Journal of Surgery* 45, 160.
5. Taylor, W. H. (1957). Management of acute renal failure following surgical operation and head injury. *Lancet* 2, 703.
6. Ladd, M. and Schreiner, G. E. (1951). Plastic tubing for intravenous alimentation. *Journal of the American Medical Association* 145, 642.
7. Shaw, G. (1959). Acute renal insufficiency treated by caval infusion of dextrose solutions of high concentration. *Lancet* 1, 15.
8. Bonner, C. D. (1951). Experience with plastic tubing in prolonged intravenous therapy. *New England Journal of Medicine* 245, 97.
9. Page, O. C. and Stephens, J. W. (1954). Prolonged intravenous alimentation: use of polyethylene tubing in inferior vena cava or common iliac veins. *Northwest Medicine* 53, 596.
10. Bansmer, G., Keith, D. and Tesluk, H. (1958). Complications following use of indwelling catheters of inferior vena cava. *Journal of the American Medical Association* 167, 1606.
11. Wilson, J. N., Grow, J. B., Demong, C. V. *et al.* (1962). Central venous pressure in optimal blood volume maintenance. *Archives of Survery* 85, 563.
12. Gilston, A. (1976). Cannulation of the femoral vessels. *British Journal of Anaesthesia* 48, 500.
13. Kantner, R. K., Zimmerman, J. J., Strauss, R. H. and Stoeckel, K. A. (1986). Central venous catheter insertion by femoral vein: safety and effectiveness for the pediatric patient. *Pediatrics* 77, 842.
14. Carter, G. A., Girod, D. A. and Hurwit, R. A. (1975). Percutaneous cardiac catheterization of the neonate. *Pediatrics* 55, 662.
15. Emerman, C. L., Bellon, E. M., Lukens, T. W., May, T. E. and Effron, D. (1990). A prospective study of femoral versus subclavian vein catheterisation during cardiac arrest. *Annals of Emergency Medicine* 19, 26.
16. Stenzel, J. P., Green, T. P., Furhman, B. P., Carlson, P. E. and Marchessault, R. P. (1989). Percutaneous femoral venous catheterizations: a prospective study of complications. *Journal of Pediatrics* 114, 411.
17. Hohn, A. R. and Lambert, E. C. (1966). Continuous venous catheterization in children. *Journal of the American Medical Association* 197, 658.
18. Curtas, S., Bonaventura, M. and Meguid, M. M. (1989). Cannulation of the inferior vena cava for long term central venous access. *Surgery, Gynecology and Obstetrics* 168, 121.
19. Nabseth, D. C. and Jones, J. E. (1962). Gangrene of the lower extremity of infants after femoral venipuncture. *New English Journal of Medicine* 268, 1003.
20. Gilston, A. (1976). Cannulation of the femoral vessels. *British Journal of Anaesthesia* 48, 500.
21. Fuller, T. J., Mahoney, J. J., Juncos, L. I. and Hawkins, R. F. (1976). Arteriovenous fistula after femoral vein catheterization. *Journal of the American Medical Association* 236, 2943.
22. Agresti, J. V., Schwartz, A. B., Chinitz, J. L., Krevolin, L. E. and Wilson, A. R. (1987). Delayed traumatic arteriovenous fistula following hemodialysis vascular catheterization. *Nephron* 46, 350.
23. Bonadio, W. A., Losek, J. D. and Melzer-Lange, M. (1988). An unusual complication from a femoral venous catheter. *Pediatric Emergency Care* 4, 27.
24. Lurie, P. R., Armer, R. M. and Klatte, E. C. (1963). Percutaneous guidewire catheterisation – diagnosis and therapy. *American Journal of Diseases of Children* 106, 189.
25. Lynn, K. L. and Maling, T. M. J. (1977). Case reports. A major pulmonary embolus as a complication of femoral vein catheterisation. *British Journal of Radiology* 50, 667.
26. Burri, C. and Ahnefeld, F. W. (1978). *The Caval Catheter.* Berlin: Springer Verlag.

PART 2

Paediatric Procedures

9

Reasons for Seeking Central Venous Access

The demands for blood sampling, short-term infusion and long-term intermittent access for corrosive or nutritive fluid therapy are facilitated by the availability of central venous access. Developments in materials and the ingenuity of recently developed devices now enable central venous access to be reliably attained in the smallest of infants.

Nevertheless, compared with the use of peripheral veins, the central venous route may involve substantially greater risk in children. Clinicians differ in the readiness with which they embark upon the central venous route. However, when the need for intravenous therapy is prolonged, central catheters may produce less problems than peripheral lines.[1,2] In more prolonged use, central catheters have greater longevity and are less likely to be associated with poor flow when compared with peripheral lines.

Long-term, continuous central venous access for parenteral nutrition has been, hitherto, largely the domain of surgical cut-down procedures for implanting Hickman or Broviac-style silicone elastomer catheters. These can now be inserted by percutaneous techniques both in children and adults[3,4] (see pp. 39 and 207).

Periodic, repetitive access to a central vein, as may be required for children who need repeated courses of antibiotic or cytotoxic medication, is almost certainly best served by the surgical introduction of an implantable infusion device connected to a central vein by a silicone elastomer catheter.[5] These devices offer the best long-term reliability, combined with low complication rate and minimal maintenance (see Chapter 3, p. 31).

Flow-directed balloon-tipped pulmonary artery catheters can be used for haemodynamic measurements in infants and children.[6] Their relatively large size makes a multi-stage vein dilatation technique obligatory.

REFERENCES

1. Ziegler, M., Jakobowski, D., Hoelzer, D., Eichenberger, M. and Koop, C. E. (1980). Route of pediatric parenteral nutrition: proposed criteria revision. *Journal of Pediatric Surgery* 15, 472.
2. Newman, B. M., Jewett, T. C. Jr, Karp, M. P. and Cooney, D. R. (1986). Percutaneous central venous catheterisation in children: first line choice for venous access. *Journal of Pediatric Surgery* 21, 685.
3. Mirro, J., Rao, B. N., Kumar, M., Rafferty, M., Hancock, M., Austin, B. A., Fairclough, D. and Lobe, T. E. (1990). A comparison of placement techniques and complications of externalized catheters and implantable ports used in children with cancer. *Journal of Pediatric Surgery* 25, 120.
4. Dudrick, S. J., O'Donnell, J. J., Englert, G. M., Matheny, R. G., Blume, E. R., Nutt, R. E., Hickey, M. S. and Barroso, A. O. (1984).100 patient-years of ambulatory home total parenteral nutrition. *Annals of Surgery* 199, 770.
5. Wallace, J. and Zeltzer, P. M. (1987). Benefits, complications and care of implantable infusion devices in 31 children with cancer. *Journal of Pediatric Surgery* 22, 833.
6. Damen, J. and Wever, J. E. A. T. (1987). The use of balloon tipped pulmonary artery catheters in children undergoing cardiac surgery. *Intensive Care Medicine* 13, 266.

10

Choosing the Vein

ANATOMICAL CONSIDERATIONS

The smaller dimensions of blood vessels in infancy and the relatively extreme contours of their routes make advancing a catheter, which has been successfully introduced into the vein, much more difficult.

PERIPHERAL ARM VEINS

As in adults, the advantage of peripheral veins is that they can be seen or at least palpated. In neonates, the median basilic vein can be difficult to cannulate. The available catheters tend to totally fill the vein. If the vein goes into spasm during insertion, advancement of the catheter is impeded. These limitations disappear as children become larger and approach the adult anatomy. Nevertheless, fine silicone catheters can be advanced successfully from a variety of peripheral veins.[1] The proximal basilic vein is often not visible or palpable in infants even when distended by axillary compression.[2] Obviously, injury to nerves may complicate blind cannulation of this vein.

AXILLARY VEIN

The axillary vein is accessible to catheterisation from its origin, as the basilic vein passes over the inferior border of the teres major muscle to the point at which it becomes obscured by the pectoralis major. Throughout its course it is closely related to the axillary artery and the branches of the brachial plexus within a neurovascular bundle. It is therefore desirable to identify the axillary or proximal basilic vein either visually or by palpation before making any attempt to puncture the vein in order to minimise accidental arterial puncture or nerve injury. Obviously, identification of the vein is much more difficult in infants and small children but if the dangers are borne in mind, the method is an alternative to other peripheral and deep veins. The route is probably unsuitable for operators with limited experience, especially when dealing with infants.

EXTERNAL JUGULAR VEIN

This vein offers the advantage of being visible and palpable. Serious traumatic complications are therefore unusual. Unfortunately, the distal course of the vein is tortuous (Figure 10.1) which makes the passage of stiff catheters into a central vein almost impossible. Nevertheless, highly flexible catheters can traverse the vein. It is the favoured vein for inserting a flexible silicone elastomer catheter through a metal winged needle.[3] It is usually of an adequate calibre for the passage of a narrow catheter and external jugular venous catheterisation bears little risk of iatrogenic complications. The several valves in the lower portion of the external jugular vein frequently offer obstruction to the easy passage of a catheter. Once past these valves, a catheter inserted through the right external jugular vein runs what should be a straight course to the right atrium; however, experience shows that the catheter tip may still find its way into unsatisfactory positions. A catheter inserted from the left side traverses the left innominate vein to meet the right innominate vein at an angle which encourages its passage into the right atrium.

INTERNAL JUGULAR VEIN

The internal jugular vein is intimately related to the carotid artery throughout its course. It lies deep to the sternomastoid muscle, presenting to the outer margin of the triangle formed by the sternal and clavicular heads of that muscle. When the head is turned towards the opposite side, the vein tends to be just covered by the medial margin of the clavicular head of the muscle. A catheter inserted through the right internal jugular vein runs an almost straight course through the right innominate vein and superior vena cava into the right atrium. On the other hand, the left internal jugular vein joins the left innominate vein which has an almost horizontal course to the point at which it meets the confluence of the right innominate vein and the superior vena cava at virtually a right angle. For this reason, cannulation of the right side is preferred for central venous catheterisation through the internal jugular veins.[5]

Cannulation of the internal jugular vein is often considered to be facilitated by some degree of neck extension combined with rotation of the head away from the side of cannulation. In infants and young children, the relatively large size of the head makes it necessary to lift the chest by means of a pad under the shoulders or extension of the head over the edge of the table. It should be remembered that extreme lateral rotation of the head tends to make the sternomastoid muscle move further over the vein and to compress it. If the child is anaesthetised, the sternomastoid muscle can be relaxed, reducing the tendency for the vein to be compressed, whilst positive pressure ventilation can increase the venous pressure making the vein more prominent. Sustained positive pressure applied to the airway, though, produces a Valsalva effect which tends to move the apex of the lung further through the thoracic inlet, making injury to the lung from an exploring needle more likely.

SUBCLAVIAN VEIN

The subclavian vein tends to arch higher into the neck in infants than in adults. This is more pronounced on the right side causing the right subclavian vein to join the innominate vein at a right angle. Because of this, guide wires and catheters inserted through this vein tend to be directed up into the neck rather than into the superior vena cava (Figure 10.1). Beyond the age of 1 year, as in adults, both right and left subclavian veins have an almost horizontal course.

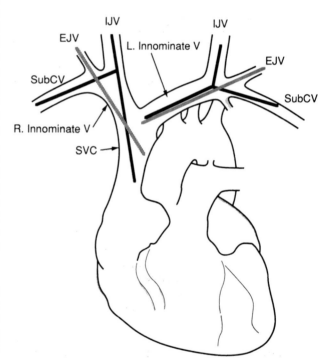

Figure 10.1. The axes of the various venous approaches to the superior vena cava in infants. Modified from Cobb *et al.* (1987).[4]

The subclavian vein route is more hazardous than the internal or external jugular techniques because of the proximity of the adjacent artery which cannot be palpated and the close relation of the pleura. Furthermore if severe bleeding is accidentally produced, haemostasis by the application of pressure to the vessel is virtually impossible because of the overlying clavicle. An alternative route should be considered in an infant with coagulopathy.

FEMORAL VEIN

Because of the proximity of the perineum, the risk of infection through the cannulation site is always a concern when this route is used. The presence of a femoral hernia would contraindicate the use of this site.

The femoral vein is usually medial to the femoral artery although it can sometimes lie directly behind it.[6] Ultrasound imaging can be helpful in identifying the position and patency of the femoral vein relative to the palpable adjacent artery.[7] Ultrasound imaging reveals a close correlation between femoral artery diameter and patient's weight. The femoral vein is often larger than the artery, particularly in infants, and is subject to great variation in size with the respiratory cycle. The vein expands to double its 'resting' size when a Valsalva manoeuvre is induced.

Because the vein is relatively remote from the thorax, radiological confirmation of the position of the catheter tip is essential.[8]

REFERENCES

1. Durand, M., Ramanathan, R., Martinelli, B. and Tollentino, M. (1986). Prospective evaluation of percutaneous central venous silastic catheters in newborn infants with birth weights of 510 to 3920g. *Pediatrics* 78, 245.
2. Ayim, E. N. (1977). Percutaneous catheterisation of the axillary vein and proximal basilic vein. *Anaesthesia* 32, 753.
3. Dolcourt, J. L. and Bose, C. L. (1982). Percutaneous insertion of silastic central venous catheters in newborn infants. *Pediatrics* 70, 484.
4. Cobb *et al.* (1987). The central venous anatomy in infants. *Surgery, Gynecology and Obstetrics* 165, 230.
5. English, I. C. W., Frew, R. M. and Piggott, J. F. (1969). Percutaneous catheterisation of the internal jugular vein. *Anaesthesia* 24, 521.
6. Bosch, G. T., Kengeter, J. P. and Beling, C. A. (1950). Femoral venepuncture. *American Journal of Surgery* 79, 722.
7. Sahn, D. J., Goldberg, S. J., Allen H. D., Valdez-Cruz, L. M., Canale, J. M., Lange, L. and Friedman, M. J. (1982). A new technique for non-invasive evaluation of femoral arterial and venous anatomy before and after percutaneous cardiac catheterization in children and infants. *American Journal of Cardiology* 49, 349.
8. Kelly, M. A., Finer, N. N. and Dunbar, L. G. (1984). Fatal neurologic complication of parenteral feeding through a central vein catheter. *American Journal of Diseases of Children* 138, 352.

11

Choosing the Equipment

There are two important considerations in choosing equipment for central venous catheterisation in very small patients. The first consideration is an immediate one: how best to successfully puncture the chosen vein and advance a catheter whilst minimising traumatic complications. Equipment must be scaled down to accommodate the smaller dimensions and thinner walls of the infant vein. The catheter must be capable of negotiating curves of a much tighter radius than in adults without kinking. The second consideration is how to reduce the longer term complications of catheterisation. In this respect, the importance of catheter material is highlighted.

DIMENSIONAL CONSIDERATIONS

It is useful to consider the implications of scaling. The full-term neonate (3 kg) is approximately one-third of the length, one-ninth of the surface area and one-twenty-fourth of the weight of a 70 kg adult. If it is (reasonably) assumed that all linear dimensions will be similarly reduced a 12 mm diameter internal jugular vein in the adult will be 4 mm in a neonate. A 14 gauge cannula (2·1 mm O.D.) is considered large in an adult; its equivalent in a neonate would be 22 gauge (0·71 mm O.D.). However, catheters as large as 1·6 mm O.D. (5 French Gauge) have been passed percutaneously into the pulmonary artery in infants.[1] Such catheters must virtually fill the cannulated vein.

A perhaps more important consideration is the need for catheters to negotiate, without kinking, curves of much smaller radius than in adults, and also to do so without exerting excessive pressure on the infant vein wall. Applying the scaling concept, a catheter inserted into an infant must have an elastic recoil of much smaller value than that which would be acceptable in adults in order to avoid excessive and damaging pressure on the intima of the vein as the catheter negotiates a curve.

It is not surprising that the incidence of catheter-related damage is higher in infants. The catheter material must provide great flexibility with little force. At body temperature it must be something of a 'wet noodle'.

CATHETER MATERIALS

Silicone elastomer

Silicone elastomer is a natural choice for central venous catheters. It is a chemically and biologically inert material which has the facility to recover its shape readily after being deformed when the deforming force is removed. Catheters made of this material tolerate repeated bending and kinking without any tendency to weaken and to kink again at the same point. Radio-opaque marker material renders silicone elastomer an opaque white. Fluid, particulate matter and gas bubbles within the tubing cannot therefore be observed. The disadvantages of silicone elastomer are that it is difficult to fashion into a tapered point and it tends not to thread easily over a guide wire. Therefore, catheters of this material are either inserted surgically or through a needle or cannula which has been previously inserted into the vein.

If the introducer is to be removed intact, the catheter cannot be provided with a connector bonded on to its proximal end. At one time, it was common practice to provide a makeshift connector by pushing the catheter over the tip of a winged needle. Such a technique was sure to produce an incidence of accidental shearing of the catheter with subsequent migration of the catheter into the heart and beyond. This danger could be reduced by deliberately blunting the needle tip before attaching the catheter.[2] The Tuohy Borst adaptor is unsuitable as a connector because it compresses and occludes a silicone rubber catheter without achieving a secure grip. If a Tuohy Borst adaptor is to be used it is necessary to feed the catheter over some form of stiffener tube before applying compression to the catheter. These problems have been overcome by the introduction of the 'peel away' introducer. Once the catheter with its bonded connector has been successfully placed, the introducer cannula can be split lengthwise and removed completely.[3,4]

Polyvinyl chloride

PVC plastics are made more flexible by the addition of plasticisers. These additives tend to leach out of the material with the passage of time so that such catheters become harder. They are therefore unsuitable for long-term use (i.e. several weeks or months). The tendency for PVC to soften when warm makes it possible to formulate a material which is sufficiently stiff for it to be readily inserted over a guide wire but which softens effectively at body temperature.

Polyethylene and PTFE

These plastics are relatively stiff and are readily tapered to conform over guide wires. Suitably lubricated, they are easily advanced into a vein. Catheters made from these materials have a tendency to kink repeatedly at the same site and to eventually weaken and fracture. They are therefore relatively unsuitable for use in infants unless the chosen vein has a straight course.

Polyurethane copolymers

These recently introduced plastics represent a significant advance. They can be formulated to produce diverse material characteristics ranging from the very flexible silicone elastomer to the near

rigid vein dilator devices whilst retaining the ease with which tip contours can be constructed for easy insertion and minimum tip trauma. They tend to soften considerably when warmed from room to body temperature.

SURFACE CHARACTERISTICS

The ideal surface characteristic of an indwelling catheter is that it should be biologically inert and 'invisible' to platelets. Failing this it should be so 'slippery' that platelets, having aggregated, cannot organise a firm thrombus sheath around the material.

The surface characteristics of catheters made of various plastics vary. With silicone elastomer, polyethylene and PTFE, a fibrin sheath forms after about 24 hours use. Some polyurethane formulations appear to have the best surface characteristics.

If heparin is bonded to the surface, fibrin sheath formation is minimised.[5] The value of heparin coating diminishes as the heparin is lost from the catheter, although some recent techniques of heparin bonding can extend the period of protection from fibrin sheath formation to 9–10 days.

An alternative to heparin bonding is to coat the catheter with a hydrophilic substance, i.e. having the property of attracting water molecules to its surface. Platelets can then 'see nothing' foreign to cause them to initiate the clotting mechanism. The Viggo Hydrocath ® (Viggo-Spectramed, Swindon, UK) is coated with hydromer. These catheters become very slippery when wetted because of their hydrophilic characteristic. The hydromer coating is delicate when wetted and easily damaged by rough handling during catheter insertion.

NEEDLES, CATHETERS AND GUIDE WIRES

The introducing needle and cannula

It is commonly believed that the use of an introducing needle for a Seldinger wire is less traumatic than an introducing cannula because of its thinner wall. It should be remembered that the needle which has a lumen just sufficient for the passage of the wire will create a track through the superficial tissues and through the vessel wall which is smaller than the external diameter of the catheter. The catheter may then be difficult to pass into the lumen of the vessel and may cause the vessel wall to tear. This is particularly true of multilumen catheters and is the reason for which these devices require the intermediate step of introducing a vein dilator. If a cannula-over-needle device is used for the introduction of the guide wire, the needle diameter needs to be no larger than the wire itself, minimising exploratory trauma, while the cannula, doubling as a vein dilator, provides a better track through which the catheter may be introduced. The introducing cannula, once safely introduced into the vessel with the needle removed, forms a secure access for the insertion of the wire when compared with the potential for posterior vessel wall puncture which always accompanies the use of a rigid needle introducer.

When using a cannula-over-needle device, the cannula tip must be in the lumen of the vessel before it is advanced. In confined circumstances, it may be necessary to transfix the vessel, then retract the introducer needle from the cannula before withdrawing the cannula tip back into the lumen and advancing it in the vessel. Whichever device is chosen as the introducer, the catheter must be positioned with minimum damage to the vessel wall. With all but the most flexible catheters, this is best achieved using a suitable guide wire.

J-wire

The success of central venous cannulation via the external jugular vein is greatly enhanced by the use of a 'J'-ended Seldinger wire which assists in negotiating the tortuous pathway of the vein as it joins the subclavian vein.[6] It has been suggested that the relatively poor success of the external jugular vein approach to the central veins in infants and children is related to the excessive radius of the curve of the tip of the J-wire. This is consistent with the finding that the technique becomes progressively less successful with reducing age[7].

Length of catheter

The head grows very quickly in early life, reaching very nearly its final dimensions by the age of 3 years. This largely explains the disproportionate rate of increase of the full and sitting heights with increasing age. Height is a reasonably linear predictor of intravenous catheter length. Figure 11.1 has been drawn on the assumption that there is a perfect direct relationship between standing height and catheter lengths. Clearly, the disproportionate rate of head growth would make this assumption untrue for fine-bore flotation catheters introduced to a central vein from a scalp vein, but for catheters approaching a central vein from elsewhere, the assumption is reasonably useful.

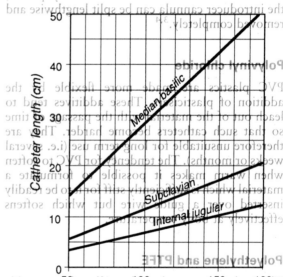

Figure 11.1. Predicted catheter length versus height of the child.

Figure 11.2 relates catheter length and weight of child. The graph can be used to serve as a guide for ordering purposes, but is not an alternative to direct surface measurement and radiological confirmation in determining the correct catheter length in an individual patient.

Figure 11.3 shows the relationship which exists between the various measurement units used for needle and catheter size. Charrier and French gauge are numerically the same, representing the circumference of a tubular material. Thus, a 2 mm catheter is $2 \times \pi = 2 \times 3.14 = 6.3$ Ch. or F.G.

Standard Wire Gauge (S.W.G.)	Diameter (mm)	French Gauge or Charrier
30	0.31	0.99
29	0.34	1.08
28	0.38	1.18
27	0.42	1.31
26	0.46	1.43
25	0.51	1.59
24	0.56	1.75
23	0.61	1.91
22	0.71	2.23
21	0.81	2.55
20	0.91	2.87
19	1.02	3.20
18	1.22	3.83
17	1.42	4.46
16	1.63	5.12
15	1.83	5.75
14	2.02	3.20
13	2.34	7.35
12	2.64	8.29
11	2.95	9.26
10	3.25	10.20

Figure 11.3. Equivalent values of various catheter size units.

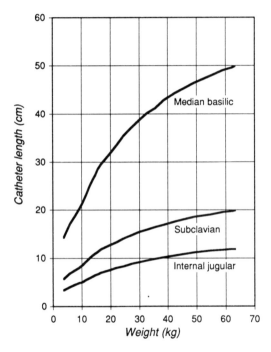

Figure 11.2. Catheter length versus weight of the child. Drawn partly from data presented by Stuart and Stevenson in Nelson (1959)[8] based on measurements of two groups of children in the United States of almost exclusively Western European descent.

Cannulae and catheters

Implantable silicone elastomer catheters were introduced in 1973 by Broviac[9] for the prolonged administration of total parenteral nutrition solutions. The catheter bears a Dacron ® felt cuff which is embedded within a subcutaneous tunnel. As time passes, the material becomes infiltrated by fibroblasts and is incorporated into the fibrous lining of the tissue conduit which forms around the catheter. The cuff forms an obstruction to fluid passing along the outside of the catheter and anchors the device, making skin anchorage unnecessary. These devices have tended to be inserted by surgical cut-down because of concern for the difficulty in controlling haemorrhage, particularly in patients with malignancy and thrombocytopenia. However, satisfactory results can be obtained by percutaneous insertion. In one series in which Broviac catheters were inserted percutaneously into 37 patients with thrombocytopenia (including five children with ages ranging from 1 month to 16 years) a 10% incidence of relatively trivial complications resulted. There were three arterial punctures (without sequelae) and one cervical haematoma.[10] These results compare favourably with some studies where catheters inserted by surgical cut-down have produced a 20% incidence of subcutaneous tract haematomas in one series[11] and a 6% incidence of significant postoperative bleeding in another.[12]

Multilumen catheters

Multilumen catheters in sizes which are sufficiently small to be introduced into infants are now available. They tend to be rather less flexible than single lumen devices and are therefore more likely to become associated with vein trauma. Nevertheless, their use greatly facilitates the simultaneous administration of incompatible solutions and blood sampling. The percutaneous route may also be used for inserting haemodialysis catheters in small infants, though the device may require extensive modification.[13]

REFERENCES

1. Pollack, M. M., Reed, T. P., Holbrook, P. R. and Fields, A. I. (1980). Bedside pulmonary artery catheterization in pediatrics. *Journal of Pediatrics* **96**, 274.
2. Cockington, R. A. (1979). Silicone elastomer for naso-jejunal intubation and central venous cannulation in neonates. *Anaesthesia and Intensive Care* **7**, 248.
3. Kirkemo, A. and Johnstone, M. R. (1982). Percutaneous subclavian vein placement of the Hickman catheter. *Surgery* **91**, 349.
4. Dudrick, S. J., O'Donnell, J. J., Englert, G. M., Matheny, R. G., Blume, E. R., Nutt, R. E., Hickey, M. S. and Barroso, A. O. (1984). 100 patient-years of ambulatory home total parenteral nutrition. *Annals of Surgery* **199**, 770.
5. Curnow, A., Idowu, J., Behrens, E. *et al.* (1985). Urokinase therapy for Silastic catheter-induced intravascular thrombi in infants and children. *Archives of Surgery* **120**, 1237.
6. Blitt, C. D. (1974). Central venous catheterization via the external jugular vein: a technique employing the 'J' wire. *Journal of the American Medical Association* **229**, 817.
7. Nicolson, S. C., Sweeney, M. F., Moore, R. A. and Jobes, D. R. (1985). Comparison of internal and external jugular cannulation of the central circulation in the pediatric patient. *Critical Care Medicine* **13**, 747.
8. Nelson, W. E. (ed.) (1959) *Textbook of Pediatrics*, 7th Edn, pp. 50–61. Philadelphia: W. B. Saunders.
9. Broviac, J. W., Cole, J. J. and Scribner, B. H. (1973). A silicone rubber atrial catheter for prolonged parenteral alimentation. *Surgery, Gynecology and Obstetrics* **136**, 602.
10. Stellato, T. A., Gauderer, M. W., Lazarus, H. M. and Herzig, R. H. (1985). Percutaneous silastic catheter insertion in patients with thrombocytopenia. *Cancer* **56**, 2691.
11. Adami, G. F., Bacigulupo, A. and Bonalumi, U. (1981). Use of Hickman right atrial catheter for vascular access in marrow transplant recipients (letter). *Archives of Surgery* **116**, 1099.
12. Reed, W. P., Newman, K. A., de Jongh, C. *et al.* (1983). Prolonged venous access for chemotherapy by means of the Hickman catheter. *Cancer* **52**, 185–92.
13. Weiss, M. and Sutherland, D. E. (1984). Percutaneous subclavian vein catheterisation for haemodialysis in small children. *Surgery* **95**, 353–4.

12

Practical Aspects of Technique

The reader is directed to Chapter 3 (p. 31) where many additional practical considerations in the insertion and maintenance of central venous lines are discussed.

SEDATION AND ANAESTHESIA

The uncooperativeness of many small patients to attempts at venous access can result in a thoroughly unpleasant experience for both patient and the clinician. Several approaches have been employed to overcome this problem.

'Pin down' techniques

The literature on securing venous access in small children not infrequently refers to restraint, splinting of the head to the table with adhesive tape and similar undesirable stratagems.

Sedation

'Sedation' when administered to a child who is to be submitted to a painful experience is generally ineffective unless carried to a point which is virtually identical to general anaesthesia. Unfortunately, appropriate personnel and facilities, which are the prerequisites of safe anaesthetic practice may not be present when sedation is carried to this length.

Local anaesthetic

Undoubtedly, the development of a local anaesthetic cream which is effective in anaesthetising the skin represents a major advance in the field of gaining venous access in children. Emla cream 5% (TM) (Astra Pharmaceuticals Ltd, King's Langley, Herts, UK) is a eutectic mixture of lignocaine and prilocaine in an emulsion base. The widespread use of Emla (TM) is producing a generation of children who do not associate attempted venepuncture with pain.

General anaesthesia

General anaesthesia is appropriate in a number of circumstances. Its value in facilitating successful and safe cannulation of deep neck veins such as the internal jugular vein is obvious when compared with attempting venepuncture in a child who is struggling, crying, and straining. The anaesthetised child is still, the neck muscles are relaxed and a Valsalva effect to increase venous pressure in the neck and so distend the vein can easily be induced by positive pressure applied to the airway.

POSITIONING OF THE CHILD FOR CENTRAL VENOUS CATHETERISATION

The size of a child has an important influence upon the optimal positioning for central venous cannulation. When neck veins are being cannulated in adults it is customary to place the patient in a head-down position by tilting the couch or operating table in order to increase the venous pressure in the neck to above atmospheric pressure. This has the three benefits of (a) making the vein more obtrusive, (b) making the vein easier to enter rather than to tranfix with the needle and (c) being

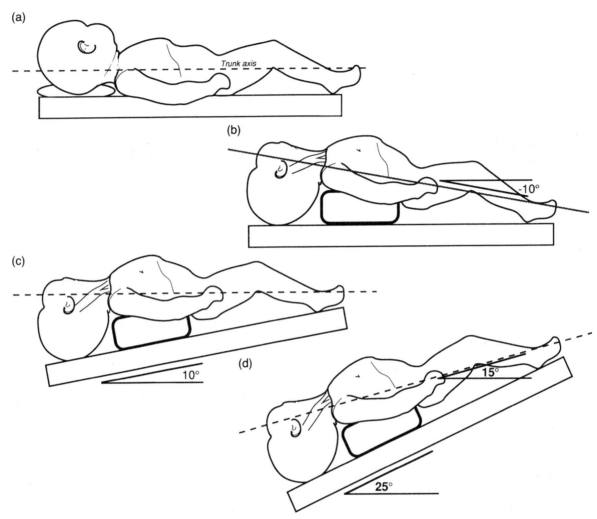

unlikely to permit air from being aspirated during the respiratory cycle.

A 15° head-down tilt in an adult may elevate the venous pressure 10–15 mmHg above atmospheric. The same tilt in an infant, one-third the length of an adult, is likely to have one-third the effect in raising the venous pressure, achieving a rise of only 3–5 mmHg. Furthermore, the relatively large head (Figure 12.1a) requires that the shoulders and chest are raised to permit the necessary extension of the neck to provide access for venepuncture. The result of these manoeuvres is actually to achieve a reverse Trendelenberg tilt (Figure 12.1b) which must then be corrected by exaggerating the tilt head down to 25° or more (Figures 12.1c and d).

Achieving this posture in an awake uncooperative child is of course not always easy. The use of general anaesthesia may well offer the best solution in these cases.

Figure 12.1. (a) The trunk axis is horizontal. An infant lying with a small pillow under the head presents no access to the neck for cannulation. (b) Effect of placing a large pad under an infant's shoulders and back to achieve full extension of the head. Note that the long axis of the trunk is now 10° head-down even though the table mattress remains horizontal. (c) As in (b) but note how 10° of head-down table tilt has been necessary to regain a horizontal axis for the trunk. (d) As in (b) but note how 25° of head-down table tilt has been necessary to achieve 15° head-down axis for the trunk.

CARE OF INFUSION SYSTEMS

Preventing blockage of the catheter with blood clot

The loss of a possibly vital central line from this cause, which may have also been difficult to obtain, is a frustrating experience.

Infusion systems which rely on the hydrostatic pressure of the fluid column as the motive force are not capable of delivering sufficient pressure to burst an obstructed vein. On the other hand the flow is easily reduced or even stopped by a modest resistance to flow resulting from thrombus developing in the vein, Valsalva manoeuvre, external compression and similar incidents. The flow of fluid may even be transiently reversed permitting reflux of blood into the catheter lumen where it may clot, causing an obstruction. As many as 44% of venous catheters may fail because of such problems.[1] These authors argued that intermittent flushing with heparin solution followed by capping of the catheter was a more reliable method of keeping long-term central venous catheters patent compared with a continuous fluid drip. The use of a volumetric pump, or at least a one-way valve, would seem to be prudent in these circumstances.

The transport of a child from area to area, e.g. ward to operating theatre, is frequently associated with failure of a precious central (or even peripheral) line unless care is exercised. With some infusion devices, if the pump is switched off and the tubing disconnected from the pump, blood may be aspirated back into the catheter where it may clot. If possible, the pump should remain connected to the catheter and the fluid flow maintained in transit.

INSERTION OF A FINE-BORE SILICONE CENTRAL VENOUS CATHETER THROUGH A WINGED INTRODUCING NEEDLE INTO ANY SUITABLE PERIPHERAL VEIN
Durand et al. *(1986)*[2]

Patient category

Infants weighing between 0·51 and 3·92 kg.

Advantages and disadvantages

Any convenient peripheral vein can be used. There is no risk of causing raised intracranial pressure with head movement as might be the case with internal jugular cannulation.[3,4]

Equipment used in original description

A winged needle from which the flexible tubing and plastic hub has been detached. A 25 gauge blunt-tipped needle and a length of Silastic ® silicone rubber tubing (Dow Corning) of 0·025 inches (0·635 mm) O.D., 0·012 inches (0·305 mm) I.D.

Advice on current equipment

The 'Epicutaneo Cave' kit of component parts is available from Vygon (Vygon UK Ltd, Cirencester, Gloucestershire, GL17 1PT, UK).

Anatomical landmarks

Visualise and identify vein directly.

Preparation

Perform the procedure under sterile conditions using local anaesthesia as indicated.

Precautions and recommendations

Suitable sites for venepuncture include the antecubital fossa, forearm, leg and scalp veins (preferably anterior to the ear).

Procedure

Puncture vein and insert the catheter for a distance which has been pre-measured so that the catheter tip will lie in a suitable central position. Withdraw and discard the needle. Attach a blunt cannula to the external end of the catheter, securing it with a suture. Confirm the catheter tip position by taking an x-ray. Clean the insertion site again with povidone iodine solution and fix the catheter to the skin using Steristrip® skin closures before covering the site with a vapour-permeable self-adhesive membrane such as OpSite (Smith & Nephew Medical Ltd, Hull, HU3 2BN, UK). Change the dressing only when necessary but change the infusates and infusion sets daily under sterile conditions. Add 1 IU/ml heparin to all infusion fluids.

Success rate

50 successful cannulations were achieved in the first 55 attempts. The mean duration that the catheter remained in position was 25.4 ± 16.7 days. There were 4 cases (6.7%) of bacteraemia. Mechanical complications occurred in 26.4% of cases, mostly blockage of catheter due to calcium phosphate precipitation.

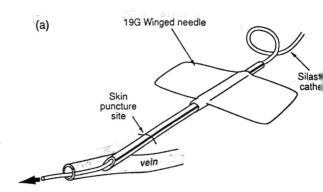

MODIFICATIONS[5] (Figure 12.2a–c)

The technique is essentially as described for Durand et al.[2] (above). An Abbott Butterfly ® (Abbott Laboratories, Hospital Products Division, Queenborough, Kent ME11 5EL, UK) 25 gauge needle whose cutting edge is first blunted using the ridged surface of a needle holder or similar surface is used as an improvised connector for the silicone rubber tubing.

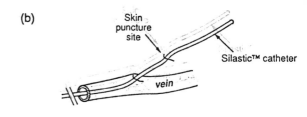

1. Introduce a Silastic feeding line (0·64 mm O.D.) through a 19 gauge winged needle from which the tubing has been removed (Figure 12.2a).
2. Remove and discard winged needle (Figure 12.2b).
3. Thread Silastic tube over 25 gauge winged needle which has been prepared as above. With the needle guard in place, the whole assembly is sandwiched between two small squares of Elastoplast® (Smith & Nephew) elastic adhesive bandage (Figure 12.2c).

The catheter recommended for insertion into the vein is a Silastic® (Catalogue Number 602.105, Dow Corning, Abco House, Reading, Berks, UK)[6] feeding line which is a silicone elastomer tube of 0·64 mm O.D., 0·3 mm I.D. The catheter can be inserted into the scalp vein, antecubital or long saphenous vein. Where possible, antecubital fossa veins are reserved for candidates for parenteral nutrition.

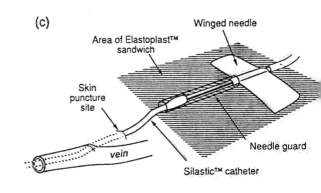

Figure 12.2. Technique described for Durand et al., 1986[2]

(a)

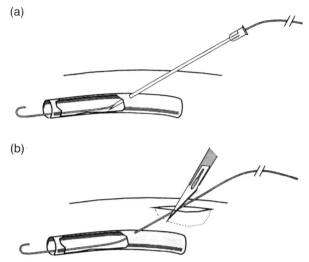

(b)

(c)

(d)

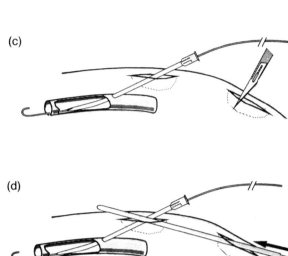

Figure 12.3. Percutaneous insertion of a Hickman line (a) Introduce J-wire after confirming position of needle in vein by aspiration, (b) make first skin incision to include J-wire point of emergence from skin, (c) insertion of vein dilator over J-wire and second skin incision for proposed site of emergence of Hickman line, (d) creation of a tunnel between the two incisions using a blunt catheter insertion device. (Dudrick *et al.*, 1984).[7]

PERCUTANEOUS INSERTION OF A SUBCUTANEOUSLY TUNNELLED HICKMAN CATHETER
Dudrick et al. (*1984*)[7]

Patient category
All ages.

Advantages and disadvantages
Avoids the need for surgical cut-down, minimising damage to the vein.

Equipment used in original description
An introducer system originally designed for the placement of pervenous cardiac pacemaker leads. The kit comprised: 18 gauge needle, 9 cm long; J-wire, 47 cm long; syringe; linearly splittable ('peel-away') winged introducer cannula of an internal diameter sufficient to pass the selected Hickman catheter; vein dilator of sufficient length and diameter to act as an obturator for the introducer.

Advice on current equipment
Any product containing these components.

Anatomical landmarks
As appropriate for chosen technique – preferably an infraclavicular subclavian cannulation technique.

Preparation
Perform puncture under sterile conditions using local anaesthesia as indicated.

Procedure
1. Introduce needle into chosen vein and check by aspiration.
2. Advance J-wire through needle until its tip lies several centimetres beyond the needle tip. Ideally, the position of the J-wire tip in the SVC should be confirmed by radiological screening (Figure 12.3a).
3. Remove needle.
4. Make a 1 cm incision in the skin to include the wire insertion site (Figure 12.3b).
5. Make a second, similar incision at the selected point of exit of the catheter. This site should provide easy access for the patient and attendants for routine wound cleaning and dressing procedures (Figure 12.3c).
6. Create a tunnel between the two incisions with a suitable, blunt shunt-passing device (Figure 12.3d).

(e)

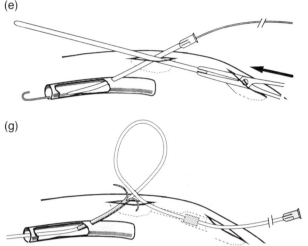

(g)

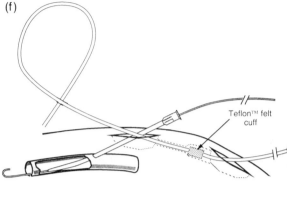

(f)

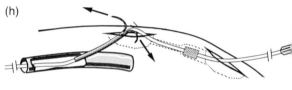

Teflon™ felt cuff

(h)

(i)

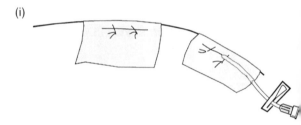

Figure 12.3   (e) Widening the tunnel at the distal end by introducing a haemostat; (f) the catheter is drawn through the tunnel using the catheter insertion device; (g) the twin dilator is removed, leaving the J-wire in place. A splittable catheter sleeve is placed over the vein dilator and the assembly is reinserted into the vein. The vein dilator is again removed, leaving the sleeve in position. The catheter, having been cut to the correct length, is advanced through this sleeve; (h) the splittable catheter introducer is removed by pulling the two split ends apart and the catheter is advanced until it lies entirely beneath the skin level. (Dudrick *et al.*, 1984).[7]

7. Widen the distal end of the tunnel using an artery forceps (haemostat) to permit entry of the Dacron cuff of the catheter (Figure 12.3e).
8. Thread the catheter through the tunnel by attaching it to the shunt-passing device and drawing it through the tunnel until the cuff is located in its final chosen position, several centimetres within the tunnel (Figure 12.3f).
9. Cut the catheter to the correct length by laying it over its proposed course and cutting it at the level of the second intercostal space adjacent to the angle of Louis.
10. Fill the catheter with heparinised saline and apply an obturator with a latex injection site to the Luer connector.
11. Thread the vein dilator over the J-wire and dilate the track into the lumen of the vein.
12. Having removed the dilator, pass it through the splittable introducer sheath and thread both (i.e. dilator and splittable introducer), assembled, over the J-wire.

13. Remove the J-wire and the vein dilator, staunching the flow of blood from the introducer with the finger of a gloved hand.
14. Introduce the cut end of the catheter through the introducer (Figure 12.3g).
15. Carefully remove the introducer by separating its wings and splitting it as it is withdrawn, taking care to prevent the catheter from being delivered with it (Figure 12.3h).
16. Close both wounds with a skin suture or an adhesive dressing (Figure 12.3i).
17. Apply rigorous antiseptic/aseptic dressing technique.

Success rate

Suitable for parenteral feeding over an extended period.

Complications

As apply to the route employed.

PERCUTANEOUS INSERTION OF A BALLOON-TIPPED PULMONARY ARTERY FLOTATION CATHETER THROUGH THE INTERNAL JUGULAR VEIN IN CHILDREN
Damen and Wever (1987)[8]

Patient category
0–15 years.

Preferred side
Right.

Equipment used in original description
Less than 20 kg – 5 French Swan–Ganz catheter (Edwards Company, Santa Anna, CA, USA) with 6 French introducer. Balloon volume 0·5 ml.
More than 20 kg – 7 or 7·5 Fr. Swan–Ganz catheter with 8 Fr. introducer. Balloon volume 1·5 ml. Introducers by Cordis Corporation, Miami, Fl, USA.

Advice on current equipment
Any equivalent product.

Preparation
Perform puncture under sterile conditions using local anaesthesia as indicated.

Precautions and recommendations
Locate the right internal jugular vein using a seeker needle of 25 or 23 gauge.

Point of insertion of needle
As appropriate for technique chosen.

Procedure
1. Having located the right internal jugular vein with the seeking needle, puncture the vessel with a 20 or 18 gauge needle and introduce a guide wire through it.
2. Advance an 18 or 16 gauge catheter over the guide wire. Replace the guide wire with a thicker one.
3. Replace the catheter with a 6 or 8 French introducer over the larger guide wire. Flush the introducer with heparinised saline before insertion.
4. In small babies, it may be necessary to shorten the catheter to the appropriate length before insertion.

5. Test the catheter balloon and fill the catheter lumens with heparinised saline.
6. When the catheter is being inserted for the purpose of management of a child undergoing corrective heart surgery, introduction of the balloon catheter into the pulmonary artery may be deferred until it is anatomically possible, either during or after corrective surgery. Place a sterile sleeve over the catheter and advance it into the introducer, using the pressure trace derived from the terminal lumen as a guide to progress and an ECG to monitor possible cardiac arrhythmias.
7. Inflate the balloon to its full diameter when the catheter passes beyond the tip of the introducer and after an acceptable right atrial pressure trace has been obtained. Advance the catheter until it can be demonstrated to have wedged in the pulmonary artery.
8. Deflate the balloon until the next estimation of pulmonary artery wedged pressure is made.

Success rate
100%. Fifty-seven out of 59 successful insertions of the introducer into the right internal jugular vein. Two out of 59 were located successfully through the left internal jugular vein.

Complications
Accidental carotid artery punctures by the seeker needle – 6 in 59 (10%); no serious haematoma or bleeding problems.
The catheter could not be wedged in only 3 instances (5%).
Balloon inflation affected the systemic pressure in 5 instances.

BLOCKAGE OF CATHETERS

Thrombolytic therapy
Thrombolytic therapy using urokinase has been employed successfully to salvage catheters occluded with thrombus in children.[9,10] Long-term catheters used for total parenteral nutrition are liable to blockage with crystalline deposits of calcium phosphate. These incidents can be minimised by carefully selecting the relative concentrations of the two ions in solutions or by arranging to prescribe calcium and phosphate sequentially.

Theoretically, the occurrence can be eliminated by using a multi-lumen catheter, with one lumen reserved for each of the supplements. Repeated irrigation with hydrochloric acid and heparin solution to dissolve catheters blocked by calcium phosphate crystals has been recommended.[11] This solution is prepared by mixing 0·1 N HCl (1 ml/kg) with 10 ml of heparin saline (10 IU/ml), 0·2 ml aliquots being used to irrigate the catheter using a to-and-fro action from a 1 ml tuberculin syringe. The process is repeated hourly, as necessary.

DETACHMENT OF CATHETER FRAGMENTS

The most common cause of embolisation of catheter fragments was, for several years, the severing of the catheter by the cutting edge of the introducing needle. More recently, alternative techniques for insertion of catheters, including Seldinger technique devices and introducer sheaths, have minimised this complication. Accidental cutting of the catheter whilst removing retaining sutures was implicated in 6 out of 8 cases of catheter embolisation recently reported.[12] Techniques in which the catheter is secured by a suture which is wrapped around it at the point of its entry through the skin, or within a tunnel track,[13] are particularly likely to be associated with accidental severance of the catheter and the subsequent loss of its distal portion into the circulation.

When catheter embolisation occurs, attempts to remove the detached component must be made since the mortality associated with retention of the fragment has been estimated as 37%.[13] There have been numerous reports of successful removal of catheter fragments using percutaneous techniques.[14–23]

PREVENTION OF INFECTION

Systemic infection is a serious limiting factor in the long-term usefulness of central venous catheters in infants and children. Catheter-induced sepsis resulting in endocarditis and subsequent mortality has been reported.[24] The incidence of catheter contamination as evidenced by positive catheter tip culture is related to the duration of use.

It is generally believed that the colonisation of the catheter tip is the result of bacteria becoming attached to, and growing upon the fibrin sheath which forms around most catheters. These organisms might arise from any number of unrelated sources, being dispersed by the circulation and infecting the catheter in much the same way as is thought to occur with other prosthetic devices such as cardiac valves. This would explain the delay which often occurs between catheter insertion and the onset of clinical symptoms. Catheter surfaces which are treated to minimise platelet adhesion and fibrin deposition should therefore be less readily involved in septicaemic incidents. Nevertheless, the nature of the organisms encountered suggests that skin-borne organisms migrate through the lumen or through the track of the catheter. Needles and catheters which are introduced over needles or guide wires are likely to be contaminated with skin pathogens on insertion. Venepuncture and catheter insertion may inoculate deeper layers of the track, facilitating the passage of organisms to the fibrin sheath. This view is supported by the finding of suppurative arthritis of the hip joint in association with femoral venepuncture.[25] The argument for tunnelling catheters is that it lengthens this path.[26] The Dacron felt cuff incorporated onto the tunnelled portion of long-term silicone catheters interrupts the continuity of the track for migrating organisms while serving also to anchor the catheter in a fibrous scar.

Staphylococcus epidermidis, once considered to be a non-pathogenic skin contaminant, has emerged as a serious pathogen in hospitalised, immunosuppressed, premature and malnourished paediatric patients. In these patients, the presence of an indwelling venous catheter greatly enhances the likelihood of infection. In one series of such patients, central venous catheters were identified as the source of 23 out of 56 cases of *Staphylococcus epidermidis* sepsis.[3]

Recommendations have been made for arbitrary removal or replacement of catheters in children after 3–7 days in order to reduce the incidence of catheter-related sepsis.[4,24,27] Such policies are totally unacceptable for patients requiring long-term central venous access for chemotherapy. In these instances, there is justification for retaining the catheter for as long as it is clinically necessary and treating any infectious incident before considering catheter removal. This applies whether or not the infection is proved to be catheter related. By this means, it has proved possible to retain suitable catheters for a year or more.

There is good evidence that percutaneously introduced Hickman and Broviac silicon elastomer catheters are less likely to be associated with subsequent obstructive or infective complications than catheters introduced by surgical cut-down.[28]

Compared with older children, infants undergoing cardiac surgery in whom an internal jugular vein catheter has been introduced seemed to be more susceptible to develop catheter-related infection in spite of prophylactic antibiotic cover. The evidence suggested that it would be safe to leave catheters *in situ* for 3 days in infants and 6 days in older children.[8] *Staphylococcus epidermidis,* an organism capable of causing endocarditis, was the organism most commonly found on the catheter tips in this series. Opsonins, necessary to coat the organisms to make phagocytosis possible, are much depleted in infants compared with adults,[29] and the levels are further reduced by anaesthesia and surgery[6] and by cardiopulmonary bypass.[30]

There appears to be no consistent relationship between positive tip cultures and the duration of insertion of the catheter. There is some evidence that catheters introduced through the basilic vein become less frequently infected than those introduced through the internal or external jugular veins.[31]

Femoral venepuncture has been implicated in several incidents of suppurative arthritis of the hip joint in infants.[32,33] This is hardly surprising when one recommended technique includes advancing the needle until the bone is felt before aspirating gently on withdrawal. Clavicular periostitis has also been reported as a complication of central venous cannulation.[34]

REFERENCES

1. Ladd, M. and Schreiner, G. E. (1951). Plastic tubing for intravenous alimentation. *Journal of the American Medical Association* 145, 642.
2. Durand, M., Ramanathan, R., Martinelli, B. and Tollentino, M. (1986). Prospective evaluation of percutaneous central venous silastic catheters in newborn infants with birth weights of 510 to 3920 g. *Pediatrics* 78, 245.
3. Scherer, L. R., West, K. W., Weber, T. R., Teiman, M. and Grosfeld, J. L. (1984). *Staphylococcus epidermidis* in pediatric patients: clinical and therapeutic considerations. *Journal of Pediatric Surgery* 19, 358.
4. Rao, T. L., Wong, A. Y. and Salem, M. R. (1977). A new approach to the percutaneous catheterisation of the internal jugular vein. *Anesthesiology* 46, 362.

5. Puntis, J. W. (1986). Percutaneous insertion of central venous feeding catheters. *Archives of Disease in Childhood* 61, 1138.
6. Perttila, J., Lilius, E-M. and Salo, M. (1986). Effects of anaesthesia and surgery on serum opsonic capacity. *Acta Anaesthesiologica Scandinavica* 30, 173.
7. Dudrick, S. J., O'Donnell, J. J., Englert, G. M., Matheny, R. G., Blume, E. R., Hickey, M. S. and Barroso, A. O. (1984). 100 patient-years of ambulatory home total parenteral nutrition. *Annals of Surgery* 199, 770.
8. Damen, J. and Wever, J. E. A. T. (1987). The use of balloon tipped pulmonary artery catheters in children undergoing cardiac surgery. *Intensive Care Medicine* 13, 266.
9. Winthrop, A. L. and Wesson, D. E. (1984). Urokinase in the treatment of central venous catheters in children. *Journal of Pediatric Surgery* 19, 536.
10. Curnow, A., Idowu, J., Behrens, E. *et al.* (1985). Urokinase therapy for Silastic catheter-induced thrombi in infants and children. *Archives of Surgery* 120, 1237.
11. Breaux Jr, C., Duke, D., Georgeson, K. E. and Mestre, J. R. (1987). Calcium phosphate occlusion of central venous catheters used for total parenteral nutrition in infants and children: Prevention and treatment. *Journal of Pediatric Surgery* 22, 829.
12. Grabenwoeger, F., Bardach, G., Dock, W. and Pinterits, P. (1989). Percutaneous extraction of centrally embolised foreign bodies: a report of 16 cases. *British Journal of Radiology* 61, 1014.
13. Alfieris, G. M., Wing, C. W. and Hoy, G. R. (1987). Securing Broviac catheters in children. *Journal of Pediatric Surgery* 22, 825.
14. Moncada, R. and Demos, T. C. (1977). Iatrogenic cardiovascular foreign bodies. *Review Interam Radiology* 2, 205.
15. Fisher, R. G. and Mattox, K. L. (1978). Percutaneous extraction of an embolised hyperalimentation catheter fragment. *Southern Medical Journal* 71, 1438.
16. Millan, V. G. (1978). Retrieval of intravascular foreign bodies using a modified bronchoscopic forceps. *Radiology* 129, 587.
17. Chung, K. J., Chernoff, H. L., Leape, L. L. and Kreidberg, M. B. (1980). Transfemoral snaring of broken catheters from the right heart in small infants. *Catheterization and Cardiovascular Diagnosis* 6, 331.
18. Weber, J. and Sartor K. (1980). Percut. removal of intravascular fragments from infusion, angiographic, and CSF drainage caths. with the loop-snare technic. *Chirurgie* 51, 711.
19. Endrys, J., Rubacek, M. and Podrabski, P. (1985). Percutaneous retrieval of foreign bodies from the cardiovascular system. *Coret Vasa* 27, 36.
20. Uflacker, R., Lima, S. and Melichar, A. C. (1986). Intravascular foreign bodies: percutaneous retrieval. *Radiology* 160, 731.
21. Alzen, G., Mertens, R. and Gunther, R. (1987). Percutaneous catheter extraction of a ruptured Portacath in a small child. *Klinische Paediatrie* 199, 296.
22. Gross, D. M., Cox, M. A., Denson, S. B. and Ferguson, L. (1987). Unique use of a tip-deflecting guide wire in removing a catheter embolus from an infant. *Pediatric Cardiology* 8, 117.

23. Engelhardt, W., Muhler, E., Lang, D. and von Bernuth, G. (1989). Percutaneous removal of embolised catheters from pulmonary arteries or the right heart in children. *Klinische Pediatrie* **200**, 444.

24. Stanton, B. F., Baltimore, R. S. and Clemens, J. D. (1984). Changing spectrum of infective endocarditis in children. An analysis of 26 cases, 1970–1979. *American Journal of Diseases of Children* **138**, 720.

25. Asnes, R. S. and Arendar, G. M. (1966). Septic arthritis of the hip: a complication of femoral venepuncture. *Pediatrics* **38**, 837.

26. Dudrick, S. J., Groff, D. B. and Wilmore, D. W. (1969). Long term venous catheterisation in infants. *Surgery, Gynecology and Obstetrics* **129**, 805.

27. Notterman, D. A. (1985). Invasive haemodynamic monitoring. In *Critical Care Paediatrics* edited by S. S. Zimmerman and J. H. Gidea, p. 43. Philadelphia: W. B. Saunders.

28. Mirro, J., Rao, B. N., Kumar, M., Rafferty, M., Hancock, M., Austin, B. A., Fairclough, D. and Lobe, T. E. (1990). A comparison of placement techniques and complications of externalized catheters and implantable ports used in children with cancer. *Journal of Pediatric Surgery* **25**, 120.

29. Fleer, A., Gerards, L. J., Aerts, P., Westerdaal, N. A. C., Senders, R. C., Van Dijk, H. and Verhoef, J. (1985). Opsonic defence to *Staphylococcus epidermidis* in the premature neonate. *Journal of Infectious Disease* **152**, 930.

30. Jones, H. M., Matthews, N., Vaughan, R. S. and Stark, J. M. (1982). Cardiopulmonary bypass and complement activation. *Anaesthesia* **37**, 629–33.

31. Gertner, J., Herman, B., Pescio, M. D. and Wolff, M. A. (1979). Risk of infection in prolonged central venous catheterization. *Surgery, Gynecology and Obstetrics* **149**, 567.

32. Samilson, R. L., Bersani, F. A. and Watkins, M. G. (1958). Acute suppurative arthritis in infants and children. *Pediatrics* **21**, 798.

33. Baitch, A. (1962). Recent observations of acute suppurative arthritis. *Clinical Orthopaedics* **22**, 157.

34. Marty, F. and Truong, P. (1983). Clavicular periostitis: an unusual complication of percutaneous subclavian venous catheterization. *Radiology* **64**, 139.

13

Choice of a Technique

GENERAL

The many factors to be taken into account when choosing a particular route for central venous catheterisation are discussed in Chapter 1 (p. 3).

Some reviews of published data concerning intravenous alimentation in paediatric patients have concluded that the jugular veins offer the best means of access in infants, with the catheter tunnelled subcutaneously to an exit point behind and above the right ear. The technique of floating a fine silicone elastomer catheter, particularly through the basilic vein, is best suited to older infants and small children. The subclavian route is more appropriate in larger children. The femoral vein is best avoided because of the increased infection risk.[1]

PERIPHERAL VEINS

Flexible silicone catheters, inserted through thin wall needles, are usually employed to gain central venous access through peripheral veins. Their bore is necessarily fine and therefore susceptible to blockage by clot and calcium phosphate crystals from parenteral nutrition solutions.[2] These catheters can accommodate a maximum flow rate of 50 ml/h.[3] Several studies in infants show conclusively that percutaneous central venous catheterisation compares favourably with insertion of silastic catheters (sometimes of a large diameter) by surgical cut-down on deeper veins.[3–8]

AXILLARY VEIN

Central venous catheterisation through the axillary vein route avoids the potentially serious complications associated with catheterisation of the deep neck veins.[9,10] The relatively short catheter needed for the axillary vein route is easier to pass centrally, in comparison with catheters inserted through more peripheral veins.

Two techniques are detailed below. The technique described by Oriot and Defawe[11] seeks to identify the vein directly whilst that of Metz et al.[12] identifies the axillary artery and defines its relation to the vein. The advantages of the latter method are its application to children with an impalpable vein and the reduced risk of arterial puncture. A third technique (described by Nickalls in 1987 and Taylor and Yellowlees in 1990) for use in adults and infants (see Chapter 4, p. 53), seeks to access the middle part of the axillary artery by using indirect landmarks. Of the three methods, it is probably the least appropriate for infants.

TECHNIQUE FOR INSERTING A SILICONE CATHETER THROUGH AN INTRODUCING NEEDLE INTO THE AXILLARY VEIN
Oriot and Defawe (1988)[11]

Patient category

Low birth weight neonates.

Advantages and disadvantages

Facility and comparatively low incidence of complications.

Preferred side

None.

Position of patient

Supine with arm abducted to 120° (Figure 13.1a). The humerus is maximally externally rotated.

Position of operator

Not stated.

Equipment used in original description

19 gauge thin-wall needle (Vygon). 30 cm, 24 gauge silicone elastomer micro-catheter (Vygon).

Anatomical landmarks

With the arm abducted away from the side of the body, palpate the axillary artery (Figure 13.1a). This lies between the medial side of the head of the humerus and the small tuberosity of the humerus. The axillary vein lies medial (i.e. on the chest side) to the axillary artery. On low birth weight neonates, the vein is frequently visible.

Preparation

Perform the puncture under sterile conditions using
local anaesthesia as indicated.

Precautions and recommendations

Infusions should contain 1 IU heparin/ml, up to 100 IU/day.

Point of insertion of needle (Figure 13.1b)

Insert the needle subcutaneously, 1 cm below the small tuberosity of the humerus.

Direction of the needle and procedure

Advance the needle in a line parallel to the axis of the humerus slowly, aspirating gently until flash-back of blood signals entry into the vein (Figure 13.1b,c). With fine forceps, insert the catheter into the needle shaft and advance to a predetermined length such that the tip lies in the superior vena cava. Withdraw the needle from the vein. Immobilise the arm with a small board acting as a splint.

Attach the catheter to an appropriate infusion system and fix the portion of the catheter outside the skin entry site to the arm. Confirm the correct positioning of the catheter tip by x-ray, having firstly filled the catheter with radio-opaque dye.

Success rate

217 successful with 226 attempts (96%). 187 neonates had a birth weight less than 1·5 kg.

Complications

Three cases of catheter-related sepsis with positive blood and catheter tip-related cultures. Eight cases of shoulder oedema which subsided when the catheter was removed. Examination after 6 months revealed no vascular or limb abnormalities.

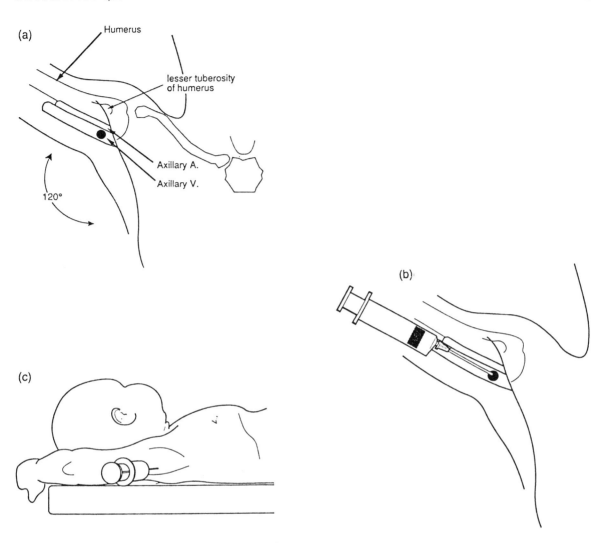

Figure 13.1. Inserting a silicone catheter through an interducing needle into the axillary vein (Oriot and Defawe, 1988).

TECHNIQUE FOR CENTRAL VENOUS CANNULATION VIA THE AXILLARY VEIN, USING THE AXILLARY ARTERY AS A LANDMARK

Metz et al. *(1990)*[12]

Similar to the technique described by Gouin *et al.*[35] for adults (see Chapter 4, p. 53).

Patient category

4 days–12 years (3–59 kg), median age 0·9 years (median weight 7 kg).

Advantages and disadvantages

Favourable complication rate.

Preferred side

Not stated.

Position of patient

Trendelenberg position when possible, with the arm abducted 100–130° and rotated externally (Figure 13.2a,b).

Position of operator

Not stated.

Equipment used in original description:

22 gauge short (2·5 cm) cannula-over-needle device or a thin-walled needle for insertion of a Seldinger wire introducer for a suitable single, double or triple lumen catheter device.

Advice on current equipment

Use a flexible catheter introduced over a Seldinger wire. Estimate length to be inserted by measuring the distance from axilla to sternal notch.

Anatomical landmarks

Palpate the axillary artery (Figure 13.2c).

Preparation

Perform procedure under sterile conditions using local anaesthesia as indicated.

Point of insertion of needle

In the axilla, parallel and inferior (i.e. on the chest wall side) to the axillary artery (Figure 13.2c).

Direction of needle and procedure

Palpate the axillary artery (Figure 13.2d,e). Insert the needle into the vein by assuming it lies immediately caudal (i.e. on the chest side) to the artery. Confirm entry into the vein by aspirating blood. Thread the catheter or guide wire centrally.

Success rate

79% – 41 out of 52 attempts. 33% of catheter tips were located in the SVC. 61% reached the subclavian vein. 5·6% terminated in the axillary/subclavian junction. Duration of catheterisation was 2–22 days (median 8 days).

Complications

Catheters became dislodged, with subsequent tissue infiltration in 10%, or were accidentally removed in a further 4 cases. Catheter occlusion occurred in 7% and there were solitary instances of venous thrombosis, venous stasis and suspected sepsis. There was 1 pneumothorax, and 1 axillary haematoma due to accidental axillary artery puncture.

SUBCLAVIAN VEIN

Reports of central venous catheterisation through the subclavian vein in infants are confined to the infraclavicular approach, presumably because of fear of inflicting serious trauma to the lung and other vital structures associated with the supraclavicular method.

Some workers warn against the subclavian route in infants of less than 4·5 kg.[13,14] Other reports though, describe the method in very small children of weights between 0·6 and 5 kg.[9,10] Nevertheless, the reported incidence of serious complications cannot be escaped. Careful consideration should therefore be exercised before choosing the subclavian vein route in very small patients. The subclavian approach should not be attempted by the inexperienced without appropriate supervision.

Puncture of the subclavian vein is necessarily a 'blind' procedure. In most techniques the needle is inserted below the mid-point of the clavicle and identifying the direction in which the needle is advanced by aiming for a target in the suprasternal notch.[9,14,34] Both Filston and Grant[10] and Eichelberger *et al.*[15] recommend the deltopectoral groove as an additional landmark.

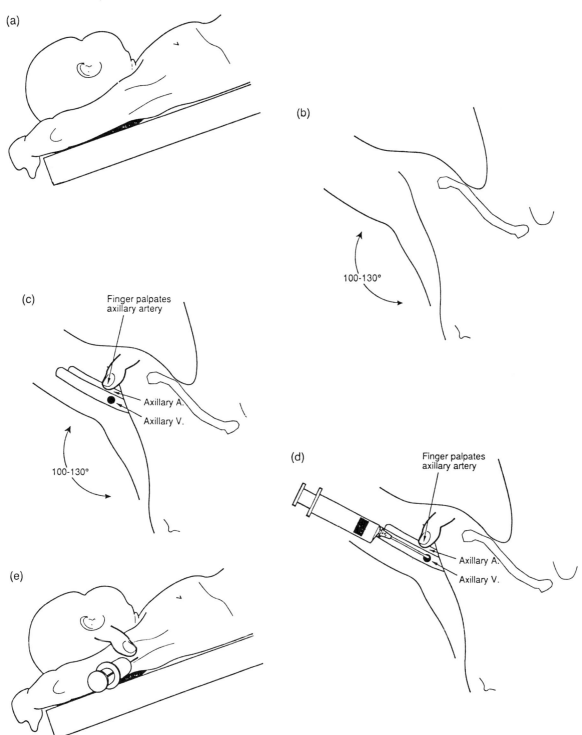

Figure 13.2.   Central venous cannulation via the axillary vein, using the axillary artery as a landmark (Metz *et al.*, 1990).

TECHNIQUE FOR CENTRAL VENOUS ACCESS VIA THE INFRACLAVICULAR PORTION OF THE SUBCLAVIAN VEIN

Dudrick et al. *(1969)*[14]

Patient category

Adults and infants over 4·5 kg.

Advantages and disadvantages

Catheter exit site easy to manage.

Preferred side

Not stated.

Position of patient (Figure 13.3a,b)

Place the patient in a 25° head-down position. Throw the child's shoulders back maximally or hyperextend over a roll placed beneath the vertebral column. Rotate the head to the opposite side.

Position of operator

Not stated.

Equipment used in original description

(a) Longdwel (Becton Dickinson) PTFE catheter (size not specified for infants).
(b) Deseret Angiocath (C. R. Bard).

Advice on current equipment

Any catheter-through-needle, catheter-through-cannula or catheter-over-guide wire of suitable size.

Anatomical landmarks

Mid-point of inferior border of clavicle; suprasternal notch (Figure 13.3c).

Preparation

Perform the procedure under sterile conditions using local anaesthesia as indicated.

Point of insertion of needle

Immediately below the mid-point of the inferior border of the clavicle (Figure 13.3c,d).

Direction of needle and procedure

Place the point of the needle on the entry site and swing the syringe and needle laterally so that the needle is directed towards a finger tip pressed firmly

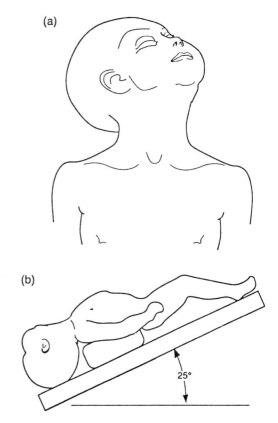

Figure 13.3. (a,b). Position with head hyperextended and rotated (Dudrick *et al.*, 1969).

in the suprasternal notch (A→B) (Figure 13.3d,e). Advance the tip of the needle maintaining gentle aspiration all the time and keeping the syringe and needle parallel to the coronal plane of the patient. A flashback signals entry into the vein; advance the needle or cannula 2–3 mm more to ensure complete entry of the tip into the vein. Remove the syringe and introduce the catheter to the required distance. Ensure that blood can be freely aspirated from the catheter before it is connected to an appropriate infusion system. Secure and apply a suitable sterile dressing. Take a chest x-ray to confirm the position of the catheter tip and to exclude a pneumothorax.

Success rate

Not stated but authors recommend that infants below 4·5 kg are better catheterised by a cut-down technique, utilising the internal or external jugular vein.

Complications

Not stated.

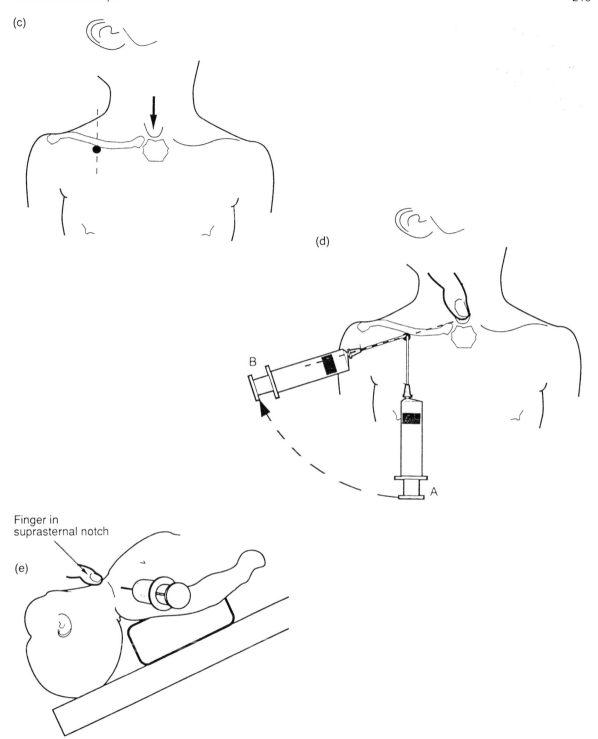

Figure 13.3 (c). Mid point of sternum and suprasternal notch, (d,e) axis of needle insertion (Dudrick *et al.*, 1969).

TECHNIQUE FOR CENTRAL VENOUS ACCESS VIA THE INFRACLAVICULAR PORTION OF THE SUBCLAVIAN VEIN; AN EXTENSION OF THE TECHNIQUE DESCRIBED BY DUDRICK *ET AL.*[13]

Groff and Ahmed (1974)[9]

These authors used the technique described by Dudrick *et al.*[13] but added a number of salient points.

This description should be read in conjunction with the figures accompanying that of Dudrick *et al* (see above).

Patient category

Patients under 2 years.

Preferred side

Not stated.

Position of patient (Figure 13.4a)

Carefully restrain if the patient is conscious. Turn the head away from the side of the procedure. Head-down position is optional.

Equipment used in original description

19 gauge thin wall, 1·5 inch needle with Bardic- or Deseret-type catheters (the use of a 14 gauge needle for this purpose has been reported in infants[9]. A syringe attached to the needle hub is advised to prevent air embolism.

Advice on current equipment

Catheter-through-needle device with removable catheter so that syringe can be attached directly, catheter – through – cannula or catheter over-guide-wire of suitable size.

Point of insertion of needle (Figure 13.4c,d)

Mid-point of the lower border of the clavicle.

Direction of needle and procedure

The needle MUST be inserted and withdrawn in a straight line because searching for the vein beneath the clavicle is dangerous. As many as 6 or 7 insertions can be made in this way.

Place the point of the needle on the entry site and swing the syringe and needle laterally (A→B) so that the needle is directed towards a finger tip pressed firmly in the suprasternal notch (Figure

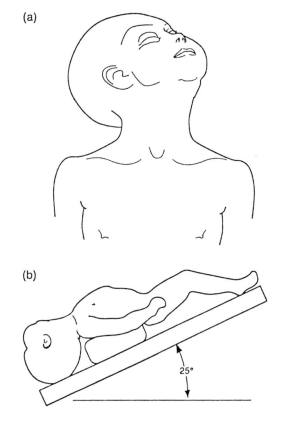

(a)

(b)

Figure 13.4. (a,b). Position with head hyper-extended and rotated (Groff and Ahmed, 1974).

13.4d,e). Advance the tip of the needle maintaining gentle aspiration all the time and keeping the syringe and needle parallel to the coronal plane of the patient. A flashback signals entry into the vein; advance the needle 2–3 mm more to ensure complete entry of the tip into the vein. If blood does not enter syringe during the initial passage beneath the clavicle, slowly withdraw the needle along the same track, aspirating gently. The lumen of the vein is often identified by this procedure. Remove the syringe and introduce the catheter to the required distance. Ensure that blood can be freely aspirated from the catheter before it is connected to an appropriate infusion system. Secure and apply a suitable sterile dressing. Take a chest x-ray to confirm the position of the catheter tip and to exclude a pneumothorax.

It is often necessary to manipulate the catheter to make it pass from the subclavian to the superior vena cava. This is in contrast to adults where the catheter is almost always easily inserted after the needle is positioned in the vein. If the catheter binds on the needle, the catheter and needle are

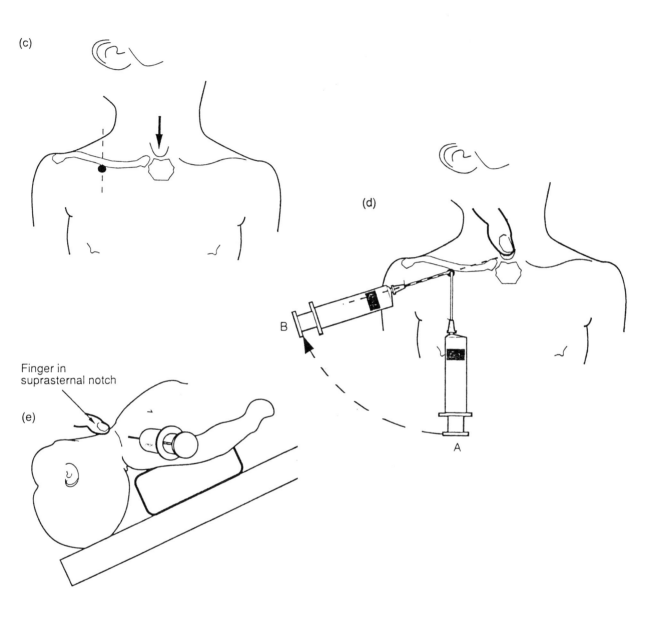

Figure 13.4 (c). Mid point of sternum and suprasternal notch, (d,e) axis of needle insertion (Groff and Ahmed, 1974).

withdrawn together to avoid severing the catheter on the sharp needle bevel.

Success rate

Each catheter insertion required, on average, three needle insertions (range 1–8).

Complications

One pneumothorax, 2 hydrothoraces (1 died), 1 haemothorax, 6 catheter sepsis, 1 uncontrolled bleeding (died).

INFRACLAVICULAR APPROACH TO THE SUBCLAVIAN VEIN USING THE DELTOPECTORAL GROOVE AS A LANDMARK

Filston and Grant (1979)[10]

Patient category

Ages from 1 day to 6 months; weight 690–5270 g.

Advantages and disadvantages

Deltopectoral groove usually easily identified.

Preferred side

Left side preferred. In this series 7% required cannulation on right side after failure on the left.

Position of patient

Tie down hands and feet (conscious patient) and tape the head so that it faces forward with the neck extended (Figure 13.5a,b). Tilt the table head down.

Position of operator

Not stated.

Equipment used in original description

Catheter-through-cannula device (Argyl Intramedicut Catheter, Sherwood Medical Industries).

Advice on current equipment

Catheter-through-cannula device or guide wire technique.

Anatomical landmarks

Mid-point of lower border of clavicle; deltopectoral groove; suprasternal notch (Figure 13.5c).

Preparation

Perform the procedure under sterile conditions using local anaesthesia as indicated.

Point of insertion of needle

Infraclavicularly, just lateral to the mid-point of the clavicle (Figure 13.5c,d).

Direction of needle and procedure

Place the needle point on the site of insertion and swing needle and syringe laterally (A→B) until they lie along the line which aims the tip of the needle towards a point 1–1·5 cm above the suprasternal notch (Figure 13.5d,e). The syringe and needle should now lie along the deltopectoral groove.

Elevate the needle and syringe 45° above the coronal plane (Figure 13.5) at first. This enables the needle to pass under the clavicle (d,f). This angle is then reduced to 15–20° above the coronal plane (Figure 13). If the patient has a prominent pectoral region, the needle is flattened against the chest wall. Advance the needle into the vein.

When the blood is aspirated, withdraw 0·5 ml blood and inject it forcefully, advancing the needle a few millimetres further into the vein.

Success rate

95% in 80 patients.

Complications

Malpositioned catheter 4%, arterial puncture 2%, hydrothorax 1%, pneumothorax 1%, pneumomediastinum 1%, haemorrhage 1%, hydrothorax due to catheter migration 1%, arm swelling 1%, catheter fault – broken hub 1%, septicaemia related to central line 2·5%.

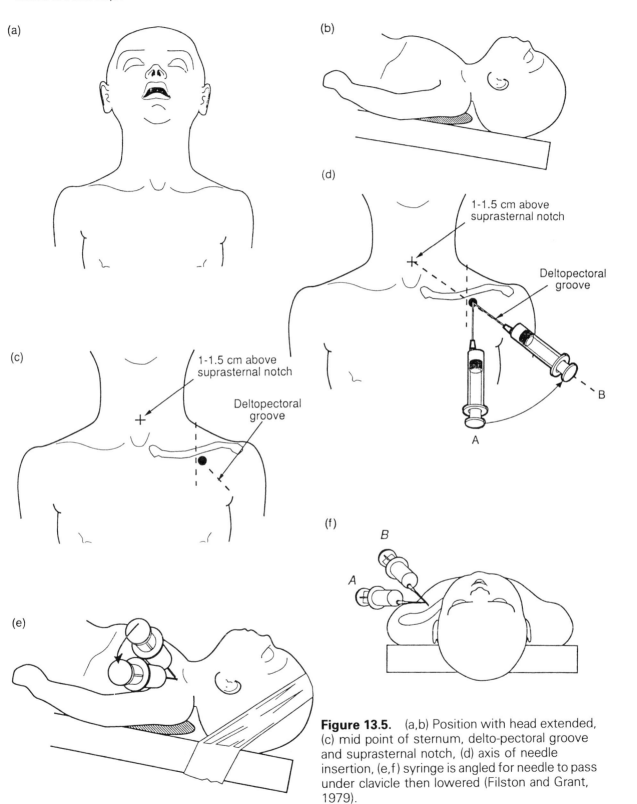

(a)

(b)

(c) 1-1.5 cm above suprasternal notch

Deltopectoral groove

(d) 1-1.5 cm above suprasternal notch

Deltopectoral groove

B

A

(e)

(f)

B

A

Figure 13.5. (a,b) Position with head extended, (c) mid point of sternum, delto-pectoral groove and suprasternal notch, (d) axis of needle insertion, (e,f) syringe is angled for needle to pass under clavicle then lowered (Filston and Grant, 1979).

INFRACLAVICULAR APPROACH TO THE SUBCLAVIAN VEIN USING THE DELTOPECTORAL GROOVE AS A LANDMARK
Eichelberger et al. *(1981)*[15]

This technique represents a modification of that described by Filston *et al.* (see above p. 222).

Patient category
Infants and small children.

Advantages and disadvantages
Puncture site easy to manage. No major complications.

Preferred side
None stated.

Position of patient
Supine (with restraint if conscious). Place a cylindrical roll of 4 × 4 gauze longitudinally in the interscapular region to enhance the backward lie of the shoulders (Figure 13.6a,b). The head is maintained in the looking straight ahead position by means of a piece of adhesive tape strapped across the forehead. Tilt the table head down.

Position of operator
Not stated.

Equipment used in original description
18 or 20 gauge PVC catheter-through-cannula (Argyl Intramedicut).

Advice on current equipment
Silicone elastomer or similarly flexible catheter, introduced through a cannula.

Anatomical landmarks
Deltopectoral groove; lower border of clavicle; suprasternal notch (Figure 13.6c).

Preparation
Perform the procedure under sterile conditions using local anaesthesia as indicated.

Precautions and recommendations
Use a fenestrated translucent self-adhesive drape so that the child can be easily seen through it.

Point of insertion of needle
In the deltopectoral groove, 2 cm from the lower margin of the clavicle (Figure 13.6d,e).

Direction of the needle and procedure
Identify the palpable deltopectoral groove where the clavicle crosses the first rib and insert the needle at the point of insertion. Swing the syringe and needle laterally to lie in the deltopectoral groove (A–B), keeping the needle in the coronal plane (Figure 13.6d,e). Advance the needle tip, bevel down, until aspiration of blood confirms entry into the subclavian vein as the latter passes between the clavicle and first rib. Immediately redirect the syringe so that the needle is aimed at a point above the suprasternal notch (C–D). This point should be 1 cm above the notch but in children older than 1 year, the point should be less than 1 cm.

Advance the needle a few millimetres into the vein and if a cannula-over-needle is being used, advance the cannula into the vein and remove the needle. The catheter is introduced through the cannula and advanced to the superior vena cava. The cannula is then withdrawn along the catheter. This is important since, if the cannula were to remain in the vein, accidental extraction of the catheter would leave the cannula open to atmosphere with the attendant grave risk of air embolism or haemorrhage.

Success rate
191 catheters inserted into 135 patients. Of these, 34·6% were conducted on neonates, another 34·6% on 1 to 12-month-old infants and the remainder (30·8%) were 1–18 years old. Mean duration of catheter usage was 23·7 days. Failed catheter insertions are not identified.

Complications
There were no incidents of pneumothorax, haemopneumothorax, haemorrhage, superior vena cava obstruction or facial oedema. 60 cases (31·4%) suffered catheter-related sepsis though the catheter was considered to be the primary cause in only 3·4% of children over 12 months of age and in 6·8% of younger children. Routine blood cultures are essential to monitor for infection and all catheter tips should be sent for culture. There were 3 cases (1·6%) of pleural effusion, 2 instances (1%) of subclavian vein thrombosis and 9 lines (4·7%) became blocked. The line or its hub cracked in 14 cases (7·3%).

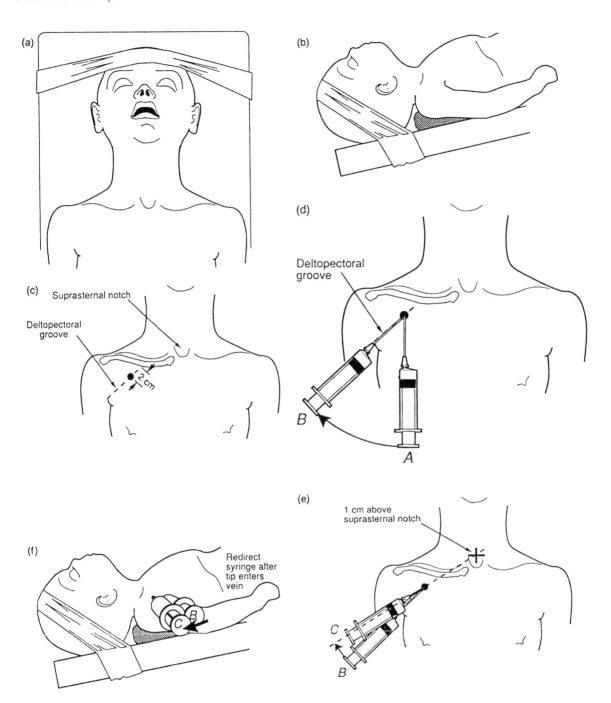

Figure 13.6 (a) Position with head restrained and extended, (b) Head down tilt, (c) Deltopectoral groove, lower border of clavicle, suprasternal notch, (d) Swing syringe to align with deltopectoral groove, (e,f) Redirect needle towards suprasternal notch after achieving venepuncture.

INTERNAL JUGULAR VEIN

English *et al.*[16] described two alternative techniques for central venous cannulation via the internal jugular vein and reported the results of 500 attempted cannulations which included 85 children and infants. Their 'elective' technique is unique in that it demands that the internal jugular vein is positively identified by palpation. For those patients, particularly small children and infants, where this is not possible, the authors described an 'alternative' technique, using the clavicular head of the sternomastoid as the sole identifier of the location of the internal jugular vein.

Long-term cannulation of the internal jugular vein for parenteral nutrition in infants and children was first described by Dudrick *et al.*[14] They and several other groups of workers [17–20] advocated tunnelling the catheter to a point behind the ear as a means of limiting infection problems. Although a Broviac catheter with its Dacron wool cuff can be used in full-term infants and children, premature babies requiring nutrition have insufficiently large veins for the use of this device. Pereyra *et al.*[21] have described a novel technique in which a plain silicone central venous catheter is introduced surgically into the internal jugular vein and then tunnelled to the preferred position of the chest wall where it is fixed by cementing silicone sheet material to the catheter material and sewing this to the skin. This technique could be used to enhance the fixation of percutaneously introduced silicone catheters.

The internal jugular vein can be approached at one of three levels. English *et al.*[16] seek to identify the vein by palpation (high approach) while three groups (English *et al.*,[16] Hall and Geefhuysen[22] and Korshin *et al.*[23]) exploit the relationship of the vein with the triangle formed by the two heads of the sternomastoid muscle and the clavicle (low approach). Korshin *et al.* also describe a method of identifying the carotid artery and deflecting it medially in order to minimise accidental arterial puncture (high approach). This technique is described below. Rao *et al.*[24] favour identifying a 'notch' on the upper border of the clavicle (very low approach). Most of these authors recommend a steep angle between the needle and the skin in order to minimise the risk of traumatising the adjacent apex of the lung. Korshin *et al.* do not subscribe to this precaution. Two techniques (Krausz *et al.*[25] and Hall and Geefhuysen[22]) approach the vein at an extreme angle from behind the lateral margin of the sternomastoid muscle, minimising lung trauma at the expense of inheriting some inevitable difficulty in causing the wire or catheter to advance into a central vein.

Most of the recommendations which are made in the chapter on internal jugular vein catheterisation (p. 115), which seek to maximise the success rate and minimise complications, are as pertinent to children as they are to adults. High techniques are preferable to low approaches. The number of stabs at a given vein should be limited. The large head and short neck in the infant and very small child can make adequate access to the neck difficult. A high priority should therefore be given to careful positioning of the patient prior to attempting venepuncture. Equipment of appropriate design and scaled-down dimensions can influence the success and complication rate.

Central venous catheterisation in infants and very small children should ideally be carried out only by those whose work regularly involves performing these techniques in children.

Techniques which can be used in children are described in detail in Chapter 6 (p. 115) which deals with the internal jugular vein route in depth. Two methods which are not included in Chapter 6 are decribed below.

HIGH TECHNIQUE: MEDIAL APPROACH – CAROTID ARTERY METHOD
Korshin et al. *(1978)*[23]

Patient category
Ages from 4 months to 81 years.

Advantages and disadvantages
Positively identifies carotid artery and seeks to avoid it.

Preferred side
Right side.

Position of patient
Place table with a 10–15° head-down tilt. Hyperextend the head and turn towards the contralateral side (Figure 13.7a,b).

Position of operator
Not stated.

Equipment used in original description

Bardic Intracath (a catheter-through-needle device). 16 gauge, 12 inch catheter with 14 gauge needle for larger children, 19 gauge, 12 inch catheter with 17 gauge needle for infants and children.

Advice on current equipment

Any suitable guide wire device.

Anatomical landmarks

Mid-neck technique: palpate the common carotid artery at the level of the cricoid cartilage (Figure 13.7c).

Preparation

Perform puncture under sterile conditions using local anaesthesia as indicated.

Precautions and recommendations

If the patient is breathing spontaneously, whether anaesthetised or awake, advance the needle only during expiration.

(a)

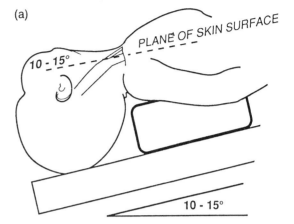

(b)

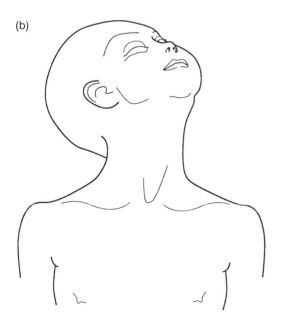

(c)

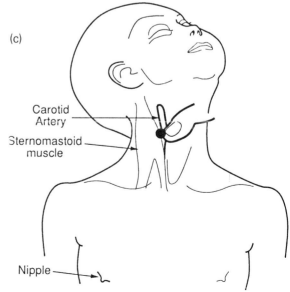

Figure 13.7. (a,b) Position with head extended and rotated away from side of venepuncture, (c) technique.

Point of insertion of needle

The needle is inserted immediately lateral to the carotid artery and medial to the border of the sternomastoid muscle at the level of the cricoid cartilage (Figure 13.7d).

Direction of needle and procedure

Palpate the carotid artery with the left hand and retract the artery slightly medially (Figure 13.7d). Place the point of the needle on the skin and point the syringe caudally (A). Swing the syringe and needle so that it points 'slightly laterally' (A to B). Elevate the syringe 10–15° above the skin surface (B to C). Point the needle towards the junction of the first and middle thirds of the ipsilateral clavicle, which usually positions the needle pointing more or less towards the ipsilateral nipple. Advance the needle into the vein. Confirm correct positioning of the catheter tip by taking a chest x-ray.

Success rate

The results of the carotid artery technique are presented together with an alternative method using the triangle formed by the two heads of the sternomastoid muscle and clavicle as a guide (see below). A total of 162 patients were involved of whom 54 were infants and children (median age = 5 years). The overall success rate was 86·4%. Four catheters (7·4%) were found to be malpositioned.

Complications

1 puncture of right pleural dome. Accidental carotid puncture also occurred.

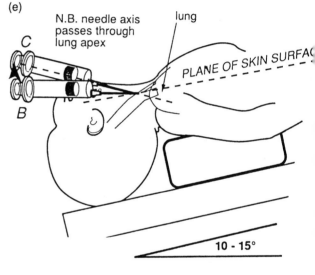

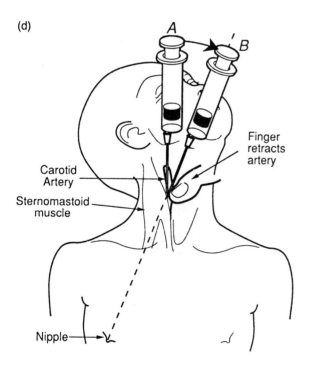

Figure 13.7 (d) palpating the carotid artery, and sighting the ipsilateral nipple, (e) rotate needle into a plane which includes the ipsilateral nipple. (Korshin *et al.*, 1978).

HIGH TECHNIQUE: CENTRAL APPROACH – ALTERNATIVE (TRIANGLE) METHOD
Korshin et al. *(1978)*[23]

Patient category
All ages.

Advantages and disadvantages
The triangle formed by the two heads of the sternomastoid are not always easy to demonstrate.

Preferred side
Right side.

Position of patient (Figure 13.8a)
Place table with a 10–15° head-down tilt. Hyperextend the head and turn towards the contralateral side.

Position of operator
Not stated.

Equipment used in original description
Bardic Intracath (a catheter-through-needle device). 16 gauge, 12 inch catheter with 14 gauge needle for larger children, 19 gauge, 12 inch catheter with 17 gauge needle for infants and children.

Advice on current equipment
Any suitable guide wire device.

Anatomical landmarks
Identify both sternal and clavicular heads of the sternomastoid muscle and the medial head of the clavicle (Figure 13.8b).

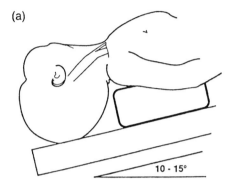

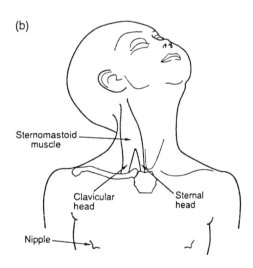

Figure 13.8 Alternative (Triangle) method (a) Position with head extended and rotated away from the side of venepuncture, (b) showing two heads of sternomastoid.

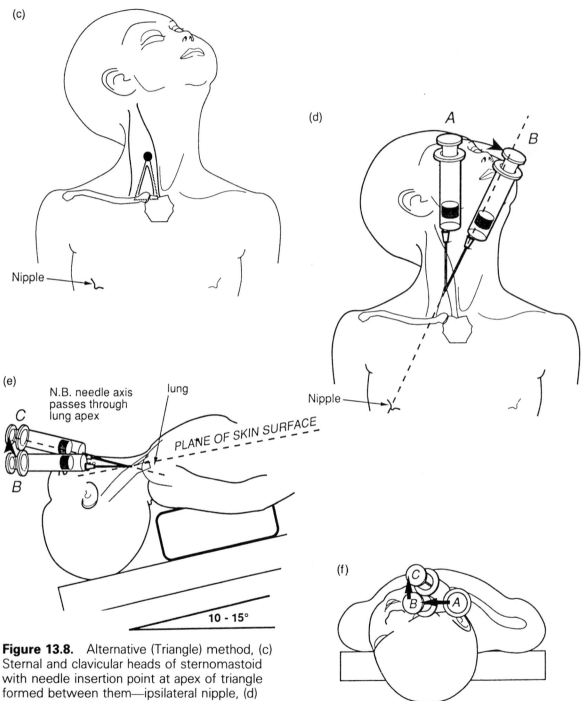

Figure 13.8. Alternative (Triangle) method, (c)
Sternal and clavicular heads of sternomastoid
with needle insertion point at apex of triangle
formed between them—ipsilateral nipple, (d)
introduce needle and swing into place which
includes ipsilateral nipple, (e) Raise barrel of
syringe to form 15° angle with skin, (f) top view
(Korshin *et al.*, 1978).

Preparation

Perform puncture under sterile conditions using local anaesthesia as indicated.

Precautions and recommendations

If the patient is breathing spontaneously, whether anaesthetised or awake, advance the needle only during expiration.

Point of insertion of needle

At the apex of the triangle formed by the two heads of the sternomastoid muscle (Figure 13.8c).

Direction of needle and procedure

Palpate the carotid artery with the left hand and retract the artery slightly medially. Place the point of the needle on the skin and point the syringe caudally (A) (Figure 13.8d). Swing the syringe and needle so that it points 'slightly laterally' (A to B). Elevate the syringe 10–15° above the skin surface (B to C) (Figure 13.8e,f). Point the needle towards the junction of the first and middle thirds of the ipsilateral clavicle, which usually positions the needle pointing more or less towards the ipsilateral nipple. Advance the needle into the vein. Confirm correct positioning of the catheter tip by taking a chest x-ray.

Success and complication rates

See under 'carotid' method above.

EXTERNAL JUGULAR VEIN

The superficial nature of the external jugular vein has made it a favoured site for surgical access for the insertion of long-term silicone elastomer catheters[26] since these are sufficiently pliable to follow the tortuous route by which the vein reaches the subclavian vein.

FEMORAL VEIN

Of the routes available for central venous catheterisation, there appears to have been a reluctance to use the femoral vein on the basis of a small number of reported serious complications which have included two instances of gangrene of the extremities after femoral venepuncture.[27,28] The high incidence of catheter-related thrombus formation (20–46% in adults) which has been found at autopsy in patients who had had central venous catheters inserted through the femoral vein is disturbing.[29,30] However, this incidence still compares favourably with an incidence of 67% with internal jugular catheters[31] and 61% with umbilical artery catheters.[32]

A prospective analysis has shown that central venous catheterisation through the femoral vein for the purpose of haemodynamic monitoring is safe and effective and a reasonable method to teach to paediatric trainees.[27]

When attempting femoral venepuncture, there is a risk of entering the capsule of the hip joint and striking the femoral head with the possibility of producing a subsequent suppurative arthritis. This risk is obviously increased in infants and very small children.[33]

FEMORAL VEIN
Kanter et al. *(1986)*[27]

Patient category
All children requiring haemodynamic monitoring.

Advantages and disadvantages
Safe and effective technique which can be effectively taught to all trainees.

Preferred side
Not stated.

Position of patient
Supine and immobilised (Figure 13.9a).

Position of operator
Not stated.

Equipment used in original description
Seldinger guide wire technique using 19 gauge needle, 0·025 inch (0·635 mm) wire and PVC or polyethylene 19 gauge pulmonary artery catheter.

Advice on current equipment
Any flexible catheter introduced over a Seldinger wire. A J-wire may be unsuitable in infants because the radius of the curved tip could be too great in such a small vessel.

Anatomical landmarks
Identify the inguinal ligament. Palpate the femoral artery; the vein lies immediately medial to the artery (Figure 13.9b).

Preparation
Perform puncture under sterile conditions using local anaesthesia as indicated.

Point of insertion of needle
Just medial to the palpated femoral artery, 2–3 cm inferior to the inguinal ligament (Figure 13.9b).

Direction of needle and procedure
Place the point of the needle at the entry site (A). Swing the needle slightly laterally (A to B) (Figure 13.9c). Elevate the syringe above the skin surface 15–30° (B to C) (Figure 13.9d); this helps to avoid the risk of puncturing the capsule of the hip joint. Advance the needle whilst aspirating gently on the attached syringe. If the vein is not immediately entered, withdraw the needle tip to the skin surface before redirecting it in order to minimise the risk of lacerating the vein. In infants and very small children, advance the needle very slowly and to a depth of 0·5–0·75 cm only to avoid entering the hip joint. Advance the tip a further 1 mm into the vein after withdrawing blood. Introduce the guide wire and advance it 5–10 mm into the vein before removing the needle. Insert the catheter over the wire. In the event of inadvertent arterial puncture, withdraw the needle and apply firm pressure for 5 minutes. Advance sufficient length of catheter so that its tip lies in the intrathoracic portion of the inferior vena cava and not in the right atrium. Confirm correct positioning of the tip with an x-ray.

Success rate
Successful cannulation was achieved in 25 of 29 (86%) patients. Ten of the patients weighed less than 10 kg and 14 were 'in shock' at the time of cannulation. Trainees were successful in cannulating 17 of 25 patients presented (68%)

Complications
Inadvertent femoral artery puncture occurred in 4 of the 29 patients (14%) and 4 patients (14%) experienced leg swelling which resolved when the catheter was removed. A catheter thrombus was found in one child at autopsy. There had been no associated signs in this case.

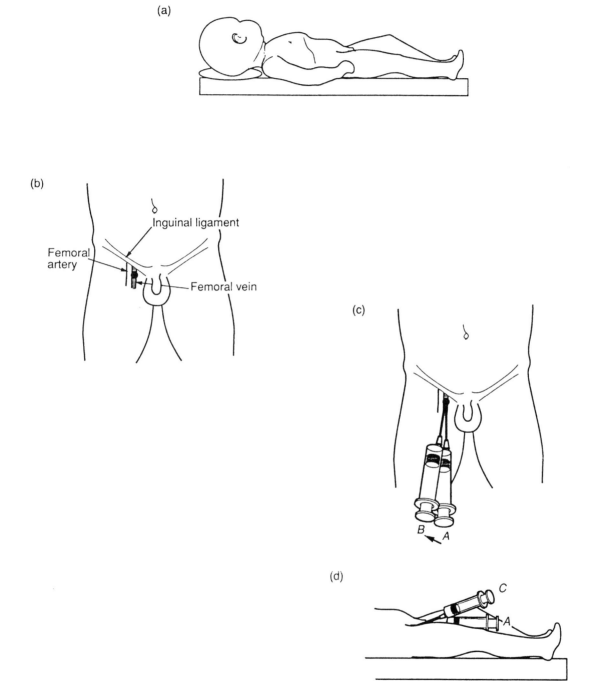

Figure 13.9. Central venous catheterisation
(Kanter *et al.*, 1986).

REFERENCES

1. Heird, W. C., Driscoll, J. M., Schullinger, J. N., Grebin, B. and Winters, R. W. (1972). Intravenous alimentation in pediatric patients. *Journal of Pediatrics* **80**, 351.
2. Eggert, L. D., Rusho, W. J., MacKay, M. *et al.* (1982). Calcium and phosphorus compatibility in parenteral nutrition solutions for neonates. *American Journal of Hospital Pharmacy* **39**, 49.
3. Puntis, J. W. (1986). Percutaneous insertion of central venous feeding catheters. *Archives of Disease in Childhood* **61**, 1138.
4. Dolcourt, J. L. and Bose, C. L. (1982). Percutaneous insertion of silastic central venous catheters in newborn infants. *Pediatrics* **70**, 484.
5. Shulman, R. J., Pokorny, W. J., Martin, C. G., Petitt, R., Baldaia, L. and Roney, D. (1986). Comparison of percutaneous and surgical placement of central venous catheters in neonates. *Journal of Pediatric Surgery* **21**, 348.
6. Evans, J. R., Allen, A. C. and Stinson, D. A. (1983). Percutaneous insertion of central venous catheters (letter). *Pediatrics* **71**, 668.
7. Carrera, G. and Liberatore, A. (1985). Percutaneous silicone catheters in the newborn infant. *Pediatrie* **40**, 285.
8. Carrera, G., Coccia, C., Coppalini, B., Liberatore, A. and Minoli, I. (1987). Percutaneous central venous silastic catheters in newborn infants. *Pediatrics* **79**, 837.
9. Groff, D. B. and Ahmed, N. O. (1974). Subclavian vein catheterisation in the infant. *Journal of Pediatric Surgery* **9**, 171.
10. Filston, H. C. and Grant, J. P. (1979). A safer system for percutaneous subclavian venous catheterisation in newborn infants. *Journal of Pediatric Surgery* **14**, 564.
11. Oriot, D. and Defawe, G (1988). Percutaneous catheterisation of the axillary vein in neonates. *Critical Care Medicine* **16**, 285.
12. Metz, R. I., Lucking, S. E., Chaten, F. C., Williams, T. M. and Mickell, J. J. (1990). Percutaneous catheterization of the axillary vein in infants and children. *Pediatrics* **85**, 531.
13. Dudrick, S. J., Groff, D. B. and Wilmore, D. W. (1969). Long term venous catheterisation in infants. *Surgery, Gynecology and Obstetrics* **129**, 805.
14. Dudrick, S. J. D., Wilmore, D. W., Vars, H. M. and Rhoads, J. E. (1969). Can intravenous feeding as the sole means of nutrition support growth in the child and restore weight loss in the adult? An affirmative answer. *Annals of Surgery* **169**, 974.
15. Eichelberger, M. R., Rous, P. G., Hoelzer, D. J., Garcia, V. F. and Koop, C. E. (1981). Percutaneous, subclavian venous catheters in neonates and children. *Journal of Pediatric Surgery (Supplement 1)* **16**, 547.
16. English, I. C. W., Frew, R. M. and Piggott, J. F. (1969). Percutaneous catheterisation of the internal jugular vein. *Anaesthesia* **24**, 521.
17. Filler, R. M. and Coran, A. G. (1976). Total parenteral nutrition in infants and children: central and peripheral approaches. *Surgical Clinics of North America* **56**, 395.
18. Feliciano, D. V. and Telander, R. L. (1976). Total parenteral nutrition in infants and children. *Mayo Clinic Proceedings* **51**, 647.
19. Zumbro, G., Mullin, M. and Neilson, T. (1971). Catheter placement in infants needing parenteral nutrition using common facial vein. *Annals of Surgery* **102**, 71.
20. Kosloske, A. M. and Klein, M. D. (1982). Techniques of central venous access for long term parenteral nutrition in infants. *Surgery, Gynecology and Obstetrics* **154**, 395.
21. Pereyra, R., Andrassy, R. J. and Mahour, G. H. (1980). Central venous cannulation in neonates. *Surgery, Gynecology Obstetrics* **151**, 253.
22. Hall, D. M. and Geefhuysen, J. (1977). Percutaneous catheterisation of the internal jugular vein in infants and children. *Journal of Pediatric Surgery* **12**, 719.
23. Korshin, J., Klauber, P. V., Christensen, V. and Skovsted, P. (1978). Percutaneous catheterisation of the internal jugular vein. *Acta Anaesthesiologica Scandinavica, Supplementum* **1978**, 27.
24. Rao, T. L., Wong, A. Y. and Salem, M. R. (1977). A new approach to the percutaneous catheterisation of the internal jugular vein. *Anesthesiology* **46**, 362.
25. Krausz, M. M., Berlatzky, Y., Ayalon, A., Freund, H. and Schiller, M. (1979). Percutaneous cannulation of the internal jugular vein in infants and children. *Surgery, Gynecology and Obstetrics* **148**, 591.
26. Krul, E. J., van Leeuwen, E. F., Vos, A. and Voute, P. A. (1986). Continuous venous access in children for long-term chemotherapy by means of an implantable system. *Journal of Pediatric Surgery* **21**, 689.
27. Kanter, R. K., Zimmerman, J. J., Strauss, R. H. and Stoeckel, K. A. (1986). Central venous catheter insertion by femoral vein: safety and effectiveness for the pediatric patient. *Pediatrics* **77**, 842.
28. Nabseth, D. C. and Jones, J. E. (1963). Gangrene of the lower extremities of infants after femoral venepuncture. *New England Journal of Medicine* **268**, 1003.
29. Moncrief, J. A. (1958). Femoral catheters. *Annals of Surgery* **147**, 166.
30. Bansmer, G., Keith, D. and Tesluk, H. (1958). Complications following use of indwelling catheters of inferior vena cava. *Journal of the American Medical Association* **167**, 1606.
31. Chastre, J., Cornud, F., Bouchama, A. *et al.* (1982). Thrombus as a complication of pulmonary artery catheterization via the internal jugular vein. *New England Journal of Medicine* **306**, 278.
32. Symansky, M. R. and Fox, H. A. (1972). Umbilical vessel catheterization. *Journal of Pediatrics* **80**, 820.
33. Asnes, R. S. and Arendar, G. M. (1966). Septic arthritis of the hip: a complication of femoral venepuncture. *Pediatrics* **38**, 837.

14

Results and Complications

The wide range of successful cannulation rates and reported complications occurring in both adults and children are described in detail in the relevant adult chapters as well as in Table 14.1 which concentrates on those particularly related to paediatric practice.

The complications of central venous catheterisation can be divided into two groups. First, those which are encountered at the time of cannulation and consist of trauma to surrounding vital structures. The incidence and severity of injuries are much higher when 'blind' puncture of deep neck veins is attempted compared with cannulation of visible and palpable peripheral veins.

The second group of complications are manifest at some later stage and are the consequence of intravascular accidents and catheter-related infection.

Most complications are applicable to both adult and paediatric practice. Nevertheless, some problems are peculiar to infants and small children. Particular care must be exercised when attempting to cannulate veins in children with suspected or known cardiovascular abnormalities. For instance, the absence of a right superior vena cava, with the persistence of a left superior vena cava, occurs in 0·2% of the population. This congenital anomaly can be responsible for failure to cannulate the right internal jugular vein.[1] The catheter which was introduced into the right subclavian vein crossed the mid-line to terminate in the left superior vena cava. In another incident, multiple attempts to cannulate the right internal jugular vein resulted in the puncture of a 6 cm Gore-text shunt between the right subclavian artery and the right pulmonary artery.[2] Both patients were suffering from Fallot's tetralogy.

PERIPHERAL ARM VEINS

Not surprisingly, complications are rarely encountered in catheterisation of these veins.

Reports of experience with techniques utilising the axillary vein are few. Clearly, the method requires more skill than venepuncture of visible or palpable arm veins.

JUGULAR VEINS

Catheterisation through the external jugular vein is safer than through the internal jugular vein but successful cannulation is less predictable than through the internal jugular vein.[3,4] In contrast to the internal jugular vein approach where age appears to play no part, when a J-wire is used in the external jugular vein route in children, successful cannulation increases with advancing age. The poorer performance in small children has been attributed to the inappropriately large radius of curvature of the J-tipped wire.[3]

Success rates with the internal jugular vein route are consistently good. Comparing complications arising with techniques using the high approach, the clinical significance of sequelae associated with the low approach would tend to caution against its use.[5].

Table 14.1 Results and complications.

Author(s) and year	Vein	Technique insertion point	Side	Skin>V (mm)	Age range	Successes/ patients (%)	Complications	%	Personnel	Comments	Conscious?
Oriot and Defawe (1988)[30]	AxV	Axilla	Either	10	Neonates	217/226 (94%)	Shoulder oedema catheter sepsis	3.5 1.3	?	?	?
Nicolson et al. (1985)[3]	EJV	Visualise and cannulate vessel using Seldinger technique with J-wire	R then L	–	< 1 month 1 month–1 year 1–5 years > 5 years	1/1 (100%) 6/17 (35%) 13/22 (59%) 56/77 (73%)	Failed CV access	14.5	Trainees and consultants	15–20° trend. head extended away from puncture side	GA
Krul et al. (1986)[23]	EJV	Surgical cut-down of implantable closed system – Abbott 'Portacath'	R side preferred	–	0–16 years	33/42	Innominate v. placement Wound dehiscence Haematoma Catheter disconnection Catheter occlusion Catheter-related sepsis	21 2.4 2.4 4.8 9.5 4.8	?Authors	Authors conclude that this is the preferred method for long-term venous access	Unknown
Hohn and Lambert (1966)[8]	FV	PTFE catheter over nylon monofilament (modified Seldinger technique)	–	–	3–15 years	8/8 (100%)	Clot within tube	25.0	?	IVC access	?
Kanter et al. (1986)[22]	FV	'Percutaneous, Seldinger' training programme	–	–	Paediatric	25/29 (86%)	Arterial puncture Leg swelling	14.0 14.0	Mostly trainees	Technique easy to teach	Yes
English et al. (1969)[9]	IJV	2 techniques: (a) palpate IJV or, if fail, (b) blind. 500 cases inc. 85 children	R	–	<1–15 years	0–1 year, 11/12 1–5 years, 23/27 5–15 years, 43/46	Pneumothorax Arterial puncture Misplaced tip	0.2 0.6 0.2	Consultants and trainees	Complication rate for all cases	Most GA
Prince et al. (1976)[10]	IJV	Skin puncture at apex of triangle formed by 2 heads of sterno-mastoid and clavicle. Needle at 45° to skin towards nipple	R then L	1–2	6 weeks–14 years	40/52 on R side 77%	Carotid artery puncture Horner's syndrome Haematoma	23.0 3.8 5.8	Trainees	15–20° trend. head extended away from punct.side	GA
Hall and Geefhuysen (1977)[11]	IJV	(a) Enter at apex of sternomastoid triangle Advance at 30° to skin slightly laterally or (b) posterior edge of sternomastoid	Either	–	2 weeks–9 years	>90/100	None serious Arterial puncture Troublesome bleeding	4 –	–	Head extended over edge of bed and away from site	Yes
Rao et al. (1977)[12]	IJV	Needle in palpable notch 0.25–1 cm from sternal end of clavicle parallel to sagittal plane and at 30–40° to coronal plane	Mostly R	–	0–11 years	180/192(94%) on 1st attempt and 97% at 2nd on same side	2/23 on L side punctured Th. duct Carotid artery puncture	9.0 0.8	Trainees and consultants	25° trendel. head extended slightly away from punct. side	GA
Korshin et al. (1978)[13]	IJV	(a) Lateral to carotid A (b) Apex of triangle	Mostly R	–	0–14 years	86.4% in 54 cases	Punctured lung apex Carotid artery puncture	1.8 ?	Consultants (naive)	–	GA
Coté et al. (1979)[5]	IJV	'Rao (low)'. Needle at 30–45°	R	28	0–19 years	38/51 (74%)	Haematoma Pneumothorax	3.9 2.0	Authors		GA

Reference	Route	Technique	R/L	No.	Age range	Success	Complications	%	Operator	Comments	GA
Coté et al. (1979)[5]	IJV	'Prince (high)', needle at 30–45°	R	22	0–19 years	59/71 (83%)	Haematoma Carotid artery puncture	4.2 8.5	Authors	Intracath used. Extreme head-down tilt with legs elevated vertically	no
Krausz et al. (1979)[14]	IJV	Posterior edge of sternomastoid muscle	Either	10–20	0–12 years	201/206 (97.6%)	Mediastinal extravasation SVC obstruction Pneumothorax Tracheal puncture R hydrothorax Catheter sepsis	1.5 1 0.5 0.5 0.5 10.6	?Authors		GA
Nicolson et al. (1985)[3]	IJV	Confluence of two heads of 'sternomastoid m., towards' nipple and at 30–45° to skin. Seldinger technique	R then L	–	<1 month 1 month–1 year 1–5 years >5 years	4/5 (80%) 32/38 (84%) 24/28 (86%) 49/57 (86%)	Failed CV access Carotid artery puncture	0.9 8.0	Trainees and consultants	15–20° trend. head extended away from puncture side	GA
Damen and Wever (1987)[28]	IJV	Balloon-tipped PA catheters, 6 and 8F introducers	R	–	24 <1 year 34 >1 year	58/58 (100%)	Carotid puncture Catheter sepsis	10 4	Consultant	Wedge success 92%	All GA
Evans et al. (1983)[18]	Peripheral	Silicone catheter-through-needle	–	–	Infants	18/20 (90%)	Septicaemia	11	Authors	E.JV, Bas V., AxV Superficial Temp V used	?
Durand et al. (1986)[21]	PV	'Percutaneous, scalp or limb' vein access with floated Silicone catheter through needle	–	–	newborn 0.51–3.9 kg	50/55 (91%) (1st attempt)	Sepsis Occlusion Dislodgement Fluid extravasation	7.0 15.0 8.0 4.0	–	Indwelling for 25 (2–80) days	Yes
Puntis (1986)[25]	PV	'Percutaneous, scalp or limb' vein access with floated Silicone catheter	–	–	(1–7 kg)	41/57 (72%)	Sepsis Blockage Limb swelling	10 17 10	Consultant	Indwelling for 17 days average. 'Scalp, long' saphenous and antecubital v.s	Restraint
Carrera et al. (1987)[27]	PV	Fine-bore silicone catheters, various veins	–	–	Neonates	555 (?100%)	Infection Dislodgement Extravasation Occlusion Thrombosis Pulm. oedema	0.2 18 16 10 0.7 0.5	?	Electively used for mean of 16 days	?
Eichelberger et al. (1981)[15]	SCV	Infraclavicular using delto-pect. groove	–	20	–	191/?	clotted line SVC thrombus migration and pleural effusion arm swelling sepsis	4.7 1 1.6 1.6 31	–	success not stated	(GA if not co-operative
Scherer et al. (1984)[19]	SCV	All cases with Staph. epidermidis septicaemia	–	–	2 weeks–15 years	–	Infected catheters	35.0	–		
Stellato et al. (1983)[20]	SCV	Percutaneous Broviac for thrombocytopenia	–	–	1 month–16 years	5/5 (100%)	Arterial puncture Haematoma	8.0 2.7	?	5 children in series of 199	GA
Pollack et al. (1980)[15]	FV(6) IJV(5) ACV(8)	PA balloon catheter at bedside without fluoroscopy	–	–	2 days–19 years	22/22 (100%) (6/22 = cut-down)	Pneumothorax IJV Bleeding FV BP down at PAWP	4.5 4.5 4.5	Supervised by consultants	'PA, 4-lumen' Swan-Ganz catheter 5–7 Fr.	LA at bedside

Table 14.1 Continued

Author(s) and year	Vein	Technique insertion point	Side	Skin>V (mm)	Age range	Successes/ patients (%)	Complications	%	Personnel	Comments	Conscious?
Ziegler et al. (1980)[16]	SCV and I&EJV	Infraclavicular	—	—	Neonates and children	SCV 118/? I&EJV 82/?	Pleural effusion Central v. thrombosis catheter sepsis	2.5 1 10.5	Consultants and trainees	Using Filston's technique	Sedation
Dolcourt and Bose (1982)[17]	Basilic or EJV	Silicone catheter-through-needle		—	27–35 weeks gestation	15/17	Accidental removal Ca3(PO4)2 blockage	20 7	Authors	No infection observed	Yes
Kanter et al. (1986)[22]	FV	All percutaneous	—	—	Paediatric	44/?	Leg swelling Transient cyanosis	7.0 5.0	— —	Review of 161 catheters indwelling 1–15 days (median 3 days)	Yes Yes
	SCV	Infraclavicular	—		Paediatric	37/?	Cellulitis	1.0	—		Yes
	IJV		—		Paediatric	48/?	Sepsis	3.0	—		Yes
	EJV		—		Paediatric	4/?	None/48	0.0	—		Yes
	ACV	Percutaneous and cut-down	—		Paediatric	23/?	None/4 'Arm, neck swelling' Sepsis Bleeding	0.0 9.0 4.0 4.0	— — — —		Yes Yes Yes
Newman et al. (1986)[24]	IJV SCV FV	XRO polyethylene catheters used in a comparison of central and peripheral venous lines for access	—		1 day–17 years	77/83 (93%)	Arterial puncture Catheter slippage Poor flow	3.0 5.0 3.0	Senior staff	Percutaneous technique	Restraint LA
	PV	PVs all cut-down techniques				40/49 (82%)	Poor flow Infiltration Phlebitis	65.0 37.5 27.5	Senior staff	Cut-down technique	Restraint LA
Shulman et al. (1986)[26]	PV	Floated silicone catheter from ACV vs.	—	—	Neonates	29/28 (100%)	Displacement Malposition Block – clotted Block – precip. Brachial V. thromb.	17 7 14 7 4	?Consultants only	0.635 mm O.D. × 0.305 mm I.D. float catheter	Conscious 'bedside technique'
	JV	Cut-down technique with 4–5 cm tunnel			Neonates	25/25 (100%)	Displacement Difficult removal Blocked – clotted Blocked – precip. SVC syndrome	12 7 4 0 4		16-gauge silicone catheter	?GA in operating theatre
Wallace and Zeltzer (1987)[29]	CFV JV	Cut-down insertion of implanted ports	—	—	5 months– 16 years	?100%	Positive blood culture Extravasation Spontaneous extrusion	6.5 6.5 3.2	Surgeon	Catheters survived 163 ± 149 days	All GA
Stenzel et al. (1989)[7]	FV	'Percutaneous, Seldinger'	—	—	<18 months	92/?	Infectious	5.4	All specialists		
		'Percutaneous, Seldinger'			<18 months	92/?	thrombosis	2.2	All specialists		
		'Percutaneous, Seldinger'			1.5–6 years	48/?	Infectious	2.1	All specialists		
		'Percutaneous, Seldinger'			1.5–6 years	48/?	thrombosis and embolism	4.2	All specialists		
		'Percutaneous, Seldinger'			>6 years	22/?	Infectious	0.0	All specialists		
		'Percutaneous, Seldinger'			>6 years	22/?	Non-infectious	0.0	All specialists		
	nonFV	'Percutaneous, Seldinger'			<18 months	116/?	Infectious	8.6	All specialists		
		'Percutaneous, Seldinger'			<18 months	116/?	Non-infectious	0.0	All specialists		

	Vein	Technique	Age	Success	Complication	%	Operators	Comments	
		'Percutaneous, Seldinger'	1.5–6 years	46/?	Infectious	6.5	All specialists		
		'Percutaneous, Seldinger'	1.5–6 years	46/?	Perforation	2.1	All specialists		
		'Percutaneous, Seldinger'	1.5–6 years	46?	Bleeding	4.3	All specialists		
		'Percutaneous, Seldinger'	<6 years	71/?	Infectious	8.7	All specialists		
		'Percutaneous, Seldinger'	>6 years	71/?	Thrombosis	1.4	All specialists	?	
Metz et al. (1990)[31]	AxV	Medial to Ax.A. Seldinger technique via needle or cannula	4 days– 12 years	41/52 (79%)	Ax.A. haematoma	1/41	Mostly consultants plus five trainees		
					Pneumothorax	1/41			
					Tissue infiltration	4/41			
					Venous thrombosis	1/41			
Mirro et al. (1990)[32]	CV	(a) Percutaneous, Seldinger; (b) Surgical via ceph. V (c) Implanted Port device	'Children' 'Children' 'Children'	69/70 195/196 92/93	Pneumothorax	1.5	Specialist	Ports better long term.	GA
					Migration	0.35	Specialists	Catheter: Percut. less	GA
						0.0	Specialists	problems than surgery	GA
Taylor and Yellowlees (1990)[33]	AxV	'Percutaneous, Seldinger'	Mostly adult	98/102 (96%)	Malposition	6.0	Consultants and trainees		Some GA
					Arterial puncture	5.0			Some GA
					Transnt. paraesthesia	2.0			Some GA
					Pneumothorax	1.0			Some GA

Periph, peripheral vein; IJV, internal jugular vein; CFV, ?; JV, jugular vein; AxV, axillary vein; FV, femoral vein; SCV, subclavian vein; SVC, superior vena cava; Ceph.V, cephalic vein; R, right side; L, left side; GA, general anaesthetic.

SUBCLAVIAN VEIN

Good results with few complications have been reported with this technique in infants and small children[6] but a review of the literature confirms that subclavian venepuncture should be undertaken only when there is a valid indication. Supervision of the inexperienced attempting this technique in the paediatric patient is obviously highly advisable.

FEMORAL VEIN

Fear of infective complications has been a deterrent in the use of the femoral vein for central venous catheterisation. However, in a recent study the femoral vein has been recommended as a safe route for central venous catheterisation in the infant and small child. There were no significant differences in infectious or other sequelae when compared with those of catheterisation through other routes.[7]

REFERENCES

1. Mehta, Y., Bhavani, S. S. and Sharma, K. K. (1990). A difficult cannulation of the right internal jugular vein (letter). *Anaesthesia* 45, 1087.
2. Watson, D. and Simpson, J. C. (1984). Yet another hazard of percutaneous central venous cannulation (letter). *Anesthesiology* 60, 524.
3. Nicolson, S. C., Sweeney, M. F., Moore, R. A. and Jobes, D. R. (1985). Comparison of internal and external jugular cannulation of the central circulation in the pediatric patient. *Critical Care Medicine* 13, 747.
4. Belani, K. G., Buckley, J. J., Gordon, J. R. and Castaneda, W. (1980). Percutaneous cervical central vein placement: a comparison of the internal and external jugular vein routes. *Anesthesia Analgesia* 59, 40.
5. Coté, C. J., Jobes, D. R., Schwartz, A. J. and Ellison, N. (1979). Two approaches to the cannulation of a child's internal jugular vein. *Anesthesiology* 50, 371.
6. Morgan, W. W. and Harkins, G. A. (1972). Percutaneous introduction of long-term in dwelling venous catheters in infants. *Journal of Pediatric Surgery* 7, 538.
7. Stenzel, J. P., Green, T. P., Fuhrman, J. B., Carlson, P. E. and Marchessault, R. P. (1989). Percutaneous femoral venous catheterisations: a prospective study of complications. *Journal of Pediatrics* 114, 411.
8. Hohn, A. R. and Lambert, E. C. (1966). Continuous venous

catheterisation in children. *Journal of the American Medical Association* 197, 658.
9. English, I. C. W., Frew, R. M. and Piggott, J. F. (1969). Percutaneous catheterisation of the internal jugular vein. *Anaesthesia* 24, 521.
10. Prince, S. R., Sullivan, R. L. and Hackel, A. (1976). Percutaneous catheterisation of the internal jugular vein in infants and children. *Anesthesiology* 44, 170.
11. Hall, D. M. and Geefhuysen, J. (1977). Percutaneous catheterisation of the internal jugular vein in infants and children. *Journal of Pediatric Surgery* 12, 719.
12. Rao, T. L., Wong, A. Y. and Salem, M. R. (1977). A new approach to the percutaneous catheterisation of the internal jugular vein. *Anesthesiology* 46, 362.
13. Korshin, J., Klauber, P. V., Christensen, V. and Skorsted, P. (1978). Percutaneous catheterisation of the internal jugular vein. *Acta Anaesthesiologica Scandinavica, Supplementum* 1978, 27.
14. Krausz, M. M., Berlatzky, Y., Ayalon, A., Freund, H. and Schiller, M. (1979). Percutaneous cannulation of the internal jugular vein in infants and children. *Surgery, Gynecology and Obstetrics* 148, 591.
15. Pollack, M. M., Reed, T. P., Holbrook, P. R. and Fields, A. I. (1980). Bedside pulmonary artery catheterization in pediatrics. *Journal of Pediatrics* 96, 274.
16. Ziegler, M., Jakobowski, D., Hoelzer, D., Eichenberger, M. and Koop, C. E. (1980). Route of pediatric parenteral nutrition: proposed criteria revision. *Journal of Pediatric Surgery* 15, 472.
17. Dolcourt, J. L. and Bose, C. L. (1982). Percutaneous insertion of silastic central venous catheters in newborn infants. *Pediatrics* 70, 484.
18. Evans, J. R., Allen, A. C. and Stinson, D. A. (1983). Percutaneous insertion of central venous catheters (letter). *Pediatrics* 71, 668.
19. Scherer, L. R., West, K. W., Weber, T. R., Teiman, M. and Grosfeld, J. L. (1984). *Staphylococcus epidermidis* in pediatric patients: clinical and therapeutic considerations. *Journal of Pediatric Surgery* 19, 358.
20. Stellato, T. A., Gauderer, M. W., Lazarus, H. M. and Herzig, R. H. (1985). Percutaneous silastic catheter insertion in patients with thrombocytopenia. *Cancer* 56, 2691.
21. Durand, M., Ramanathan, R., Martinelli, B. and Tollentino, M. (1986). Prospective evaluation of percutaneous central venous silastic catheters in newborn infants with birth weights of 510 to 3920g. *Pediatrics* 78, 245.
22. Kanter, R. K., Zimmerman, J. J., Strauss, R. H. and Stoeckel, K. A. (1986). Central venous catheter insertion by femoral vein: safety and effectiveness for the pediatric patient. *Pediatrics* 77, 842.
23. Krul, E. J., van Leeuwen, E. F., Vos, A. and Voute, P. A. (1986). Continuous venous access in children for long-term chemotherapy by means of an implantable system. *Journal of Pediatric Surgery* 21, 689.
24. Newman, B. M., Jewett, T. C. Jr, Karp, M. P. and Cooney, D. R. (1986). Percutaneous central venous catheterisation in children: first line choice for venous access. *Journal of Pediatric Surgery* 21, 685.
25. Puntis, J. W. (1986). Percutaneous insertion of central

venous feeding catheters. *Archives of Disease in Childhood* **61**, 1138.

26. Schulman, R. J., Pokorny, W. J., Martin, C. G., Petitt, R., Baldaia, L. and Roney, D. (1986). Comparison of percutaneous and surgical placement of central venous catheters in neonates. *Journal of Pediatric Surgery* **21**, 348.

27. Carrera, G., Coccia, C., Coppalini, B., Liberatore, A. and Minoli, I. (1987). Percutaneous central venous silastic catheters in newborn infants. *Pediatrics* **79**, 837.

28. Damen, J. and Wever, J. E. A. T. (1987). The use of balloon tipped pulmonary artery catheters in children undergoing cardiac surgery. *Intensive Care Medicine* **13**, 266.

29. Wallace, J. and Zelter, P. M. (1987). Benefits, complications and care of implantable diffusion devices in 31 children with cancer. *Journal of Pediatric Surgery* **22**, 833.

30. Oriot, D. and Defawe, G. (1988). Percutaneous catheterisation of the axillary vein in neonates. *Critical Care Medicine* **16**, 285.

31. Metz, R. I., Lucking, S. E., Chaten, F. C., Williams, T. M. and Mickell, J. J. (1990). Percutaneous catheterization of the axillary vein in infants and children. *Pediatrics* **85**, 531.

32. Mirro, J., Rao, B. N., Kumar, M., Rafferty, M., Hancock, M., Austin, B. A., Fairclough, D. and Lobe, T. E. (1990). A comparison of placement techniques and complications of externalized catheters and implantable parts used in children with cancer. *Journal of Pediatric Surgery* **25**, 120.

33. Taylor, B. L. and Yellowlees, I. (1990). Central venous cannulation using the infraclavicular axillary vein. *Anesthesiology* **72**, 55.

34. Morgan, W. W. and Harkins, G. A. (1972). Percutaneous introduction of long-term indwelling venous catheters in infants. *Journal of Pediatric Surgery* **7**, 538.

35. Gouin, F., Martin, C. and Saux, P. (1985). Central venous and pulmonary artery catheterizations via the axillary vein. *Acta Anaesthesiologica Scandinavica, Supplementum* **81**, 27.

Index